Advances in Diagnosis and Therapy of Pancreatic Cystic Neoplasms

Editor

TAMAS A. GONDA

GASTROINTESTINAL ENDOSCOPY CLINICS OF NORTH AMERICA

www.giendo.theclinics.com

Consulting Editor
CHARLES J. LIGHTDALE

July 2023 • Volume 33 • Number 3

ELSEVIER

1600 John F. Kennedy Boulevard ● Suite 1800 ● Philadelphia, Pennsylvania, 19103-2899

http://www.theclinics.com

**GASTROINTESTINAL ENDOSCOPY CLINICS OF NORTH AMERICA Volume 33, Number 3
July 2023 ISSN 1052-5157, ISBN-13: 978-0-443-18201-3**

Editor: Kerry Holland
Developmental Editor: Jessica Cañaberal

Gastrointestinal Endoscopy Clinics of North America (ISSN 1052-5157) is published quarterly by Elsevier Inc., 360 Park Avenue South, New York, NY 10010-1710. Months of issue are January, April, July, and October. Business and Editorial Offices: 1600 John F. Kennedy Blvd., Suite 1800, Philadelphia, PA, 19103-2899. Periodicals postage paid at New York, NY and additional mailing offices. Subscription prices are $381.00 per year for US individuals, $703.00 per year for US institutions, $100.00 per year for US and Canadian students/residents, $419.00 per year for Canadian individuals, $830.00 per year for Canadian institutions, $501.00 per year for international individuals, $830.00 per year for international institutions, and $245.00 per year for international students/residents. To receive student/resident rate, orders must be accompanied by name of affiliated institution, date of term, and the *signature* of program/residency coordinator on institution letterhead. Orders will be billed at individual rate until proof of status is received. Foreign air speed delivery is included in all *Clinics* subscription prices. All prices are subject to change without notice. **POSTMASTER:** Send address change to *Gastrointestinal Endoscopy Clinics of North America*, Elsevier Health Sciences Division, Subscription Customer Service, 3251 Riverport Lane, Maryland Heights, MO 63043. **Customer Service: 1-800-654-2452 (US). From outside the United States, call 1-314-447-8871. Fax: 1-314-447-8029. E-mail: JournalsCustomerService-usa@elsevier.com (for print support) or JournalsOnlineSupport-usa@elsevier.com (for online support).**

Reprints. For copies of 100 or more, of articles in this publication, please contact the Commercial Reprints Department, Elsevier Inc., 360 Park Avenue South, New York, NY 10010-1710. Tel. 212-633-3874; Fax: 212-633-3820; E-mail: reprints@elsevier.com.

Gastrointestinal Endoscopy Clinics of North America is covered in *Excerpta Medica, MEDLINE/PubMed (Index Medicus), and MEDLINE/MEDLARS.*

Contributors

CONSULTING EDITOR

CHARLES J. LIGHTDALE, MD
Professor of Medicine, Division of Digestive and Liver Diseases, Columbia University Medical Center, New York, New York, USA

EDITOR

TAMAS A. GONDA, MD
Associate Professor of Medicine, Director, Pancreatic Disease Program, Chief of Endoscopy, Division of Gastroenterology and Hepatology, Department of Medicine, NYU Grossman School of Medicine, New York, New York, USA

AUTHORS

AHMAD M. AL-TAEE, MD
Carle Illinois College of Medicine, University of Illinois Urbana-Champaign, Digestive Health Institute, Urbana, Illinois, USA

CANDICE W. BOLAN, MD
Department of Radiology, Mayo Clinic, Jacksonville, Florida, USA

RANDALL BRAND, MD
Professor of Medicine, Academic Director, GI Division, UPMC Shadyside, Director, GI Malignancy Early Detection, Diagnosis and Prevention Program, UPMC Division of Gastroenterology, Hepatology, and Nutrition, Pittsburgh, Pennsylvania, USA

ALICE CATTELANI, MD
Department of General and Pancreatic Surgery, The Pancreas Institute, University of Verona Hospital Trust, Verona, Italy

JOHN A. CHABOT, MD
David V. Habif Professor of Surgery, Chief, Division of GI/Endocrine Surgery, Department of Surgery, Herbert Irving Pavilion, Columbia University Irving Medical Center, Columbia University Vagelos College of Physicians and Surgeons, New York, New York, USA

HERSH CHANDARANA, MD
Department of Radiology, NYU Grossman School of Medicine, New York, New York, USA

ANKIT CHHODA, MD
Clinical Fellow in Pancreatic Diseases, Division of Gastroenterology, Beth Israel Deaconess Medical Center, Boston, Massachusetts, USA

SUMIT CHOPRA, PhD
Department of Radiology, NYU Grossman School of Medicine, New York, New York, USA

STEFANO FRANCESCO CRINÒ, MD
Gastroenterology and Digestive Endoscopy Unit, The Pancreas Institute, G.B. Rossi University Hospital, Verona, Italy

KOUSHIK K. DAS, MD
Associate Professor of Medicine, Division of Gastroenterology, Siteman Cancer Center, Washington University School of Medicine, St Louis, Missouri, USA

SHENIN DETTWYLER, MS, CGC
Perlmutter Cancer Center, NYU Langone Health, New York, New York, USA

JESSICA EVERETT, MS, CGC
Clinical Assistant Professor of Medicine, Perlmutter Cancer Center, NYU Langone Health, New York, New York, USA

JAMES J. FARRELL, MD
Professor of Medicine and Surgery, Director, Center for Pancreatic Diseases, Section of Digestive Diseases, Yale School of Medicine, Yale University, New Haven, Connecticut, USA

IDO HAIMI, MD
Department of Surgery, NYU Langone Health, New York, New York, USA

NASSIER HARFOUCH, MD
Department of Radiology, NYU Grossman School of Medicine, New York, New York, USA

ELIZABETH M. HECHT, MD
Department of Radiology, NewYork-Presbyterian–Weill Cornell Medicine, New York, New York, USA

CHENCHAN HUANG, MD
Department of Radiology, NYU Grossman School of Medicine, New York, New York, USA

MICHAEL D. KLUGER, MD, MPH
Associate Professor, Division of GI/Endocrine Surgery, Department of Surgery, Herbert Irving Pavilion, Columbia University Irving Medical Center, Columbia University Vagelos College of Physicians and Surgeons, New York, New York, USA

GRACE C. LO, MD
Department of Radiology, NewYork-Presbyterian–Weill Cornell Medicine, New York, New York, USA

GIOVANNI MARCHEGIANI, MD, PhD, Department of General and Pancreatic Surgery, The Pancreas Institute, University of Verona Hospital Trust, Verona, Italy

ALEC J. MEGIBOW, MD, MPH, FACR
Professor of Radiology and Surgery, Department of Radiology, NYU Langone Health, NYU Grossman School of Medicine, New York, New York, USA

WALTER G. PARK, MD, MS
Associate Professor of Medicine, Division of Gastroenterology and Hepatology, Stanford University, Stanford, California, USA

MATTHEW T. PELLER, MD
Advanced Endoscopy Fellow and Clinical Instructor of Medicine, Division of Gastroenterology, Washington University School of Medicine, St Louis, Missouri, USA

GIAMPAOLO PERRI, MD
Department of General and Pancreatic Surgery, The Pancreas Institute, University of
Verona Hospital Trust, Verona, Italy

STEPHANIE ROMUTIS, MD
Clinical Assistant Professor of Medicine, UPMC Division of Gastroenterology,
Hepatology, and Nutrition, Pittsburgh, Pennsylvania, USA

ROBERTO SALVIA, MD, PhD
Department of General and Pancreatic Surgery, The Pancreas Institute, University of
Verona Hospital Trust, Verona, Italy

LAUREN E. SCHLEIMER, MD
Resident, Department of Surgery, Columbia University Irving Medical Center, New York,
New York, USA

JULIE SCHMIDT, APRN
Section of Digestive Disease, Yale Multidisciplinary Pancreatic Cyst Clinic (Yale MPaCC),
Center for Pancreatic Diseases, Section of Digestive Disease, Yale School of Medicine,
New Haven, Connecticut, USA

PRADEEP K. SIDDAPPA, MBBS
Division of Gastroenterology and Hepatology, Stanford University, Stanford, California,
USA

DIANE M. SIMEONE, MD
Associate Director, Department of Surgery, Perlmutter Cancer Center, NYU Langone
Health, Laura and Isaac Perlmutter Professor of Surgery and Pathology, Director,
Pancreatic Cancer Center, New York, New York, USA

MICHIO TAYA, MD
Department of Radiology, New York Presbyterian e Weill Cornell Medicine, New York,
New York, USA

JASON R. TAYLOR, MD
St Luke's Hospital, Chesterfield, Missouri, USA

Contents

> Pancreatic cysts are an increasingly identified entity with significant health care implications. Although some cysts present with concurrent symptoms that often require operative intervention, the advent of improved cross-sectional imaging has heralded an era of increased incidentally detected pancreatic cysts. Although the rate of malignant progression in pancreatic cysts remains low, the poor prognosis of pancreatic malignancy has driven recommendations for ongoing surveillance. A uniform consensus has not been reached on the management and surveillance of pancreatic cysts leading clinicians to grapple with the burden of how best to approach pancreatic cysts from a health, psychosocial, and cost perspective.

> The detection of incidental pancreatic cystic lesions has increased over time. It is crucial to separate benign from potentially malignant or malignant lesions to guide management and reduce morbidity and mortality. The key imaging features used to fully characterize cystic lesions are optimally assessed by contrast-enhanced magnetic resonance imaging/magnetic resonance cholangiopancreatography, with pancreas protocol computed tomography offering a complementary role. While some imaging features have high specificity for a particular diagnosis, overlapping imaging features between diagnoses may require further investigation with follow-up diagnostic imaging or tissue sampling.

> This article reviews the types of pancreatic cysts encountered in Radiologic practice. It summarizes the malignancy risk of each of the following: serous cystadenoma, mucinous cystic tumor, intraductal papillary mucinous neoplasm main duct and side branch, and some miscellaneous cysts such as neuroendocrine tumor and solid pseudopapillary epithelial neoplasm. Specific reporting recommendations are given. The choice between radiology follow-up versus endoscopic analysis is discussed.

This review focuses on endoscopic imaging of PCLs including endoscopic and endosonographic features and fine needle aspiration. We then review the role of adjunct techniques, such as microforceps, contrast-enhanced endoscopic ultrasound, pancreatoscopy, and confocal laser endomicroscopy.

Pancreatic cyst fluid analysis can help diagnose pancreatic cyst type and the risk of high-grade dysplasia and cancer. Recent evidence from molecular analysis of cyst fluid has revolutionized the field with multiple markers showing promise in accurate diagnosis and prognostication of pancreatic cysts. The availability of multi-analyte panels has great potential for more accurate prediction of cancer.

Pancreatic cystic neoplasms (PCNs) are increasingly detected because of the widespread use of cross-sectional imaging and overall aging population. While the majority of these cysts are benign, some can progress to advanced neoplasia (defined as high-grade dysplasia and invasive cancer). As the only widely accepted treatment for PCNs with advanced neoplasia is surgical resection, accurate preoperative diagnosis, and stratification of malignant potential for deciding about surgery, surveillance or doing nothing remains a clinical challenge. Surveillance strategies for pancreatic cysts (PCNs) combine clinical evaluation and imaging to assess changes in cyst morphology and symptoms that may indicate advanced neoplasia. PCN surveillance heavily relies on various consensus clinical guidelines that focus on high-risk morphology, surgical indications, and surveillance intervals and modalities. This review will focus on current concepts in the surveillance of newly diagnosed PCNs, especially on low-risk presumed intraductal papillary mucinous neoplasms (those without worrisome features and high-risk stigmata), and appraise current clinical surveillance guidelines.

The overall prevalence of pancreatic cysts (PCs) is high in the general population. In clinical practice PCs are often incidentally discovered and are classified into benign, premalignant, and malignant lesions according to the World Health Organization. For this reason, in the absence of reliable biomarkers, to date clinical decision-making relies mostly on risk models based on morphological features. The aim of this narrative review is to present the current knowledge regarding PC's morphologic features with related estimated risk of malignancy and discuss available diagnostic tools to minimize clinically relevant diagnostic errors.

> Historically, the management of pancreatic cystic neoplasms (PCN) has been operative. Early intervention for premalignant lesions, including intraductal papillary mucinous neoplasms (IPMN) and mucinous cystic neoplasms (MCN), offers an opportunity to prevent pancreatic cancer—with potential decrement to patients' short-term and long-term health. The operations performed have remained fundamentally the same, with most patients undergoing pancreatoduodenectomy or distal pancreatectomy using oncologic principles. The role of parenchymal-sparing resection and total pancreatectomy remains controversial. We review innovations in the surgical management of PCN, focusing on the evolution of evidence-based guidelines, short-term and long-term outcomes, and individualized risk–benefit assessment.

GASTROINTESTINAL ENDOSCOPY CLINICS OF NORTH AMERICA

SERIES OF RELATED INTEREST

Gastroenterology Clinics
(www.gastro.theclinics.com)
Clinics in Liver Disease
(www.liver.theclinics.com)

THE CLINICS ARE AVAILABLE ONLINE!
Access your subscription at:
www.theclinics.com

GASTROINTESTINAL ENDOSCOPY CLINICS
OF NORTH AMERICA

FORTHCOMING ISSUES

October 2023
Updates in my Barrett's Esophagus
D. Nageshwar Reddy and
Rupjyoti Talukdar, Editors

January 2024
The Endoscopic Oncologist
Kenneth J. Chang and Jason B.
Samarasena, Editor

April 2024
Cardiac Annual Meeting
Ali A. Siddiqui, Editor

RECENT ISSUES

April 2023
Pediatric Endoscopy
Catharine M. Walsh, Editor

January 2023
Endoscopic Gastrointestinal Submucosal
Dissection and Third Space Endoscopy
Amrita Sethi, Editor

October 2022
Endoscopic Therapies for the GI system
Endoscopic Treatment of Early Luminal
Neoplasia

SERIES OF RELATED INTEREST

Gastroenterology Clinics
Available at: https://www.gastro.theclinics.com
Clinics in Liver Disease
Available at: https://www.liver.theclinics.com

Foreword

Incidental Pancreatic Cysts: What to Do

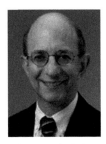

Charles J. Lightdale, MD
Consulting Editor

With the widespread use of chest and abdominal imaging using computed tomography or MRI, the incidental finding of pancreatic cysts has become commonplace. Herein lies the rub. While the great majority of these cysts are benign or indolent, a small minority may offer the chance to prevent or cure a potentially lethal pancreatic cancer. What to do?

Dr Tamas A. Gonda, an expert pancreatologist, and the Editor for this issue of the *Gastrointestinal Endoscopy Clinics of North America*, has long been a leader in answering this question. He has selected a broad range of topics with a strong cast of specialist authors in radiology, gastroenterology, gastrointestinal endoscopy, and surgery to present "Advances in the Diagnosis and Treatment of Pancreatic Cystic Neoplasms." This is a state-of-the-art issue for those in the clinical trenches having to deal with anxious patients and provides a strong glimpse into the future as research progresses.

Charles J. Lightdale, MD
Department of Medicine
Columbia University Medical Center
161 Fort Washington Avenue
New York, NY 10032, USA

E-mail address:
CJL18@columbia.edu

Gastrointest Endoscopy Clin N Am 33 (2023) xiii
https://doi.org/10.1016/j.giec.2023.04.009
1052-5157/23/© 2023 Published by Elsevier Inc.

giendo.theclinics.com

Preface

Advances in the Diagnosis and Treatment of Pancreatic Cystic Neoplasms

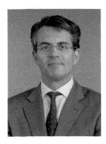

Tamas A. Gonda, MD
Editor

Pancreatic cystic lesions are increasingly recognized through broad use of cross-sectional imaging and may also be increasing in prevalence. Although the majority of these lesions are either benign or will not progress to an invasive cancer, a subset of them represents a unique opportunity to detect an early and curable precursor to pancreatic cancer. Since the recognition of these cystic precursors and the development of the early guidelines for management of pancreatic cysts, significant advances have been made in the understanding of the epidemiology, radiologic classification, endoscopic imaging, and biomarkers.

When the first guidelines for pancreatic cysts were written, few recommendations existed for screening for pancreatic cancer at all. The recognition of both familial pancreatic cancer and risk associated with a number of germline mutations led to the evolution of pancreatic screening programs that now often lead to the diagnosis of cystic lesions.

Although the guidelines have incorporated many of these important discoveries, it is recent advances in radiomics, molecular biomarkers in blood or cyst fluid, and risk modeling using machine learning and artificial intelligence that are likely to most profoundly impact the management of pancreatic cysts.

Treatment strategies have also evolved. Surgical resection remains the standard of care, but advances in surgical technique lead to safer and more parenchyma-preserving approaches. Ablation of pancreatic cysts is emerging as an important and much less invasive modality that is increasingly demonstrating efficacy and safety.

In this issue, five articles review in detail the current epidemiologic data ("Burden of New Pancreatic Cyst Diagnosis" By Romutis and Brand), radiologic testing and reporting ("Pancreatic Cystic Lesions: Imaging Techniques and Diagnostic Features" by Taya

Gastrointest Endoscopy Clin N Am 33 (2023) xv–xvi
https://doi.org/10.1016/j.giec.2023.04.008
1052-5157/23/© 2023 Published by Elsevier Inc.

and colleagues and "Pancreatic Cysts: Radiology" by Megibow), and endoscopic imaging ("Endoscopic Imaging of Pancreatic Cysts" by Taylor and Al-Taee). These articles are coupled with three others that explore the evolving new approaches in each discipline to improve the diagnostic accuracy using radiomics ("Pancreatic Cystic Lesions: Next Generation of Radiologic Assessment" by Huang and colleagues) and blood- or cyst fluid-based biomarkers ("Blood-based Biomarkers in the Diagnosis and Risk Stratification of Pancreatic Cysts" by Peller and Das and "Pancreatic Cyst Fluid Analysis" by Siddappa and Park). Four additional sections focus on some of the most difficult management questions, such as individuals at high risk of pancreatic cancer with cysts ("Are All Cysts Created Equal? Pancreatic Cystic Neoplasms in Patients with Familial or Genetic Risk Factors for Pancreatic Cancer" by Haimi and colleagues), surveillance of cysts ("Surveillance of Pancreatic Cystic Neoplasms" by Farrell and colleagues), and risk stratification and approach to surgery ("Risk Models for Pancreatic Cyst Diagnosis" by Cattelani and colleagues and "Innovation in the Surgical Management of Pancreatic Cystic Neoplasms: Same Operations, Narrower Indications, and an Individualized Approach to Decision Making" by Schleimer and colleagues).

Our issue combines a comprehensive review of what is known today and how novel approaches and ongoing studies may impact management tomorrow. We focus on some of the most challenging and important questions of surveillance, therapy, and risk assessment. Although the field is rapidly changing, we hope this issue provides our readers a valuable summary of the state-of-the-art in pancreatic cysts in 2023.

Tamas A. Gonda, MD
Pancreatic Disease Program
Division of Gastroenterology and Hepatology
Department of Medicine
New York University Grossman School of Medicine
240 East 38th Street
New York, NY 10032, USA

E-mail address:
tamas.gonda@nyulangone.org

Burden of New Pancreatic Cyst Diagnosis

Stephanie Romutis, MD*, Randall Brand, MD

KEYWORDS

- Pancreatic cysts • Pancreatic cystic neoplasm
- Intraductal papillary mucinous neoplasm (IPMN) • Prevalence • Psychosocial burden
- Cost-effectiveness

KEY POINTS

- Improvements in cross-sectional imaging along with an aging population have led to an increase in incidental pancreatic cyst findings.
- The overall risk of malignant progression of asymptomatic pancreatic cysts remains low at 0.24%/year.
- Several guidelines exist to govern the management of pancreatic cysts; however, there is no clear consensus on how long surveillance should last.
- The diagnosis of a pancreatic cyst can lead to significant psychosocial burden for the patient and potential significant costs for the health care system.

BACKGROUND

Pancreatic cysts can arise following episodes of pancreatitis or pancreatic injury; however, most lesions are asymptomatic and detected incidentally on cross-sectional imaging performed for other indications. Cysts can be further classified based on their appearance, malignant potential, or mucinous versus non-mucinous properties. Determining a cyst subtype is paramount as the risk for malignancy varies among cyst types. Pancreatic pseudocysts arise following pancreatic injury (either secondary to pancreatitis or pancreatic duct injury) and are not felt to carry a risk for malignancy. Pancreatic cystic neoplasms (PCN) include a number of cyst subtypes with varying degrees of malignant potential. Serous cyst adenomas (SCA) are slow-growing, benign tumors with a female sex predominance. Mucinous cystic neoplasms (MCN) also have a female sex predominance; however, like other mucinous cysts, they are felt to harbor an increased risk for malignant progression. Intraductal papillary mucinous neoplasms (IPMN) can be seen in a branch-duct (BD-IPMN), main-duct

UPMC Division of Gastroenterology, Hepatology, and Nutrition, 200 Lothrop Street, Mezzanine Level C-wing, Pittsburgh, PA 15213, USA
* Corresponding author.
E-mail address: romutissl@upmc.edu

Gastrointest Endoscopy Clin N Am 33 (2023) 487–495
https://doi.org/10.1016/j.giec.2023.03.001
1052-5157/23/Published by Elsevier Inc.
giendo.theclinics.com

(MD-IPMN), or mixed variety with a risk of malignant progression greater in cysts involving the main pancreatic duct. Less commonly, pancreatic cysts may represent solid pseudopapillary neoplasm (SPN) or cystic pancreatic endocrine neoplasms.[1-3]

Determining pancreatic cyst subtype based on imaging alone remains an ongoing burden of great significance, as the malignant potential of different cysts helps drive recommendations for cyst management. The increasing incidence of pancreatic cysts has generated significant clinical burden regarding how best to manage these often asymptomatic lesions over the long term (**Box 1**).

DISCUSSION
Burden of Increased Incidental Findings

Continued improvement in cross-sectional imaging has led to an explosion in the number of incidental findings including asymptomatic pancreatic cystic lesions. Incidental pancreatic cysts have an estimated prevalence of 2% to 15% on cross-sectional imaging[1,4,5]; however, autopsy studies have demonstrated pancreatic cyst prevalence approaching 50%, particularly in the aging population.[6] In a meta-analysis encompassing 48,860 patients from 2008 to 2018, the prevalence of incidentally noted pancreatic cysts was found to range from 0.2% - 45.9% across abdominal imaging modalities with a pooled prevalence of 8%.[7] The 2018 European Society guidelines on the management of pancreatic cysts note that PCN have been demonstrated to have a prevalence of 2.1% to 2.6% on computerized tomography (CT) imaging and 13.5% to 45% on MRI.[8] In a retrospective review of 8052 patient records from a tertiary care center of 10 years, incidental pancreatic cysts were found in 2034 patients (25.3%), 1524 of which were detected by CT imaging and 510 detected by MRI.[9] In a prospective study involving the Study of Health in Pomerania (SHIP) cohort from Northeast Germany, Kromery and colleagues reviewed 1077 participants who underwent MRI and magnetic resonance cholangiopancreatography (MRCP) as part of a comprehensive health examination. A total of 494 unique participants were found to have incidental pancreatic cysts with a weighted cyst prevalence of 49.1%. From the 1077 participants from the SHIP cohort, 676 participants who subsequently

---

Box 1
Potential burdens of pancreatic cysts

Burden of cyst detection
  Incidental findings
  Differentiating cyst subtype
  Determining malignant potential
  Comorbid conditions associated with pancreatic cysts

Burden of cyst management
  Surveillance vs surgical resection
  Optimal surveillance timeline
  Cost of surveillance vs resection

Burden faced by patients
  Psychological burden
  Socioeconomic and racial disparities in cyst management

Areas requiring further research
  Cost-effective cyst management strategies
  Serum-based testing for cyst characterization
  Improved predictors of cyst malignant potential
  Impact of socioeconomic status and race on cyst outcomes

underwent repeat MRI and MRCP were analyzed and demonstrated an incidence of asymptomatic pancreatic cysts of 12.9% at a 5-year follow-up.[6]

Despite the increase in incidental pancreatic cyst findings, there are limited data regarding the global distribution of pancreatic cyst burden. One meta-analysis suggested that patients within an Asian population had a higher incidence of asymptomatic pancreatic cysts (OR 3.69), although the authors reported that this finding was based on limited data.[10] Although data in the global stratification of cyst burden is limited, studies have noted that the prevalence of pancreatic cysts increases with patient age. This was further highlighted in the comprehensive review provided by Farrell, where it was noted that incidental pancreatic cysts had a prevalence of 2.5% on CT imaging which increased to 10% in patients aged 70 or older. Similar to what has been demonstrated in previous studies, the review noted a prevalence of asymptomatic pancreatic cysts on MRI ranging from 2% to 38%.[2] With an increasingly aging population, incidental detection of asymptomatic pancreatic cysts is expected to continue to rise. Incidental discovery of pancreatic cysts places considerable burden on clinicians, patients, and health systems as they navigate how best to manage these cysts moving forward.

Burden of Differentiating Cyst Subtype

Differentiating subtypes of pancreatic cysts based on imaging findings alone is a burden in itself. Although it was previously thought that the majority of incidentally noted pancreatic cysts represented asymptomatic pseudocysts, recent studies have shown that of the cysts identified, up to 95% are likely PCN.[9,11] Further subclassification of PCN into SCA, MCN, IPMN, or SPN is limited by imaging characteristics alone and surgical pathology remains the gold standard for cyst classification. In a retrospective study, de Pretis *and colleagues* reviewed 174 patient cases who underwent surgery for pancreatic cysts at a single tertiary care center between 2000 and 2012. Overall, the accuracy of pre-operative diagnosis (based on CT, MR, and/or endoscopic ultrasound [EUS] imaging findings) was 69%. Although this finding was in keeping with the reported 68% to 78% accuracy of pre-operative cyst classification based on imaging, the authors noted that there was wide variation in the accuracy of determining different cyst subtypes. Of the 174 patients included in the study, 24% (n = 41) were ultimately found to have a benign cyst; classified as SCA (n = 17), pseudocyst (n = 15), simple cyst (n = 8), or lymphangioma (n = 1). Of the remaining cysts, surgical pathology confirmed pre-operative diagnosis for 87.5% of presumed SCA, 80% of presumed pseudocysts, 73.3% of branch-duct IPMN, and only 53.6% of MCN.[12] The authors did note that increased cyst size seemed to correlate with presumed pre-operative diagnosis; however, they noted that relying on imaging characteristics alone could lead to inappropriate resection of otherwise benign lesions.

In an effort to improve incidental cyst classification and subsequent management plans, more invasive testing involving EUS-guided fine needle aspiration (FNA) has emerged. Although EUS-FNA cytology can help differentiate cyst types, further fluid analysis studies including biochemistry profiles and genetic testing are under investigation to see if they can help not only identify cyst type but also help determine a cyst risk profile. Current guidelines aim to provide cyst management recommendations based on imaging characteristics in conjunction with analysis of EUS-FNA obtained cyst fluid.[1,5] However, there is no consensus on which EUS-FNA fluid studies offer the greatest diagnostic yield. Despite leading to improvements in diagnostic prognostication, fluid analysis, similar to abdominal imaging, continues to underperform in cases of high-grade dysplasia and malignancy.[1] Further, EUS-FNA is not without potential risk and may not be readily available outside of specialized care centers and accessible to all patients with incidentally noted cysts. Advances in genetic testing show promise in improving the diagnostic accuracy of EUS-FNA. Next-generation sequencing of pancreatic cyst fluid has been shown to greatly improve the specificity and sensitivity of detecting mucinous pancreatic cystic lesions and enable the detection of high-risk alterations that correspond with advanced neoplasia.[13]

Overtreatment of Pancreatic Cysts

As not all cysts harbor the same risk profile, clinicians must grapple with balancing potential surgical intervention and further invasive studies with the risk of overtreatment and unnecessary surveillance. Among the current guidelines for pancreatic cyst management, there is some consensus regarding which cysts should be referred for operative intervention. Cysts presenting with high-risk features such as concurrent jaundice, enhancing mural nodules ($\geq$5 mm), solid components, positive cytology, or main pancreatic duct dilation $\geq$ 10 mm are felt to harbor a high risk for underlying malignancy or progression to malignancy and are recommended to undergo surgical resection. Although the presence of these high-risk features supports the decision to proceed with operative resection, in cases of indeterminate-risk cysts, the decision to proceed with surgery is much more convoluted. As de Pretis and colleagues demonstrated, pre-operative cyst classification may overestimate a cyst risk profile and lead to unnecessary operations. The pancreaticobiliary surgical technique continues to improve, but considerable morbidity and mortality remain for pancreatic cyst resections. In a comprehensive review of pancreatic cyst management, van Huijgevoort and colleagues noted that pancreatoduodenectomy is associated with a 20% to 40% perioperative morbidity and 1% to 3% mortality rate. For those patients who undergo successful surgical resection, post-procedure complication rates approach 40% for pancreaticoduodenectomy and nearly 25% for distal pancreatectomy.[14] Complications, such as development of pancreatic fistula, new-onset diabetes mellitus, and new-onset pancreatic exocrine insufficiency, can exacerbate the cost and burden of care for incidentally noted cysts.

Despite advances in pancreatic cancer management, overall 5-year survival remains low at 12%[15–18] with a slight improvement to 15% to 25% following invasive surgery.[19] Risk of malignant progression varies greatly with cyst subtype. Both MCN and main-duct IPMN (MD-IPMN) are felt to carry a higher risk for malignancy with literature reviews citing a 10% to 39% lifetime malignancy risk for MCN and a 36% to 100% risk for MD-IPMN.[20] Given the high potential for malignancy, most MCN and MD-IPMN are recommended for surgical resection; however, some patients may opt for surveillance instead. In contrast, branch-duct IPMN (BD-IPMN) has been cited to have a malignancy risk of 10% to 39% which has driven recommendations for ongoing surveillance. In a Japanese-based cohort study involving 664 patients with pancreatic cysts who were followed for a median of 33.5 months, Ohno and colleagues noted that the cumulative incidence of pancreatic cancer was 1.2%, all in patients with suspected BD-IPMN.[15] In a separate cohort study involving 520,970 patients within the Veterans Affairs Health System, the incidence of pancreatic cancer was found to be 5.08 per 1000 person-years in pancreatic cyst patients versus 0.32 per 1000 person-years in non-cyst patients.[21] Studies have also demonstrated that patients with pancreatic cancer are more likely to have cysts relative to the remaining population. In a retrospective review of 2720 patients within a Japanese tertiary care center database, patients with pancreatic cancer had a higher prevalence of pancreatic cysts (56%) compared to a control group with no history of pancreatic disease (10%) with the majority of cysts felt to represent BD-IPMN.[22] Although there is potential for malignancy, the actual rate of malignant progression of pancreatic cysts is felt to be low, estimated at 0.24%/year (**Fig. 1**).[17] Despite this low rate of malignant progression, the poor prognosis of pancreatic malignancy is often an impetus for ongoing cyst surveillance.

Comorbid Conditions Associated with Pancreatic Cysts

In addition to incidental findings, several studies have identified extra-pancreatic conditions that are associated with pancreatic cyst presence. Further compounding the burden on clinicians, there is a paucity of data regarding how much of an impact these extra-pancreatic conditions have on cyst development and whether they warrant surveillance. In a retrospective review of 5296 individuals who underwent MRI as part of an initial comprehensive health examination, presence of a pancreatic cyst was linked with advanced age (OR 1.06), excess body mass index (BMI) greater than 25 kg/m^2 (OR 1.26), and diabetes mellitus (OR 1.39).[23] Conditions such as Peutz-Jegher, Lynch syndrome, polycystic-dominant kidney disease, and Von-Hippel Lindau (VHL) disease have been shown to be associated with pancreatic cysts, but it remains unclear if this translates to increased malignancy risk. In a review of 186 patients from a Dutch cohort database, 98 of which carried mutations for either *CDKN2A, BRCA, TP53, or LKB1/STK11* and 88 of which had a familial history of pancreatic cancer, mutation carriers were more likely to have progression of their pancreatic cysts while familial history was associated with a larger cyst size at initial presentation.[24] Although comorbid conditions can contribute to cyst presence, studies have also demonstrated that they can have significant impact on the benefit of cyst surveillance. In a retrospective, single-center study involving 440 prospectively entered individuals (excluding cases of VHL patients, serous cystadenomas, and pseudocysts), it was noted that patients

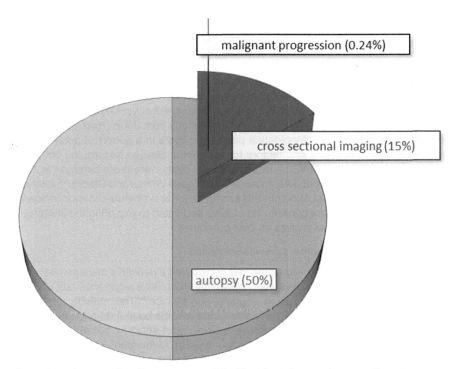

Fig. 1. Prevalence and malignancy potential of incidentally noted pancreatic cysts.

with an Age-Charlson Comorbidity Index (Age-CACI) score $\geq$ 7 had a 4-year survival rate of 40.32% which negated any benefit for cyst surveillance.[25]

Psychological Burden of Pancreatic Cyst Diagnosis

Although the risk of malignant progression in pancreatic cysts is low, the psychological burden of harboring a potential pre-malignant lesion can be extremely distressing for patients. Although a few guidelines comment on end-points for pancreatic cyst surveillance, fear of a missed malignancy may lead clinicians and patients to pursue unnecessary surveillance. In a review of the Pancreatic CYst Follow-up (PACYFIC) cohort, 109 participants completed 179 questionnaires which demonstrated that most patients felt good under a surveillance protocol due to the potential to detect cancer early. However, participants did note that undergoing surveillance did contribute to psychosocial stressors with 13% of participants reporting anxiety because of being under surveillance, 11% reporting discomfort secondary to surveillance methods, and 28% reporting that participating in surveillance was generally burdensome.[26] The psychological burden of pancreatic cyst surveillance was further highlighted in a retrospective review of pancreatic cyst patients from a tertiary care center in Italy. Patients participated in a 60-min interview which involved several psychosocial questionnaires (including the Barratt Simplified Measure of Socioeconomic Status, Brief-COPE, Perceived Stress Scale) and were subdivided into cases that underwent surgical resection of their pancreatic cysts versus patients undergoing active surveillance. Patients undergoing surveillance were more likely to report somatization and anxiety symptoms compared to patients who had undergone surgical resection and they were more likely to have a reduced perception of overall health status.[27] Although pancreatic cyst surveillance may help mitigate concerns for pancreatic malignancy development, surveillance can introduce a significant psychological burden for patients.

Socioeconomic and Racial Burden

Socioeconomic and racial factors are well-known elements that impact pancreatic cancer care. Uninsured patients and individuals from underrepresented minorities are less likely to undergo pancreatic resection or participate in clinical trials.[10,28] These factors are understudied for pancreatic cystic lesions with no available data on the relationship between socioeconomic status and pancreatic cyst outcomes. Regarding racial disparities and cyst prevalence, one small study from Johns Hopkins University looked at the prevalence of incidental pancreatic cysts in a cohort of adult patients with no history or predisposing factors for pancreatic disease undergoing outpatient multi-detector CT scan. After controlling for age, cysts were more common in Asian individuals and no statistical differences seen between Whites and Blacks.[29] Although there are several ongoing cohort studies aiming to better define outcomes in incidental pancreatic cysts, there are currently no studies dedicated to exploring the interplay of socioeconomic and racial factors on cyst outcomes.

Ambiguity Regarding Optimal Surveillance Period

Although surgical resection was previously considered a definitive management strategy for pancreatic cysts, studies have shown that PCN has a recurrence rate of 7% to 8% post-operatively necessitating ongoing surveillance.[8] The majority of current guidelines recommend ongoing cyst surveillance until the patient is no longer deemed an appropriate candidate for surgical resection. In an effort to curtail the potential expense and burden of life-long surveillance, the 2015 American Gastroenterological Association guidelines suggested that cyst surveillance could be discontinued after 5 years due to a low risk for subsequent progression to malignancy.[1] Since publishing the review, several studies have suggested that an increased malignancy risk remains and patients should continue to undergo active surveillance. In a retrospective review of a prospectively entered database spanning from 1995 to 2016, Lawrence and colleagues analyzed 3024 pancreatic cyst cases of which 596 underwent 5+ years of surveillance. The authors noted that even after 5 years of surveillance, the rate of malignancy in the pancreatic cyst group was 31.3 per 1,000,000 per year compared to 7.04 per 1,000,000 per year in the general population as calculated via Surveillance, Epidemiology, and End Results data. Given this increased risk, the authors advocated that pancreatic cyst patients warrant ongoing surveillance beyond the 5-year mark despite the known overall low risk for malignant progression.[30]

Cost Burden of Surveillance

In addition to the psychosocial and management burdens placed on patients and clinicians, incidental PCN place significant burdens on the health care system. Successful surveillance of PCN depends on a health care system's ability to accommodate repeat imaging procedures as well as potential EUS ± FNA for further investigation. Although there are limited data regarding the cost of pancreatic cyst surveillance, several studies have demonstrated that the cost of surveillance is not insignificant. Compared to no surveillance, studies have estimated a cost of $20,096 per quality-adjusted life years (QALY) for patients undergoing surveillance.[31] In a hypothetical cohort of 60-year-old patients with PCN, Markov modeling comparing based on the 2017 International Association of Pancreatology Consensus Guidelines for Management of IPMN no intervention, surgical resection, and pancreatic cyst surveillance (based on 2017 International Association of Pancreatology Consensus Guidelines for Management of IPMN), the cost of pancreatic cyst surveillance was not insignificant. One study examining the cost of short protocol MRI versus comprehensive protocol MRI noted that over a 10-year surveillance period for a 154-patient cohort, short-protocol MRI led to a cost saving of 560,000 EUR.[4] A separate study noted that in order for surveillance to be more cost-effective than surgery, the specificity of current surveillance strategies for low-grade dysplasia would need to improve. If specificity for low-grade dysplasia could improve beyond 65%, the estimated cost savings were $90,403 per QALY.[11]

SUMMARY

With an increasingly aging population, the incidence of PCN is expected to rise. Although the potential for malignant progression of PCN remains low, concerns of developing cancer remain a daunting possibility for cyst patients. Although multiple guidelines have been developed in an effort to direct the management of asymptomatic pancreatic cysts, there is no clear consensus on how best to manage these lesions. Part of the complexity of determining optimal management plans for asymptomatic cysts rests in the fact that the risk profile of cysts can vary greatly among cyst types. As the diagnosis of pancreatic cysts becomes more common, clinicians and health care systems have to grapple with the burden of balancing the cost-effectiveness and psychosocial ramifications of cyst management strategies.

CLINICS CARE POINTS

- The diagnosis of a pancreatic cyst can cause significant psychosocial stressors for a patient.
- Continued improvement in pancreatic cyst fluid analysis may help better profile the malignant potential of pancreatic cysts.

- Current data suggest that patients should continue to undergo pancreatic cyst surveillance following surgical resection.
- Given the low rate of malignant potential in pancreatic cysts, clinicians should consider comorbid conditions and the psychosocial burden of surveillance when developing management plans for patients.

DISCLOSURE

S. Romutis: no disclosures. R. Brand: Receives research funding from Immunovia and Freenome this is paid through their institution.

REFERENCES

1. DiMaio CJ. Current Guideline Controversies in the Management of Pancreatic Cystic Neoplasms. Gastrointest Endosc Clin N Am 2018;28(4):529–47.
2. Farrell JJ. Prevalence, Diagnosis and Management of Pancreatic Cystic Neoplasms: Current Status and Future Directions. Gut Liver 2015;9(5):571–89.
3. Scheiman JM, Hwang JH, Moayyedi P. American gastroenterological association technical review on the diagnosis and management of asymptomatic neoplastic pancreatic cysts. Gastroenterology 2015;148(4):824–848 e22.
4. Pozzi-Mucelli RM, Rinta-Kiikka I, Wunsche K, et al. Pancreatic MRI for the surveillance of cystic neoplasms: comparison of a short with a comprehensive imaging protocol. Eur Radiol 2017;27(1):41–50.
5. Ketwaroo GA, Mortele KJ, Sawhney MS. Pancreatic Cystic Neoplasms: An Update. Gastroenterol Clin North Am 2016;45(1):67–81.
6. Kromrey ML, Bulow R, Hubner J, et al. Prospective study on the incidence, prevalence and 5-year pancreatic-related mortality of pancreatic cysts in a population-based study. Gut 2018;67(1):138–45.
7. Zerboni G, Signoretti M, Crippa S, et al. Systematic review and meta-analysis: Prevalence of incidentally detected pancreatic cystic lesions in asymptomatic individuals. Pancreatology 2019;19(1):2–9.
8. European Study Group on Cystic Tumours of the P. European evidence-based guidelines on pancreatic cystic neoplasms. Gut 2018;67(5):789–804.
9. Chernyak V, Flusberg M, Haramati LB, et al. Incidental pancreatic cystic lesions: is there a relationship with the development of pancreatic adenocarcinoma and all-cause mortality? Radiology 2015;274(1):161–9.
10. Cervantes A, Waymouth EK, Petrov MS. African-Americans and Indigenous Peoples Have Increased Burden of Diseases of the Exocrine Pancreas: A Systematic Review and Meta-Analysis. Dig Dis Sci 2019;64(1):249–61.
11. Sharib J, Esserman L, Koay EJ, et al. Cost-effectiveness of consensus guideline based management of pancreatic cysts: The sensitivity and specificity required for guidelines to be cost-effective. Surgery 2020;168(4):601–9.
12. de Pretis N, Mukewar S, Aryal-Khanal A, et al. Pancreatic cysts: Diagnostic accuracy and risk of inappropriate resections. Pancreatology 2017;17(2):267–72.
13. Singhi AD, McGrath K, Brand RE, et al. Preoperative next-generation sequencing of pancreatic cyst fluid is highly accurate in cyst classification and detection of advanced neoplasia. Gut 2018;67(12):2131–41.
14. van Huijgevoort NCM, Del Chiaro M, Wolfgang CL, et al. Diagnosis and management of pancreatic cystic neoplasms: current evidence and guidelines. Nat Rev Gastroenterol Hepatol 2019;16(11):676–89.

15. Mizrahi JD, Surana R, Valle JW, et al. Pancreatic cancer. Lancet 2020; 395(10242):2008–20.
16. Ohno E, Hirooka Y, Kawashima H, et al. Natural history of pancreatic cystic lesions: A multicenter prospective observational study for evaluating the risk of pancreatic cancer. J Gastroenterol Hepatol 2018;33(1):320–8.
17. Xiao AY, Tan ML, Wu LM, et al. Global incidence and mortality of pancreatic diseases: a systematic review, meta-analysis, and meta-regression of population-based cohort studies. Lancet Gastroenterol Hepatol 2016;1(1):45–55.
18. Society AC. Cancer Facts & Figures 2022. 2022.
19. Kleeff J, Korc M, Apte M, et al. Pancreatic cancer. Nat Rev Dis Primers 2016;2: 16022.
20. Yoon JG, Smith D, Ojili V, et al. Pancreatic cystic neoplasms: a review of current recommendations for surveillance and management. Abdom Radiol (NY) 2021; 46(8):3946–62.
21. Munigala S, Gelrud A, Agarwal B. Risk of pancreatic cancer in patients with pancreatic cyst. Gastrointest Endosc 2016;84(1):81–6.
22. Matsubara S, Tada M, Akahane M, et al. Incidental pancreatic cysts found by magnetic resonance imaging and their relationship with pancreatic cancer. Pancreas 2012;41(8):1241–6.
23. Mizuno S, Isayama H, Nakai Y, et al. Prevalence of Pancreatic Cystic Lesions Is Associated With Diabetes Mellitus and Obesity: An Analysis of 5296 Individuals Who Underwent a Preventive Medical Examination. Pancreas 2017;46(6):801–5.
24. Konings IC, Harinck F, Poley JW, et al. Prevalence and Progression of Pancreatic Cystic Precursor Lesions Differ Between Groups at High Risk of Developing Pancreatic Cancer. Pancreas 2017;46(1):28–34.
25. Chhoda A, Yousaf MN, Madhani K, et al. Comorbidities Drive the Majority of Overall Mortality in Low-Risk Mucinous Pancreatic Cysts Under Surveillance. Clin Gastroenterol Hepatol 2022;20(3):631–640 e1.
26. Overbeek KA, Kamps A, van Riet PA, et al. Pancreatic cyst surveillance imposes low psychological burden. Pancreatology 2019;19(8):1061–6.
27. Marinelli V, Secchettin E, Andrianello S, et al. Psychological distress in patients under surveillance for intraductal papillary mucinous neoplasms of the pancreas: The "Sword of Damocles" effect calls for an integrated medical and psychological approach a prospective analysis. Pancreatology 2020;20(3):505–10.
28. Thobie A, Mulliri A, Bouvier V, et al. Same Chance of Accessing Resection? Impact of Socioeconomic Status on Resection Rates Among Patients with Pancreatic Adenocarcinoma-A Systematic Review. Health Equity 2021;5(1):143–50.
29. Laffan TA, Horton KM, Klein AP, et al. Prevalence of unsuspected pancreatic cysts on MDCT. AJR Am J Roentgenol 2008;191(3):802–7.
30. Lawrence SA, Attiyeh MA, Seier K, et al. Should Patients With Cystic Lesions of the Pancreas Undergo Long-term Radiographic Surveillance?: Results of 3024 Patients Evaluated at a Single Institution. Ann Surg 2017;266(3):536–44.
31. Maggi G, Guarneri G, Gasparini G, et al. Pancreatic cystic neoplasms: What is the most cost-effective follow-up strategy? Endosc Ultrasound 2018;7(5):319–22.

Pancreatic Cystic Lesions
Imaging Techniques and Diagnostic Features

Michio Taya, MD[a,1], Elizabeth M. Hecht, MD[a,1],
Chenchan Huang, MD[b], Grace C. Lo, MD[a],*

KEYWORDS

- Pancreatic cystic lesions • Pancreatic cystic neoplasms
- Magnetic resonance cholangiopancreatography (MRCP) • Multidetector CT

KEY POINTS

- The key imaging features used to characterize pancreatic cystic lesions are best assessed by contrast-enhanced MRI/MRCP, with pancreas protocol CT offering a complementary role.
- The role of imaging is to distinguish mucinous lesions from other pancreatic cysts, stratify malignancy risk, and detect changes that necessitate additional testing or intervention.
- Important imaging features include lesion location, size, morphology, enhancing nodules or septa, relationship to main pancreatic duct, duct size and morphology, and assessment of uninvolved parenchymal and peripancreatic tissues.
- While some imaging features have high specificity for a particular diagnosis, overlapping imaging features between diagnoses may require further investigation.

INTRODUCTION

The incidental detection of pancreatic cystic lesions has increased due to advances in imaging techniques, improvements in spatial and contrast resolution, and increasing age of the general population. In a meta-analysis with 48,860 asymptomatic patients, these pancreatic cystic lesions were seen in 8% of imaging studies. However, a wide range (0.2%–45.9%) was reported, with mucinous lesions being the most commonly detected ones.[1] While the majority of pancreatic cystic lesions are benign, it is crucial to accurately recognize the lesions that are malignant or have malignant potential to reduce morbidity and mortality. At the same time, it is equally important to spare patients from unnecessary imaging studies, invasive sampling techniques, and surgery for benign conditions. Cross-sectional imaging plays a significant role in narrowing

[a] Department of Radiology, New York Presbyterian – Weill Cornell Medicine, 520 East 70th Street, Starr 8a, New York, NY 10021, USA; [b] Department of Radiology, NYU Grossman School of Medicine, 560 1st Avenue, 2F, New York, NY 10016, USA
[1] Present address: 520 East 70th Street, Starr 8a, New York, NY 10021, USA.
* Corresponding author. 520 East 70th Street, Starr 8a, New York, NY 10021, USA.
E-mail address: gcl9003@med.cornell.edu

Gastrointest Endoscopy Clin N Am 33 (2023) 497–518
https://doi.org/10.1016/j.giec.2023.03.007
1052-5157/23/© 2023 Elsevier Inc. All rights reserved.
giendo.theclinics.com

the differential diagnosis of cystic lesions, serving to triage patients, and helping to guide management decisions. In this review, we will provide an overview of the strengths and weaknesses of cross-sectional imaging modalities for evaluating pancreatic cystic lesions, demonstrate the distinctive and overlapping imaging features for the more commonly encountered cystic lesions, and conclude by providing examples of mimics and pitfalls in the imaging workup of cystic lesions.

IMAGING MODALITIES AND PROTOCOLS
Magnetic Resonance Imaging and Magnetic Resonance Cholangiopancreatography

Diagnostic evaluation of pancreatic cystic lesions is most often performed with magnetic resonance imaging (MRI), including magnetic resonance cholangiopancreatography (MRCP) sequences, or multidetector CT (MDCT). MDCT and MRI/MRCP have comparable accuracy for characterizing pancreatic cystic lesions and estimating their aggressiveness. However, MRI can improve reader confidence in characterizing cystic pancreatic lesions and more readily determine the relationship of the lesion with the pancreatic ducts.[2,3] MRI also has the advantage of not exposing patients to radiation, which is particularly useful for serial follow-up in younger patients. For the above reasons, the American Gastroenterology Association and the Society of Abdominal Radiology's Intraductal Papillary Mucinous Neoplasm (IPMN) disease-focused panel guidelines encourage the use of MRI/MRCP for surveillance of cystic pancreatic lesions.[4,5]

Absolute contraindications to MR include implanted medical devices that are labeled MRI-unsafe. MRI/MRCP scans have long acquisition times compared to CT, which can be challenging for patients with claustrophobia, complex medical conditions, or difficulty lying flat. While both require patient cooperation with breath-hold instructions, the prolonged and repeated breath-hold instructions in MRI, depending on the number of sequences, may tire patients and reduce study quality. However, MRI can be performed with increasingly shorter acquisition times, so scans can be modified to accommodate a patient's needs. Access and scheduling barriers due to the limited availability of MRI capacity in low-resource settings are also considerations when determining the best option for imaging.

MRI/MRCP protocols
MRI/MRCP can be performed at 1.5T or 3T. Patients are typically advised to fast for 4 to 6 hours before the examination to improve gallbladder distension and reduce bowel peristalsis. At some institutions, patients are given oral contrast media just before scanning. Oral contrast agents are optional but are typically administered because they can improve image contrast by suppressing signal from overlapping fluid-filled structures in the background (hence termed "negative T2 oral contrast agent"), such as the bowel. The oral contrast allows the signal from the fluid-filled biliary tree and pancreatic ducts to be more apparent and distinct compared to the background tissue. Examples of oral contrast agents include commercially available preparations that contain gadolinium or iron or store-bought drinks (such as acai juice, black tea, pineapple juice, or blueberry juice) that naturally have a high level of manganese.

MRCP protocols can differ based on institution and vendor, but recommended sequences include axial T1 in-phase and opposed-phase gradient recalled echo (GRE) sequences, axial and coronal T2 single-shot fast spin echo breath-hold sequences, heavily T2-weighted 2D and/or 3D MRCP, and dynamic 3D fat-suppressed T1-weighted spoiled GRE axial sequences before and after administration of intravenous gadolinium contrast (**Fig. 1**).[5,6] Diffusion-weighted imaging (DWI) is typically also included (see **Fig. 1**).

T1 in- and opposed-phased GRE sequences, also called "in-phase" and "out-of-phase" imaging, help identify MR signal voids from calcification, air, and stents and, in combination with other sequences, distinguish actual pancreatic lesions from pseudo-lesions such as invaginating peripancreatic fat or duodenal diverticula. Multiplanar T2-weighted sequences are useful in differentiating cystic from solid lesions and can identify internal contents such as debris, mucin, or mural nodules.[7] These sequences can be rapidly acquired sequences with minimal motion degradation and high

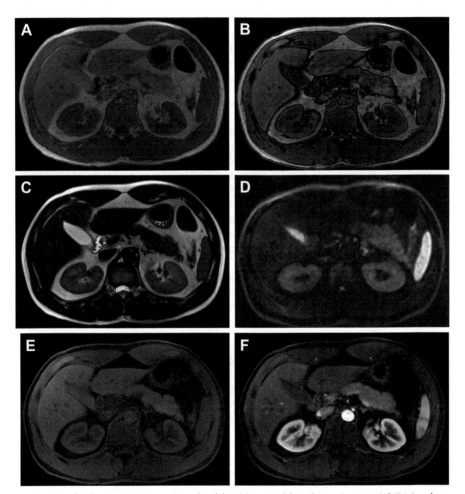

Fig. 1. Standard MRI sequences in a healthy 36-year-old male patient. Axial T1 in-phase showing normal high signal of both the visualized pancreas and surrounding visceral fat (*A*). Axial T1 opposed-phase with India-ink artifact outlining bulk fat-water interfaces (*B*). Axial T2 single-shot fast spin echo sequence [SSFSE] (*C*). High B-value diffusion weighted imaging (DWI) showing normal pancreatic tail (*D*). Fat-suppressed axial T1-weighted sequence showing a normal high parenchymal signal of liver and pancreas and nulling of subcutaneous and visceral fat (*E*). Dynamic 3D fat-suppressed T1-weighted sequence in the axial plane following timed administration of intravenous gadolinium-based contrast in the pancreatic phase (*F*).

in-plane spatial resolution. Fat-suppression techniques may be used to increase lesion conspicuity of cystic lesions and exclude mimics such as focal fat. Using various techniques to suppress the signal of peripancreatic fat (making it darker) is particularly useful because suppressing background fat increases the conspicuity of the bright T2 signal of pancreatic and peripancreatic edema that may be seen in the setting of pancreatitis.

MRCP images are heavily T2-weighted sequences performed in 2D and 3D volumetric acquisitions. These are key sequences because they highlight the biliary and pancreatic ductal anatomy. Also, 3D MRCP can achieve higher-resolution images with isotropic voxel size, which is especially useful in determining if cystic lesions of the pancreas communicate with the pancreatic ductal system and detecting very small subcentimeter cystic lesions. Finally, DWI is a sequence sensitive to Brownian motion and can increase the conspicuity of pancreatic lesions. Some studies also suggest DWI may help differentiate benign from malignant lesions in the pancreas. Additionally, it can identify subtle liver metastases.[8]

Utilization of gadolinium-based intravenous contrast agents

Intravenous contrast is recommended for initial lesion characterization, risk-stratification of IPMNs, as well as patients under surveillance for suspected IPMN, as these patients are at higher risk of pancreatic cancer, and intravenous contrast can increase the conspicuity of pancreatic cancer elsewhere in the gland.[9,10] Based on the 2017 updated Fukuoka Consensus guidelines for surveillance of IPMNs, the presence of enhancing mural nodules ≥ 5 mm is one of the three "high-risk stigmata," and cyst wall enhancement is one of the "worrisome features" of branch-duct IPMNs.[11] In retrospective studies focusing on follow-up of patients with low-risk IPMNs, MRI/MRCP without intravenous contrast has been shown to have no significant impact on management decisions compared to contrast-enhanced imaging, so some subspecialty societies suggest the use of noncontrast MRI/MRCP for follow-up of cystic lesions in lower-risk populations.[5,12] It is recommended, however, that a radiologist be consulted if there is any uncertainty when ordering an MRI/MRCP examination, as they can review prior imaging and help determine whether intravenous contrast is necessary for select patients.

MRCP with secretin

Secretin MRCP is used primarily to assess pancreatic parenchymal exocrine function and to assess for pancreatic duct anomalies or signs of strictures in patients with a history of pancreatitis. Retrospective studies show only an incremental value added in the characterization of side-branch IPMNs; therefore, it is not a recommended study for routine characterization of pancreatic cystic lesions.[5,13]

Computed Tomography

Dual-phase pancreatic protocol computed tomography (CT) is recommended for the initial evaluation of any suspected solid pancreatic mass. Sixteen-detector row CT or higher is recommended to ensure high-resolution imaging with a submillimeter isotropic voxel size. Intravenous contrast-enhanced acquisitions should be made in the pancreatic parenchymal (late-arterial) phase, typically 40 to 50 seconds after injection (depending on the scanner speed) using an injection rate of 4 to 5 mL/s (contrast concentration 300–350 mg I/mL of iodine), and in the portal venous phase at approximately 70 to 80 seconds after injection.[5,14] A precontrast phase (a.k.a. noncontrast phase) is optional but can be useful to assess for the presence of subtle calcifications or after recent instrumentation, such as surgery or stenting. Recent studies have also shown the added benefit of a delayed postcontrast phase in detecting small isodense solid masses.[15] However, this would increase the radiation dose and, therefore, is not part of the current standard protocol.[15] Coronal and sagittal multiplanar reformats are also reconstructed on most scanners or separate workstations and used for interpretation.

A single-phase CT of the abdomen and pelvis (often performed for routine nonspecific indications such as abdominal pain) is performed typically in the portal venous phase and has decreased sensitivity for detecting pancreatic parenchymal lesions.[16–18] Noncontrast CT alone is insufficient for characterizing pancreatic cystic lesions.

MRI with MRCP versus CT

While MRI/MRCP is typically preferred for the initial evaluation and follow-up of pancreatic cystic lesions, preoperative planning may be performed with contrast-enhanced CT or MR to delineate vessel anatomy and involvement, as well as to detect abdominopelvic metastasis. However, given its wide-spread availability and high resolution, CT is more commonly performed for preoperative planning. Local institutional practice and surgeon preference may dictate a preferred modality for preoperative evaluation.

Transabdominal Ultrasound

Transabdominal ultrasound (US) has been used successfully in select populations for cyst follow-up, especially in those with correlative cross-sectional imaging, with a reported detection rate as high as 88%.[19] However, this modality is not recommended for routine cyst evaluation. US can be used in select patients, but there is often incomplete visualization of the pancreas, particularly the pancreatic tail, due to body habitus and artifacts related to bowel gas. Also, quality can vary depending on the operator performing the study.

IMAGING FEATURES OF PANCREATIC CYSTIC LESIONS

When approaching a pancreatic cystic lesion, the most commonly encountered pancreatic lesions include IPMNs, serous cystic neoplasms (SCN), mucinous cystic neoplasms (MCN), and pseudocysts, with these entities accounting for the majority in a surgical series of asymptomatic patients.[20,21]

Less-common pancreatic lesions that can mimic cystic pancreatic tumors include solid pseudopapillary tumor (SPT), pancreatic neuroendocrine tumor (PNET), and highly mucinous or cystic degeneration of pancreatic ductal adenocarcinoma (PDAC). Rare benign lesions can also mimic cystic pancreatic neoplasms, such as true epithelial cysts, lymphoepithelial cysts, and mucinous nonneoplastic cysts.

Cross-sectional imaging in managing pancreatic cystic masses is to distinguish mucinous pancreatic lesions from other pancreatic cysts, stratify the risk of malignancy, and detect changes on surveillance that may necessitate additional diagnostic testing or intervention. The main imaging features that radiologists use in narrowing the differential diagnosis include lesion location, size, morphology, presence or absence of enhancing nodules or septa, relationship to the main pancreatic duct, main pancreatic duct size and morphology, and assessment of uninvolved parenchymal and peripancreatic tissues.

Intraductal Papillary Mucinous Neoplasm

IPMNs are exocrine neoplasms that arise in the mucin-producing epithelium of the pancreatic ductal system and are categorized by their involvement of the main duct, branch ducts, or a combination of the two. IPMNs are more prevalent in males than in females and are typically diagnosed in the sixth through seventh decades of life.[22] Rates of malignancy are reported at 12% to 47% for branch-duct IPMNs, in contrast with combined or main-duct IPMNs, which are observed at 38% to 65% and 38% to 68%, respectively.[23]

Main-duct IPMNs, by definition, involve the main pancreatic duct. Involvement may be segmental or diffuse, but duct dilation can also be seen in the setting of chronic pancreatitis, making it challenging to differentiate at times (**Fig. 2**). Clinical history, the presence of multifocal strictures, and the presence of an intraductal calcified stone help to favor chronic pancreatitis.[24] On the other hand, findings such as duct dilatation without stricture, bulging ampulla, and a nodule in a duct are more specific for main-duct IPMN.[24] While there are studies that try to differentiate benign from malignant pancreatic duct strictures, it cannot be stressed enough that any new focal pancreatic duct stricture or abrupt duct cutoff needs to be further investigated for an underlying mass, as this is the most reproducible sign of pancreatic cancer.

Branch-duct IPMNs can be present anywhere in the pancreas but are commonly identified in the head, with calcification being an uncommon feature.[25] Branch-duct IPMNs may present as unilocular or multilocular lesions, and they may contain thin septations and have lobulated margins. While these imaging features overlap with other cystic neoplasms, what can distinguish side-branch IPMNs is their direct communication with the main duct. This feature can be, at times, challenging to

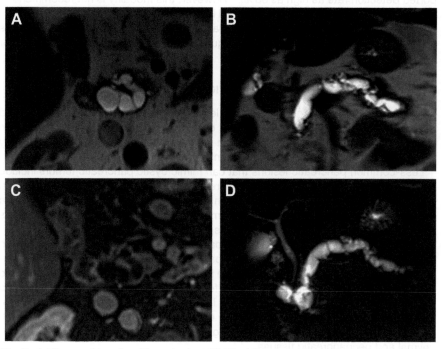

Fig. 2. A 76-year-old male with main-duct IPMN with low-grade dysplasia and no invasive carcinoma. Axial (A) and coronal (B) T2-weighted images show a diffusely dilated main pancreatic duct >5 mm in diameter with diffuse parenchymal atrophy. No enhancing mural nodule is identified on the axial fat-suppressed T1 postcontrast equilibrium phase (C). Thick-slab 2D MRCP of the same lesion (D).

identify on imaging, however. Combined-type or mixed-type IPMNs will demonstrate features of both main-duct and branch-duct IPMNs (**Fig. 3**).

IPMN size, a key imaging feature and a component of management guidelines, should be based on the single longest outer wall-to-outer wall dimension in the imaging plane with the largest measurement.[5] The presence of a solid component or an enhancing mural nodule within an IPMN is an important predictor of malignancy (**Fig. 4**). A thick enhancing wall (>2–3 mm) and enhancing thick or nodular septa are additional features associated with malignancy.[5,26]

The degree of main pancreatic ductal dilatation is an important imaging feature under the 2017 revised Fukuoka guidelines, where dilatation of 5 to 9 mm or abrupt change in caliber with distal atrophy represents a "worrisome feature," alongside six other criteria, including cyst size ≥3 cm, enhancing mural nodule less than 5 mm, thickened enhanced cyst walls, lymphadenopathy, elevated serum level of CA19-9, and rapid rate of cyst growth greater than 5 mm/2 y.[11] "Worrisome features" represent IPMNs with a relatively higher risk of malignancy than lesions without these features, although they do not represent an immediate surgical indication under these guidelines.

In contrast, a main pancreatic duct diameter of ≥10 mm is one of the "high-risk stigmata" alongside obstructive jaundice and an enhancing mural nodule ≥5 mm, representing the highest risk category where surgery should be strongly considered.[11]

While there are multiple societal consensus guidelines with variations in target cystic lesion and patient population, management recommendations all rely on a combination of the aforementioned imaging features.[11,23,27]

Serous Cystic Neoplasm

Serous cystic neoplasms (SCNs) are benign, histologically defined by cysts lined by a single uniform layer of cuboidal, glycogen-rich "serous cells."[28] There is a strong 3-to-1 female predominance, with a mean incidence in the sixth to seventh decade, hence nicknamed the "grandmother" lesion.[29] While the vast majority of lesions are isolated and sporadic, there is a reported association in patients with Von Hippel-Lindau disease.[30] Given SCNs are benign, they do not require surgical intervention or even follow-up unless they are causing symptoms.

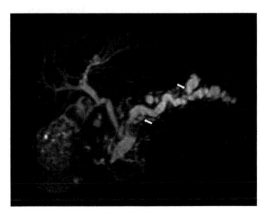

Fig. 3. A 75-year-old male with combined-type IPMN with high-grade dysplasia and no invasive carcinoma. Maximum intensity projections image from a 3D MRCP shows a diffusely enlarged main pancreatic duct >5 mm in diameter as well as several dilated branch ducts (*arrows*) that communicate with the main duct.

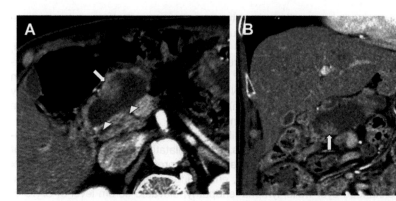

Fig. 4. A 78-year-old male with main-duct IPMN with low-grade dysplasia and no invasive carcinoma. Axial (A) and coronal (B) multidetector CT pancreatic parenchymal phases show a dilated main duct (arrowheads) containing an enhancing mural nodule (arrow).

SCNs can be located anywhere in the pancreas, although with a slight propensity for the head/uncinate (40%) compared to the tail (26%), with a presenting median tumor size of 3.1 cm.[31,32] These lesions do not communicate with the main pancreatic duct, and the surrounding pancreatic parenchyma and peripancreatic tissues are typically normal in appearance. Nonetheless, in 11% of cases, SCNs can be associated with upstream pancreatic duct dilatation, likely related to mass effect, and depending on the severity or symptoms, resection may be warranted.[32]

The classic radiologic appearance of an SCN is a well-circumscribed mass with lobulated borders and internal microcystic loculations separated by thin enhancing septations (**Fig. 5**). The microcystic variant, by definition, is composed of more than 6 cysts (or loculations), each measuring less than 2 cm, resembling the appearance of a honeycomb.[31,33–35] A central fibrous scar is often present (see **Fig. 5**).

In addition to the microcystic variant, macrocystic, mixed, and solid-appearing subtypes have also been described. In a large multi-institution retrospective cohort of 2622 SCNs diagnosed by histology or radiologic follow-up, microcystic morphology was the most common one (45%). Still, up to 32% can be macrocystic (a.k.a. cysts ≥2 cm), and 18% can have a mixed morphology. Macrocystic and unilocular SCNs can be challenging to prospectively diagnose as they mimic the appearance of other classic MCNs, pseudocysts, and IPMNs.[32] In those cases, imaging features favoring SCN include location in the pancreatic head, lobulated contours, and absence of wall enhancement.[36] Rarely, SCNs manifest as solid lesions, representing just 5% of cases in that same series. In case reports, solid SCNs are described as hypervascular solid masses with marked hyperintensity on heavily T2-weighted sequences resembling PNETs and hypervascular metastases.[36,37] Because morphologically atypical SCNs can be challenging to diagnose, tissue sampling plays a vital role in diagnosis.

Despite variability in cystic morphology, a central fibrous scar with or without calcification is highly specific for SCN and considered virtually pathognomonic although observed in only 30% of cases.[36,38–40] A central scar and thin internal vascularized septa that gradually enhance following administration of intravenous contrast are classic features. In one study of pancreatic cystic lesions detected on CT with radiology-pathology correlation, microcystic morphology was strongly and independently associated with SCNs with a positive predictive value of 88% and specificity of 98%.[40] A combination of microcystic morphology and surface lobulations had a positive predictive value and specificity of 100% for a diagnosis of SCN.

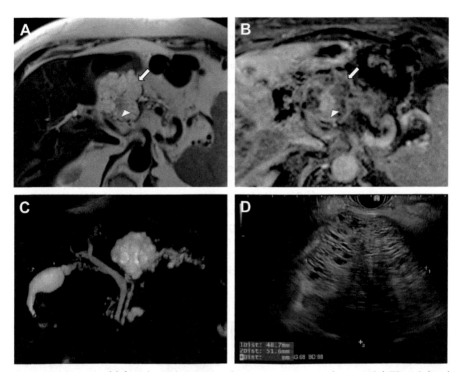

Fig. 5. An 81-year-old female with microcystic serous cystic neoplasm. Axial T2-weighted imaging (A) shows a lobulated microcystic lesion (arrow) in the pancreatic neck with a central spoke-wheel scar (arrowhead), which enhances on delayed postcontrast sequences (B). The pancreatic duct is slightly dilated, with upstream pancreatic atrophy, likely related to compression by the mass. Three-dimensional MRCP (C) shows its lobulated contour and microcystic components, as well as additional branch-duct IPMNs elsewhere in the pancreas. Endoscopic ultrasound images (D) confirm a hyperechoic microcystic mass.

Mucinous Cystic Neoplasm

Mucinous cystic neoplasms (MCNs) may be premalignant or malignant. MCNs are recognized histologically by the presence of mucin-producing epithelium amid ovarian stroma. They are almost exclusively seen in women (99.7%) in their fourth and fifth decades of life, hence the term "mother" lesion.[41] These lesions are resected because of the elevated risk of malignancy.

The origin of MCNs, which contain ovarian-type stroma, is unknown. Two hypotheses are present. With the preferential distribution of MCNs in the pancreatic body or tail (94.6%), the first hypothesis posits that in the fourth to the fifth week of embryologic development, the left primordial germ cells that eventually migrate and develop into gonads are located in proximity to the dorsal pancreatic body/tail precursor, setting the stage for the incorporation of ectopic primordial ovarian cells into the pancreas, which release hormones and growth factors locally, eventually forming cystic tumors.[42] The second hypothesis suggests that female hormones stimulate periductal endodermal immature stroma in the pancreas during embryogenesis, a theory supported by the presence of estrogen receptors and other steroidogenesis-associated proteins in MCNs.[43] While the pancreatic remnant hypothesis is favored, neither of these mechanisms explains how MCNs rarely arise in men.

Radiologically, MCNs are classically well-circumscribed round or oval lesions that are unilocular or macrocystic in morphology (**Fig. 6**), containing fewer than 6 locules, each measuring greater than 2 cm in size.[44,45] Malignancy is suspected if there is wall thickening, mural nodularity, or solid enhancing components such as papillary projections and peripheral calcifications.[39,42] In one retrospective study of 52 patients with histologically proven MCN, the simultaneous presence of all three features together, calcifications in the wall and/or septa, thick surrounding wall, and septations, was associated with a 95% probability of malignancy.[46]

Because MCNs are encapsulated lesions, unlike IPMNs, they do not typically communicate with the main pancreatic duct. MCNs are also typically quite large at initial presentation, with a mean diameter ranging from 6 to 11 cm, likely in part because they are located in the tail of the pancreas and may not elicit symptoms until they get to be quite large.[47] Given their larger size at presentation, MCNs present with obstructive pancreatitis with ductal dilatation and upstream parenchymal atrophy. Similar to cystic lesions, they are low in signal on precontrast T1-weighted sequences on MRI.[48] Pseudocysts and MCNs share many similar imaging features, so a clinical history of prior pancreatitis and imaging findings suggestive of chronic pancreatitis can be a helpful point of differentiation. However, fluid sampling may be needed for a definitive diagnosis.

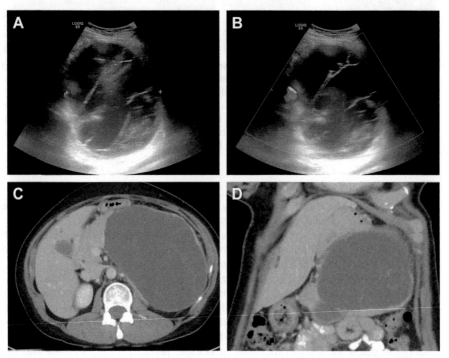

Fig. 6. A 46-year-old female with mucinous cystic neoplasm. Transverse grayscale ultrasound (A) of the left upper quadrant shows a multiseptated cystic lesion with layering internal debris. Color Doppler images (B) demonstrate no internal vascularity. Axial (C) and coronal (D) contrast-enhanced CT images show a well-circumscribed macrocystic mass arising from the pancreatic tail containing thin internal septations. No mural nodularity, solid enhancing components, or wall thickening is seen, and there is no communication with the main pancreatic duct.

Pseudocyst

Pseudocysts are the most common cystic lesions in the pancreas and, by definition, are associated with antecedent pancreatitis even if a reliable history of pancreatitis cannot be elicited from the patient.[49] Similar to pancreatitis, these lesions are more commonly encountered in men and are observed in the third to seventh decade of life.[25] Pseudocysts are not true cysts; instead, they are encapsulated collections that develop secondary to inflammation and pancreatic duct disruption. Pseudocysts can occur anywhere along the pancreas from the head to the tail and can even be found in unusual locations far from the pancreas, including rarely in the thorax.

The revised 2012 Atlanta classification provides clinical and radiologic lexica to use when describing fluid collections in the setting of pancreatitis, abandoning historically applied terminology such as acute pseudocyst and pancreatic abscess, which were confusing and inaccurate.[50] The new classification schema defines four distinct subtypes of fluid collections following pancreatitis based on the absence or presence of pancreatic necrosis and the time elapsed since the onset of symptoms from pancreatitis. In the setting of interstitial edematous pancreatitis, two fluid collections are described. Early-stage collections, within the first 4 weeks of symptoms, are called acute peripancreatic fluid collections; after 4 weeks, they are called pseudocysts. In the setting of a necrotizing pancreatitis, complex fluid collections discovered within 4 weeks of symptom onset are called acute necrotic collections (ANCs). After that time period, they are referred to as walled-off necrosis (WON). Identifying necrosis can be difficult within the first week of symptom onset, and repeat imaging at 2 weeks can be helpful to show pancreatic or peripancreatic necrosis in an ANC.[50] ANCs and WON can contain variable amounts of fluid, hemorrhage, or necrotic debris.

Typically, when these fluid collections have persisted past the 4-week mark, as in pseudocysts and WON, a more well-circumscribed, mature wall that enhances is seen along the periphery of the collection; however, no internal enhancing contents should be identified (**Fig. 7**).[49,50] Superinfection of a postpancreatitis collection is suggested by imaging when there is gas seen in the collection in the absence of a history of recent instrumentation. In chronic or recurrent pancreatitis, pseudocysts can be associated with pancreatic gland atrophy, pancreatic parenchymal calcification, and calculi within a dilated and/or strictured pancreatic duct.[39]

The term pseudocyst is used more broadly in the remainder of this section to describe mature collections with or without the presence of debris. Pseudocysts and MCNs share overlapping imaging features as they are both classically unilocular lesions with thick, enhancing walls. Aside from demographics, clinical history of pancreatitis,

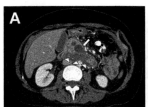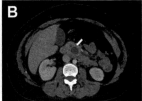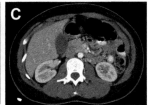

Fig. 7. A 38-year-old female with pseudocyst. On axial contrast-enhanced CT (*A*), acute pancreatitis with peripancreatic fluid (*arrowheads*) and an organizing collection (*arrow*) are visualized in the pancreatic head. Five weeks later (*B*), the pancreatic head fluid collection has organized into a pseudocyst (*arrow*), with resolution of acute peripancreatic fluid. On a comparison examination performed 13 years prior (*C*), no cystic lesion was present, helping to favor the diagnosis of pseudocyst.

and imaging stigmata of chronic pancreatitis, one helpful differentiating feature of pseudocysts is its rapid evolution over a short time.[7] Pseudocysts frequently get smaller over time or stay stable, while MCNs are expected to remain stable or slowly grow. Occasionally, pseudocysts can be seen to have a connection to the pancreatic ductal system, for example, when disconnected duct syndrome occurs secondary to pancreatic body necrosis or after necrosectomy.[50,51]

Additionally, on MRI, layering nonenhancing internal debris has shown high specificity for diagnosing pseudocysts/WON.[52] As mentioned previously, pseudocysts should never have evidence of internal enhancement. Therefore, internally enhancing soft tissue suggests the diagnosis of a cystic neoplasm until proven otherwise, and fluid or tissue sampling is recommended.[7] Finally, if present, fistulization to adjacent structures favors pseudocyst over neoplasm.

Solitary Pseudopapillary Tumor

Solitary pseudopapillary tumors (SPTs), formerly known as solid and papillary epithelial neoplasm, are sometimes referred to as "daughter" lesions because of its peak incidence in the second through fourth decade, with a female predilection (85%).[53] The tumors occur exclusively in the pancreas and have a predilection for the head or tail.[54]

Radiologically, SPTs are well-marginated, encapsulated, mixed solid and cystic masses often with central cystic or hemorrhagic degeneration and calcification (Fig. 8).[29,55,56] SPTs are typically solitary and large at presentation, with reported average tumor diameters ranging 4.9 to 9.5 cm.[57–59] Small SPTs, defined as ≤3 cm, frequently appear as purely solid tumors with a sharp margin.[60] Classically, these tumors are well circumscribed and displace rather than invade adjacent structures. They do not communicate with or obstruct the main pancreatic duct, and peripheral calcifications can be seen in 30% of cases.[61] Typically, on arterial and venous phase imaging, the capsule and solid portions of the SPT will enhance similarly to the surrounding normal pancreatic tissue.[62]

On MRI, typical SPTs demonstrate increased T2 signal, usually in the center of the mass. In contrast, the more solid tumors show only mildly increased T2 signal, with enhancement of solid components.[7] Hemorrhagic degeneration, when present, is characterized by intrinsic high signal intensity within the lesion on precontrast T1-weighted imaging or high attenuation on precontrast CT images.[63]

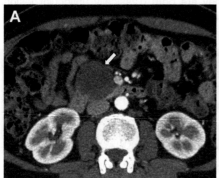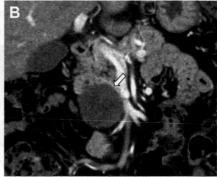

Fig. 8. A 49-year-old female with a solid pseudopapillary tumor in the uncinate process of the pancreas. Axial (A) and coronal (B) contrast-enhanced CT images in the pancreatic parenchymal phase demonstrate a well-marginated hypovascular cystic mass (arrow) with subtle internal solid components. The mass displaces, rather than invades, adjacent structures.

One distinguishing imaging feature is its fibrous capsule, which typically demonstrates early and intense enhancement relative to the the remainder of the tumor.[55] The gradual accumulation of contrast within the tumor distinguishes SPT from neuroendocrine tumors, which share similar morphologic features and demographics but, instead, characteristically demonstrate early arterial enhancement.[7] MCNs with malignant features may also share morphologic similarities with SPT. In children, the differential diagnosis can include pancreatoblastoma, another solid neoplasm.

While older age and male sex were initially reported as predictors of malignant potential, this has not been confirmed in subsequent studies.[54,59,64] In the absence of invasive margins or metastatic disease, it can be difficult to differentiate benign from malignant SPT. Imaging features that may suggest malignant transformation include eccentric lobulation and capsule discontinuity.[64] Regardless, en-bloc resection with resection of any concomitant metastases should be attempted with excellent long-term survival even in the presence of distant disease.

Cystic Pancreatic Neuroendocrine Tumor

PNETs are rare, accounting for 2% to 10% of all pancreatic neoplasms.[65] PNETs can either be functional or nonfunctional based on hormone secretion. Some are associated with inherited syndromes including multiple endocrine neoplasia type 1, von Hippel-Lindau disease, neurofibromatosis 1, and tuberous sclerosis.[66] They are slightly more common in men and are typically discovered in the sixth through eighth decade.[65]

While PNETs are classically solid pancreatic masses, they can manifest with cystic changes in 10% to 36% of cases.[67–72] Contrary to some earlier studies that suggested larger tumors were more likely to have cystic change, more recent studies have shown no significant difference in size between cystic and solid tumors although they noted that there can be discrepancies in the identification of a cystic component on imaging when compared to pathology.[68–70]

The typical appearance of a solid PNET is a solid hyperattenuating mass on arterial and portal venous phases owing to their rich capillary network (**Fig. 9**).[73] PNETs are typically well-circumscribed round or oval masses with T1 hypointensity lower than that of the adjacent pancreatic parenchyma and T2 hyperintensity higher than that of the adjacent pancreatic tissue.[73] For cystic PNETs, a hyperenhancing rim on pancreatic phase imaging can be a distinguishing feature. However, purely cystic NETs may not demonstrate more than a hairline-thin wall, rendering them indistinguishable from IPMN, MCN, or oligocystic SCN.[68]

Prognosis is variable and depends on tumor aggressiveness. Imaging features associated with a higher tumor grade and a poor prognosis include atypical enhancement with portal venous phase isoenhancement or hypoenhancement compared to adjacent pancreatic parenchyma, ductal dilatation, large size, and vascular invasion.[74–76]

Pancreatic Ductal Adenocarcinoma

PDAC accounts for 90% of all solid pancreatic neoplasms and is characterized by an infiltrative growth pattern. Patients typically present with obstructive jaundice, especially in the case of pancreatic head tumors, with a hypovascular mass (**Fig. 10**).[7] Other distinguishing features of PDAC are its infiltrative appearance and the propensity to cause abrupt duct obstruction (duct cutoff sign) and involve the adjacent vasculature.

However, PDAC can manifest with cystic features in up to 8% of cases.[77–79] Cystic features within PDAC may reflect a nonneoplastic process resulting from ductal obstruction precipitating the formation of retention cysts or pseudocysts along the periphery of the tumor. PDAC can also have a cystic appearance related to features of

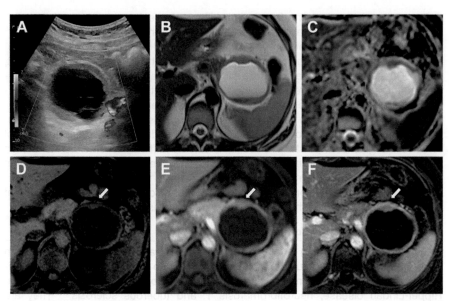

Fig. 9. A 34-year-old female with cystic PNET. Axial color Doppler US of the left upper quadrant (*A*) shows a thick-rimmed unilocular cystic lesion without internal vascularity. Axial T2-weighted image (*B*) confirms a thick-rimmed unilocular cystic lesion in the pancreatic tail. On the apparent diffusion coefficient (ADC) map (*C*), the lesion shows low signal corresponding to the outer wall, indicating diffusion restriction. On unenhanced T1-weighted imaging (*D*), there is nodular thickening along the periphery (arrow), with corresponding nodular enhancement (*arrow*) on arterial phase imaging (*E*) and delayed phase imaging (*F*).

the cancer itself, such as "large-duct-type" ectasia, increased mucinous content, or cystic necrosis.[78–80] Intratumoral cystic components secondary to "large-duct-type" PDAC are typically small, rarely exceeding 1 cm in size.[78] Colloid carcinomas have abundant mucin production mimicking the bright signal more commonly associated with fluid on T2-weighted imaging. They are more likely to present with lobulated

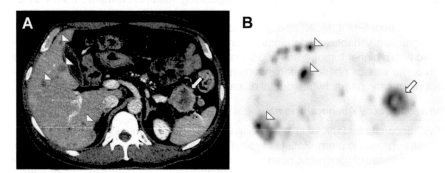

Fig. 10. A 42-year-old male with metastatic pancreatic ductal carcinoma. On contrast-enhanced axial CT image (*A*), there is an irregularly marginated mass in the tail of the pancreas with central cystic change indicating necrosis (*arrow*), as well as multiple hepatic metastases (*arrowheads*). Fludeoxyglucose positron emission tomography images (*B*) show a hypermetabolic mass in the tail of the pancreas with central photopenia (*arrow*), consistent with necrosis, as well as multiple hypermetabolic hepatic metastases (*arrowheads*).

contours, indiscrete margins, and/or a "salt-and-pepper" appearance on T2-weighted imaging.[81,82] Cystic necrosis is often irregular and can contain variable amounts of intralesional hemorrhage, which would appear T1 hyperintense.[78,79]

MIMICS AND PITFALLS

Pseudo-lesions, nonneoplastic entities, and cystic metastasis entities can occasionally mimic a cystic mass in the pancreas. Duodenal diverticula are benign outpouchings of intestinal mucosa that are usually asymptomatic and detected incidentally. However, a diverticulum located adjacent to the pancreas and completely filled with fluid can appear as a cystic mass on both CT and MRI.[83] Diverticula that appear fluid filled can be distinguished from a cystic mass if it demonstrates intraluminal air or rapid changes in size and distension from sequence to sequence compared to prior imaging studies (**Figs. 11** and **12**). On CT and fluoroscopic examinations, positive enteric contrast filling a diverticulum is definitive for diagnosis.

Intraparenchymal fat and lipomas are other pseudo-lesions that can mimic a cystic mass. The normal pancreas has a lobulated appearance surrounded by peripancreatic fat. An invagination of fat into the pancreas or a small intrapancreatic lipoma can mimic a cyst on CT (**Fig. 13**). Multiplanar reformats of CT imaging sometimes

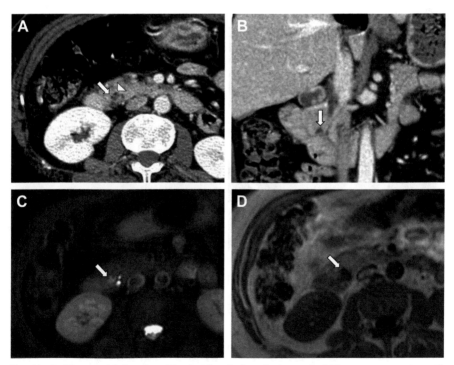

Fig. 11. A 61-year-old female with duodenal diverticulum mimicking a pancreatic cystic lesion. Axial (*A*) and coronal (*B*) contrast-enhanced CT demonstrates a periampullary cystic lesion on CT with a questionable focus of intraluminal air (*arrowhead*) on axial imaging. On MRI, the fat-suppressed T2-weighted image (*C*) shows a T2 signal intensity lesion (*arrow*) iso-intense to adjacent bowel lumen contents (not shown). In-phase gradient recalled echo (GRE) sequence (*D*) shows a focus of susceptibility artifact consistent with air, confirming the diagnosis of a duodenal diverticulum.

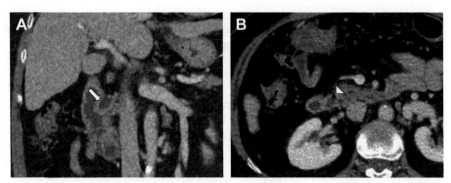

Fig. 12. A 75-year-old female with a duodenal diverticulum mimicking a pancreatic cystic lesion. On coronal contrast-enhanced CT (*A*), a cystic-appearing lesion (*arrow*) is present in the pancreatic head containing fluid. On the axial CT images (*B*), a small focus of antidependent air (*arrowhead*) confirms the diagnosis of a duodenal diverticulum.

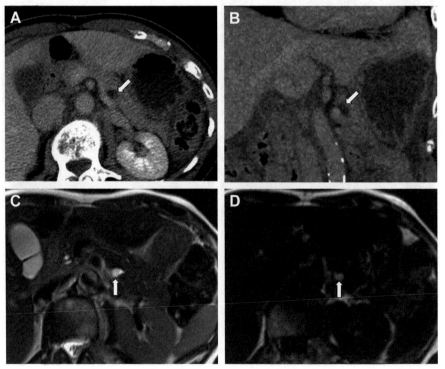

Fig. 13. A 72-year-old female with intraparenchymal fat mimicking a cystic pancreatic lesion. A low-attenuation lesion (*arrow*) is identified in the pancreatic body on axial CT (*A*) and coronal CT (*B*). Axial T2-weighted sequence (*C*) shows a T2 hyperintense lesion in the pancreatic body. T1-weighted gradient recalled echo (GRE) fat-only image (*D*) demonstrates high signal intensity confirming intraparenchymal fat.

help distinguish these pseudo-lesions, but an MRI may be needed. Differences in the precessional frequency of fat and fluid on MRI can be exploited by chemical shift sequences and help distinguish fat from fluid and pancreatic tissue.

Solid metastases to the pancreas are uncommon but are typically secondary to renal cell carcinoma or lung cancer. However, necrotic metastases with central necrosis can mimic cystic lesions in more aggressive tumors, such as sarcomas, melanomas, and ovarian carcinoma, leaving an irregular, shaggy appearance to the periphery of the lesion.[29,84] Metastases to the pancreas, however, are rare and typically occur late in the disease course of malignancy, often with multiorgan involvement observed concurrently with identification of a secondary pancreatic mass.[29] An exception to this is renal cell carcinoma, in which solitary metastatic disease can occur. Therefore, in a patient with a remote history of prior nephrectomy for renal cell carcinoma, identifying a new hyperenhancing or cystic lesion in the pancreas should raise suspicion for solitary renal cell metastasis. Comprehensive oncologic history and prior imaging availability are helpful in the diagnostic workup of a new indeterminate solitary pancreatic mass.

Other rarer mimics of cystic masses include congenital/developmental midgut duplication cysts, lymphangioma, and intrapancreatic varices.[29]

SUMMARY

Pancreatic cystic lesions are increasingly identified, and while most cystic lesions are benign, identifying potentially malignant lesions relies on imaging to narrow the differential diagnosis and guide management. The key imaging features used to characterize cystic lesions are best assessed by contrast-enhanced MRI/MRCP, the mainstay of cyst imaging and follow-up, with pancreas protocol CT offering a complementary role. While some imaging features have high specificity for a particular diagnosis, overlapping imaging features between diagnoses may require further investigation with follow-up diagnostic imaging or tissue sampling.

DISCLOSURE

The authors have nothing to disclose.

CLINICS CARE POINTS

- Contrast-enhanced MRI with magnetic resonance cholangiopancreatography (MRCP) is recommended when assessing pancreatic cystic lesions and has the advantage of no ionizing radiation for follow-up studies.
- Dual-phase pancreatic protocol CT can be also be considered and is often performed for preoperative planning.
- MRI/MRCP without intravenous contrast may be used for follow-up in lower risk patients; consultation with a radiologist is suggested to help determine whether intravenous contrast is necessary for select patients.

REFERENCES

1. Zerboni G, Signoretti M, Crippa S, et al. Systematic review and meta-analysis: Prevalence of incidentally detected pancreatic cystic lesions in asymptomatic individuals. Pancreatology 2019;19(1):2–9.

2. Sainani NI, Saokar A, Deshpande V, et al. Comparative Performance of MDCT and MRI With MR Cholangiopancreatography in Characterizing Small Pancreatic Cysts. Am J Roentgenol 2009;193(3):722–31.
3. Waters JA, Schmidt CM, Pinchot JW, et al. CT vs MRCP: Optimal classification of IPMN type and extent. J Gastrointest Surg 2008;12(1):101–9.
4. Scheiman JM, Hwang JH, Moayyedi P. American gastroenterological association technical review on the diagnosis and management of asymptomatic neoplastic pancreatic cysts. Gastroenterology 2015;148(4):824–48.e22.
5. Hecht EM, Khatri G, Morgan D, et al. Intraductal papillary mucinous neoplasm (IPMN) of the pancreas: recommendations for Standardized Imaging and Reporting from the Society of Abdominal Radiology IPMN disease focused panel. Abdom Radiol 2021;46(4):1586–606.
6. Tirkes T, Menias CO, Sandrasegaran K. MR Imaging Techniques for Pancreas. Radiol Clin North Am 2012;50(3):379–93.
7. Kalb B, Sarmiento JM, Kooby DA, et al. MR imaging of cystic lesions of the pancreas. Radiographics 2009;29(6):1749–65.
8. Jang KM, Kim SH, Min JH, et al. Value of diffusion-weighted MRI for differentiating malignant from benign intraductal papillary mucinous neoplasms of the pancreas. Am J Roentgenol 2014;203(5):992–1000.
9. Yamaguchi K. Pancreatic ductal carcinoma derived from IPMN and concomitant with IPMN. Nihon Rinsho 2015;73(4):234–9.
10. Tanno S, Nakano Y, Sugiyama Y, et al. Incidence of synchronous and metachronous pancreatic carcinoma in 168 patients with branch duct intraductal papillary mucinous neoplasm. Pancreatology 2010;10(2–3):173–8.
11. Tanaka M, Fernandez-del Castillo C, Kamisawa T, et al. Revisions of international consensus Fukuoka guidelines for the management of IPMN of the pancreas. Pancreatology 2017;17(5):738–53.
12. Pozzi-Mucelli RM, Rinta-Kiikka I, Wunsche K, et al. Pancreatic MRI for the surveillance of cystic neoplasms: comparison of a short with a comprehensive imaging protocol. Eur Radiol 2017;27(1):41–50.
13. Purysko AS, Gandhi NS, Walsh RM, et al. Does secretin stimulation add to magnetic resonance cholangiopancreatography in characterising pancreatic cystic lesions as side-branch intraductal papillary mucinous neoplasm? Eur Radiol 2014;24(12):3134–41.
14. Al-Hawary MM, Francis IR, Chari ST, et al. Pancreatic ductal adenocarcinoma radiology reporting template: Consensus statement of the society of abdominal radiology and the American pancreatic association. Gastroenterology 2014; 146(1):291–304.e1.
15. Fukukura Y, Kumagae Y, Fujisaki Y, et al. Adding delayed phase images to dual-phase contrast-enhanced CT increases sensitivity for small pancreatic ductal adenocarcinoma. Am J Roentgenol 2021;217(4):888–97.
16. Lu DSK, Vedantham S, Krasny RM, et al. Two-phase helical CT for pancreatic tumors: Pancreatic versus hepatic phase enhancement of tumor, pancreas, and vascular structures. Radiology 1996;199(3):697–701.
17. Boland G, Malley ME, Saez M, et al. Pancreatic-phase versus portal vein-phase helical CT of the pancreas: optimal temporal window for evaluation of pancreatic adenocarcinoma. Am J Roentgenol 1999;(172):605–8.
18. Fletcher JG, Wiersema MJ, Farrell MA, et al. Pancreatic malignancy: Value of arterial, pancreatic, and hepatic phase imaging with multi-detector row CT. Radiology 2003;229(1):81–90.

19. Jeon JH, Kim JH, Joo I, et al. Transabdominal ultrasound detection of pancreatic cysts incidentally detected at CT, MRI, or endoscopic ultrasound. Am J Roentgenol 2018;210(3):518–25.
20. Spinelli KS, Fromwiller TE, Daniel RA, et al. Cystic Pancreatic Neoplasms: Observe or Operate. Ann Surg 2004;239(5):651–9.
21. Fernandez-Del Castillo C, Targarona J, Thayer SP, et al. Incidental Pancreatic Cysts: Clinicopathologic Characteristics and Comparison With Symptomatic Patients. Arch Surg 2003;138(4):427–34.
22. Burk KS, Knipp D, Sahani DV. Cystic Pancreatic Tumors. Magn Reson Imaging Clin N Am 2018;26(3):405–20.
23. Megibow AJ, Baker ME, Morgan DE, et al. Management of Incidental Pancreatic Cysts: A White Paper of the ACR Incidental Findings Committee. J Am Coll Radiol 2017;14(7):911–23.
24. Kim JH, Hong SS, Kim YJ, et al. Intraductal papillary mucinous neoplasm of the pancreas: Differentiate from chronic pancreatits by MR imaging. Eur J Radiol 2012;81(4):671–6.
25. Sahani DV, Kambadakone A, MacAri M, et al. Diagnosis and management of cystic pancreatic lesions. Am J Roentgenol 2013;200(2):343–54.
26. Kim KW, Park SH, Pyo J, et al. Imaging features to distinguish malignant and benign branch-duct type intraductal papillary mucinous neoplasms of the pancreas: A meta-analysis. Ann Surg 2014;259(1):72–81.
27. Elta GH, Enestvedt BK, Sauer BG, et al. ACG Clinical Guideline: Diagnosis and Management of Pancreatic Cysts. Am J Gastroenterol 2018;113(4):464–79.
28. Adsay N.V., Cystic lesion of the pancreas. Mod Pathol, 20, 2007, S71-S93.
29. Dewhurst CE, Mortele KJ. Cystic tumors of the pancreas: imaging and management. Radiol Clin North Am 2012;50(3):467–86.
30. Buck JL, Hayes WS. From the Archives of the AFIP. Microcystic adenoma of the pancreas. Radiographics 1990;10(2):313–22.
31. Procacci C, Graziani R, Bicego E, et al. Serous cystadenoma of the pancreas: Report of 30 cases with emphasis on the imaging findings. J Comput Assist Tomogr 1997;21(3):373–82.
32. Jais B, Rebours V, Malleo G, et al. Serous cystic neoplasm of the pancreas: a multinational study of 2622 patients under the auspices of the International Association of Pancreatology and European Pancreatic Club (European Study Group on Cystic Tumors of the Pancreas). Gut 2016;65(2):305–12.
33. Curry CA, Eng J, Horton KM, et al. CT of primary cystic pancreatic neoplasms: can CT be used for patient triage and treatment? AJR Am J Roentgenol 2000;175(1):99–103.
34. Itai Y, Moss AA, Ohtomo K. Computed tomography of cystadenoma and cystadenocarcinoma of the pancreas. Radiology 1982;145(2):419–25.
35. Johnson CD, Stephens DH, Charboneau JW, et al. Cystic pancreatic tumors: CT and sonographic assessment. Am J Roentgenol 2012;151(6):1133–8.
36. Choi JY, Kim MJ, Lee JY, et al. Typical and atypical manifestations of serous cystadenoma of the pancreas: Imaging findings with pathologic correlation. Am J Roentgenol 2009;193(1):136–42.
37. Gabata T, Terayama N, Yamashiro M, et al. Solid serous cystadenoma of the pancreas: MR imaging with pathologic correlation. Abdom Imaging 2005;30(5):605–9.
38. Sakorafas GH, Smyrniotis V, Reid-Lombardo KM, et al. Primary pancreatic cystic neoplasms of the pancreas revisited. Part IV: Rare cystic neoplasms. Surg Oncol 2012;21(3):153–63.

39. Sahani DV, Kadavigere R, Saokar A, et al. Cystic pancreatic lesions: A simple imaging-based classification system for guiding management. Radiographics 2005;25(6):1471–84.

40. Shah AA, Sainani NI, Ramesh AK, et al. Predictive value of multi-detector computed tomography for accurate diagnosis of serous cystadenoma: Radiologic-pathologic correlation. World J Gastroenterol 2009;15(22):2739–47.

41. Goh BKP, Tan YM, Chung YFA, et al. A review of mucinous cystic neoplasms of the pancreas defined by ovarian-type stroma: Clinicopathological features of 344 patients. World J Surg 2006;30(12):2236–45.

42. Zamboni G, Scarpa A, Bogina G, et al. Mucinous cystic tumors of the pancreas: Clinicopathological features, prognosis, and relationship to other mucinous cystic tumors. Am J Surg Pathol 1999;23(4):410–22.

43. Fukushima N, Zamboni G. Mucinous cystic neoplasms of the pancreas: Update on the surgical pathology and molecular genetics. Semin Diagn Pathol 2014; 31(6):467–74.

44. Barral M, Soyer P, Dohan A, et al. Magnetic resonance imaging of cystic pancreatic lesions in adults: An update in current diagnostic features and management. Abdom Imaging 2014;39(1):48–65.

45. Manfredi R, Ventriglia A, Mantovani W, et al. Mucinous cystic neoplasms and serous cystadenomas arising in the body-tail of the pancreas: MR imaging characterization. Eur Radiol 2015;25(4):940–9.

46. Procacci C, Carbognin G, Accordini S, et al. CT features of malignant mucinous cystic tumors of the pancreas. Eur Radiol 2001;11(9):1626–30.

47. Buetow PC, Rao P, Thompson LDR. From the Archives of the AFIP: Mucinous Cystic Neoplasms of the Pancreas: Radiologic-Pathologic Correlation. Radiographics 1998;18(2):433–49.

48. Khan A, Khosa F, Eisenberg RL. Cystic lesions of the pancreas. Am J Roentgenol 2011;196(6):668–77.

49. Kim YH, Saini S, Sahani D, et al. Imaging diagnosis of cystic pancreatic lesions: Pseudocyst versus nonpseudocyst. Radiographics 2005;25(3):671–85.

50. Banks PA, Bollen TL, Dervenis C, et al. Classification of acute pancreatitis - 2012: Revision of the Atlanta classification and definitions by international consensus. Gut 2013;62(1):102–11.

51. Sandrasegaran K, Tann M, Gregory Jennings S, et al. Disconnection of the Pancreatic Duct: An Important But Over looked Complication of Severe Acute Pancreatitis 1 Recipient of a Certificate of Merit award for an education exhibit at the. RadioGraphics 2005;1389–401.

52. Macari M, Finn ME, Bennett GL, et al. Differentiating pancreatic cystic neoplasms from pancreatic pseudocysts at MR imaging: Value of perceived internal debris. Radiology 2009;251(1):77–84.

53. Choi JY, Kim MJ, Kim JH, et al. Solid Pseudopapillary Tumor of the Pancreas: Typical and Atypical Manifestations. Am J Roentgenol 2012;187(2).

54. Coleman KM, Doherty MC, Bigler SA. Solid-Pseudopapillary Tumor of the Pancreas. Radiographics 2003;23(6):1644–8.

55. Cantisani V, Mortele KJ, Levy A, et al. MR Imaging Features of Solid Pseudopapillary Tumor of the Pancreas in Adult and Pediatric Patients. AJR Am J Roentgenol 2012;181(2):395–401.

56. Choi BI, Kim KW, Han MC, et al. Solid and papillary epithelial neoplasms of the pancreas: CT findings. Radiology 1988;166(2):413–6.

57. Balthazar EJ, Subramanyam BR, Lefleur RS, et al. Solid and papillary epithelial neoplasm of the pancreas. Radiographic, CT, sonographic, and angiographic features. Radiology 1984;150(1):39–40.

58. Sunkara S, Williams TR, Myers DT, et al. Solid pseudopapillary tumours of the pancreas: Spectrum of imaging findings with histopathological correlation. Br J Radiol 2012;85(1019):1140–4.

59. Goh BKP, Tan YM, Cheow PC, et al. Solid pseudopapillary neoplasms of the pancreas: An updated experience. J Surg Oncol 2007;95(8):640–4.

60. Baek JH, Lee JM, Kim SH, et al. Small (≤3 cm) solid pseudopapillary tumors of the pancreas at multiphasic multidetector CT. Radiology 2010;257(1):97–106.

61. Buetow PC, Buck JL, Pantongrag-Brown L, et al. Solid and Papillary Epithelial Neoplasm of the Pancreas: Imaging-Pathologic Correlation in 56 Cases. Radiology 1996;199:707–11.

62. Butte JM, Brennan MF, Gonen M, et al. Solid pseudopapillary tumors of the pancreas. clinical features, surgical outcomes, and long-term survival in 45 consecutive patients from a single center. J Gastrointest Surg 2011;15(2):350–7.

63. Sahni VA, Mortele KJ. The bloody pancreas: MDCT and MRI features of hypervascular and hemorrhagic pancreatic conditions. Am J Roentgenol 2009;192(4):923–35.

64. Chung YE, Kim MJ, Choi JY, et al. Differentiation of benign and malignant solid pseudopapillary neoplasms of the pancreas. J Comput Assist Tomogr 2009;33(5):689–94.

65. Fraenkel M, Kim MK, Faggiano A, et al. Epidemiology of gastroenteropancreatic neuroendocrine tumours. Best Pract Res Clin Gastroenterol 2012;26(6):691–703.

66. Metz DC, Jensen RT. Gastrointestinal Neuroendocrine Tumors: Pancreatic Endocrine Tumors. Gastroenterology 2008;135(5):1469–92.

67. Nakashima Y, Ohtsuka T, Nakamura S, et al. Clinicopathological characteristics of non-functioning cystic pancreatic neuroendocrine tumors. Pancreatology 2019;19(1):50–6.

68. Kawamoto S, Johnson PT, Shi C, et al. Pancreatic neuroendocrine tumor with cystlike changes: Evaluation with MDCT. Am J Roentgenol 2013;200(3):283–90.

69. Yano M, Misra S, Salter A, et al. Assessment of disease aggression in cystic pancreatic neuroendocrine tumors: A CT and pathology correlation study. Pancreatology 2017;17(4):605–10.

70. Singhi AD, Chu LC, Tatsas AD, et al. Cystic pancreatic neuroendocrine tumors: a clinicopathologic study. Am J Surg Pathol 2012;36(11):1666–73.

71. Buetow PC, Parrino TV, Buck JL, et al. Islet cell tumors of the pancreas: Pathologic-imaging correlation among size, necrosis and cysts, calcification, malignant behavior, and functional status. Am J Roentgenol 1995;165(5):1175–9.

72. Horton KM, Hruban RH, Yeo C, et al. Multi-detector row CT of pancreatic islet cell tumors. Radiographics 2006;26(2):453–64.

73. Lewis RB, Lattin GE, Paal E. Pancreatic endocrine tumors: Radiologic-clinicopathologic correlation. Radiographics 2010;30(6):1445–64.

74. Han S, Kim JH, Yoo J, et al. Prediction of recurrence after surgery based on preoperative MRI features in patients with pancreatic neuroendocrine tumors. Eur Radiol 2022;32(4):2506–17.

75. Canellas R, Lo G, Bhowmik S, et al. Pancreatic neuroendocrine tumor: Correlations between MRI features, tumor biology, and clinical outcome after surgery. J Magn Reson Imaging 2018;47(2):425–32.

76. Kang J, Ryu JK, Son JH, et al. Association between pathologic grade and multiphase computed tomography enhancement in pancreatic neuroendocrine neoplasm. J Gastroenterol Hepatol 2018;33(9):1677–82.
77. DOnofrio M, De Robertis R, Capelli P, et al. Uncommon presentations of common pancreatic neoplasms: a pictorial essay. Abdom Imaging 2015;40(6):1629–44.
78. Yoon SE, Byun JH, Kim KA, et al. Pancreatic ductal adenocarcinoma with intratumoral cystic lesions on MRI: Correlation with histopathological findings. Br J Radiol 2010;83(988):318–26.
79. Kosmahl M, Pauser U, Anlauf M, et al. Pancreatic ductal adenocarcinomas with cystic features: neither rare nor uniform. Mod Pathol 2005;18(9):1157–64.
80. Youn SY, Rha SE, Jung ES, et al. Pancreas ductal adenocarcinoma with cystic features on cross-sectional imaging: Radiologic-pathologic correlation. Diagnostic Interv Radiol 2018;24(1):5–11.
81. Yoon MA, Lee JM, Se HK, et al. MRI features of pancreatic colloid carcinoma. Am J Roentgenol 2009;193(4). https://doi.org/10.2214/AJR.09.2347.
82. Schawkat K, Manning MA, Glickman JN, et al. Pancreatic ductal adenocarcinoma and its variants: Pearls and perils. Radiographics 2020;40(5):1219–39.
83. Macari M, Lazarus D, Israel G, et al. Original report. Duodenal diverticula mimicking cystic neoplasms of the pancreas: CT and MR imaging findings in seven patients. Am J Roentgenol 2003;180(1):195–9.
84. Ferrozzi F, Bova D, Campodonico F, et al. Pancreatic metastases: CT assessment. Eur Radiol 1997;7(2):241–5.

Pancreatic Cysts: Radiology

Alec J. Megibow, MD, MPH, FACR

KEYWORDS

- Pancreas cyst • Radiology • Malignancy determination

KEY POINTS

- Varius types of common pancreatic cysts.
- How to report pancreatic cyst.
- Follow-up protocols for radiologic evaluation of pancreatic cysts.

PREVALENCE OF PANCREATIC CYSTS

Radiologists are often the first physicians to detect pancreatic cysts, yet radiological guidelines often conflict with more established clinical and surgical guidelines (**Figs. 1–7; Table 1**). There is broad agreement about the malignancy potential of the population of pancreatic cysts controversy remains about the individual patient.[1]

In a 2013 study of the National Cancer Institute Surveillance, Epidemiology, and End Results registry, the estimated number of pancreatic cysts in the US population aged between 40 and 84 years was 3,428,874, with an overall cyst prevalence of 2.5%.[2] A second study estimated the pancreatic cyst prevalence at 2.2%.[3] Increased use of cross-sectional imaging has led to an increased detection of such cysts in recent years; 2.2% of upper abdominal computed tomographic (CT) examinations and 19.6% of MRI examinations report a pancreatic cyst.[3–5] Although commonly used management guidelines assume knowledge of a specific pancreatic cyst type,[6–8] many cysts detected at imaging are indeterminate. Therefore, radiologists cannot reliably predict an indolent versus aggressive course at the time of detection.

In patients with a family history or genetic predisposition to pancreatic ductal adenocarcinoma (PDAC), there is an increased prevalence of pancreatic cystic neoplasms.[9] In a study of 300 patients with intraductal papillary mucinous neoplasms (IPMNs) and a first-degree relative with PDAC, progression to pancreatic cancer was the same as the controls, suggesting that follow-up need not be altered for patients with cysts less than 3 cm.[10]

Types of Pancreatic Cysts

The serous cystadenoma (SCA) has 3 forms: micocystic, honeycombed, and oligocystic. There is central calcification in approximately one-third of cases. They do not

Department of Radiology, NYU-Langone Health, 550 1st Avenue, Room HCC 232, New York, NY 10016, USA
E-mail address: alec.megibow@nyulangone.org

Gastrointest Endoscopy Clin N Am 33 (2023) 519–531
https://doi.org/10.1016/j.giec.2023.03.008
1052-5157/23/© 2023 Elsevier Inc. All rights reserved.

giendo.theclinics.com

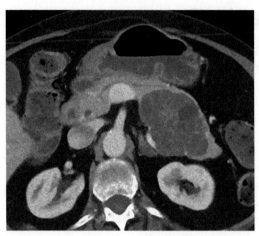

Fig. 1. Classic serous cystadenoma. Note the radiating septa toward the center of the lesion.

communicate with the main pancreatic duct (MPD). On MRI examinations, the septa within the mass may progressively enhance. They are usually benign lesions although scattered reports of malignant SCA have been reported.

The mucinous cystic tumor usually originates from the pancreatic tail and is usually seen in women. The central portion is a mucinous neoplasm but the differentiating feature is a thick wall containing ovarian stroma. When calcification is present, it is peripheral as opposed to the SCA. This lesion is considered premalignant even though the majority will never progress.

IPMN can originate from the MPD or the side branch ducts. In main duct IPMN, the entire duct or a portion of the duct may be involved. The endoscopic finding of the bulging papilla is diagnostic. The presence of enhancing mural nodules has been considered a feature of high-grade dysplasia or frank malignancy in these lesions. Malignancy is more common in those originating within the MPD with a rate of approximately 61%; further, the frequency of invasive IPMS is approximately 43%.[11]

The side branch IPMN is more confusing. Radiologists consider size of these lesions as the most important predictor of malignancy. Size is measured along the long axis of the lesion. Lesions less than 2.5 cm have a low chance of malignancy; whereas lesions

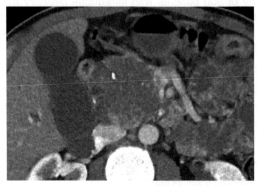

Fig. 2. Serous cystadenoma with central calcifications. Again, note the increased number of septa in the center of the lesion as opposed to the periphery.

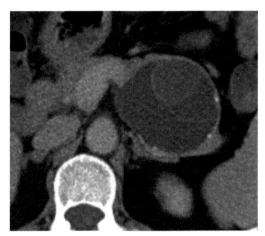

Fig. 3. Mucinous cystic tumor. Typical tumor originating in the pancreatic tail. Note the peripheral calcifications and the soft tissue mass along the ventral portion of the tumor. Both of these findings are associated with an increased malignancy potential.

greater than 2.5 cm have a progressively increased malignant risk.[12–18] A variety of ancillary diagnostic measures have been used to further characterize these lesions, the most common of which is endoscopic ultrasound (EUS). Indications for this procedure are discussed elsewhere.

Solid papillary epithelial neoplasm (SPEN) is a rarely detected mass. Most frequent in young women, this lesion is generally removed due to the small but nevertheless increasing risk of malignancy. The cystic neuroendocrine tumor occurs in approximately 5% of cases. When greater than 2 cm, the lesion is usually removed. When the size is lower, it may be removed, if it is functioning, or observed.

Pseudocysts are an important differential in these tumors. A careful history of earlier episodes of pancreatitis should be queried in every patient. If there is doubt, aspiration of amylase from the mass will be diagnostic.[4]

Challenges to the Radiologic Algorithm

Since 2010, several multi-institutional and specialty society consensus articles, meta-analyses, and large-scale observational studies have appeared[11,12,19–28] but the quality of evidence has been characterized as poor or inconclusive, and conclusions remain controversial.[25] The natural history of incidental pancreatic cysts is uncertain,

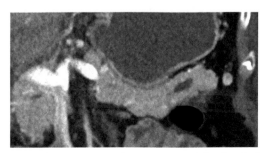

Fig. 4. Main duct IPMN. In this case, only a short segment of the duct is distended. Main duct IPMN can involve the entire duct or variable portions of the duct.

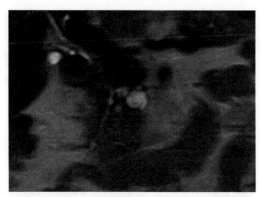

Fig. 5. Side branch IPMN. See the thin neck that attaches this lesion to the main pancreatic duct.

and our recommendations cannot be simple or entirely definitive. Physicians must discuss such uncertainty with their patients, integrating patients' risk tolerance, physicians' clinical judgment, and local expertise into management decisions. When local expertise is limited, referrals to sites of excellence in pancreatic disease are strongly encouraged.

REPORTING CONSIDERATIONS

The reporting criteria below assume that the radiologist has *no* knowledge of other parameters of the individual patient.[29]

The following 6 elements should be reported when an incidental pancreatic cyst is detected on a CT or MRI study.

1. Cyst morphology, location
2. Cyst size
3. Relation to main pancreatic duct
4. Presence of "worrisome features" and/or "high-risk stigmata"
5. Growth on follow-up examination
6. Multiplicity

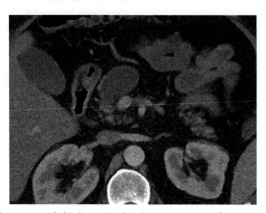

Fig. 6. Side branch IPMN with high-grade dysplasia. The size of this lesion is an indication for surgical removal. The actual histology cannot be predicted by imaging alone.

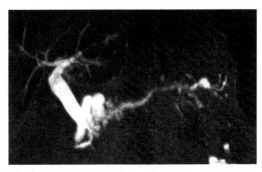

Fig. 7. MRCP revealing multiple side branch IPMNs. At least 3 IPMNs are present in this image. Radiologists are encouraged to use the largest lesion for measurement; however, cancer may develop in any of the IPMN or elsewhere in the main pancreatic duct.

Cyst Morphology and Location

As mentioned, the most frequently encountered pancreatic cysts include IPMN, SCA, MCN, SPEN, cPNET, and pseudocyst. Rare cysts include simple epithelial cyst, lymphoepithelial cyst, and mucinous nonneoplastic cyst. Cysts that are less than 10 mm are difficult or impossible to specifically characterize. Cysts measuring 1 to 3 cm are often "indeterminate" unless communication with the MPD can be established. If duct communication is established, the cyst is classified as either branch duct-IPMN (BD) or combined-type IPMN. Cysts 3 cm or greater can be classified as oligocystic, microcystic, macrocystic, unilocular, or multilocular.[30] If calcification is present within a cyst, its location should be reported. A cystic lesion with central calcification is most likely an SCA, whereas a cyst with peripheral calcification is likely an MCN or PNET. Peripheral calcification in MCNs is more strongly associated with frank malignancy.

Every attempt should be made to establish the diagnosis of SCA or pseudocyst. SCA displays characteristic features in more than 60% of cases[31] although "atypical" morphology can also be seen.[6,32] Clinical history and amylase levels in the cyst fluid of about 18,000 IU/L may help diagnose a pseudocyst; however, elevated amylase may also be seen in mucinous cysts.[33] We assume that incidental cysts that cannot be characterized when detected are likely to be mucinous (eg, IPMN). Follow-up imaging and/or EUS with fine needle aspiration (FNA) is typically needed.

Knowledge of a cyst's location (uncinate process, head, neck, body, or tail) is important when evaluating comparison studies and can also aid in differential diagnosis. For example, MCNs are commonly in the pancreatic tail, while BD-IPMNs are most frequently in the pancreatic head/uncinate process.

Table 1 Worrisome features and high-risk stigmata[a]	
Worrisome Features	**High-Risk Stigmata**
Cyst >3 cm	Obstructive jaundice with cyst in head of pancreas
Thickened or enhancing cyst wall	Enhancing or solid component within cyst
Nonenhancing mural nodule	Main pancreatic duct caliber >10 mm in absence of
Main pancreatic duct caliber >7 mm[b]	obstruction

[a] Data from Ref.[11]
[b] Data from Ref.[36]

Cyst Size

Despite the importance of a cyst's size for management decisions, there are no uni-formly accepted measurement methods, even in widely utilized consensus guide-lines.[7,11] We recommend recording *a single measurement* of the *greatest length* of the cyst in the long axis on either the axial or coronal image and also reporting the cor-responding image and series numbers. The image containing the measurement cursor must be archived. Although more precise measurements could be gleaned from 3D images, this simpler approach is more reproducible.

Relation to Main Pancreatic Duct

Radiologists should report whether there is communication between the cyst and the MPD because this is necessary for the cyst to be classified as a BD-IPMN. CT with 3D reconstructions or MRI with MRCP is excellent and equivalent to EUS to estab-lish duct communication.[33,34] However, it may not always be possible to ascertain the presence of duct communication. The importance of reporting cyst communica-tion to the MPD is that for some small BD-IPMNs, slightly less aggressive manage-ment can be pursued compared with a circumstance in which this diagnosis is less certain.

BD-IPMN should be further separated into *pure* versus *combined* forms. In the pure form, the lesion is connected to the MPD by a thin neck. In the combined form, in which the MPD is also involved, the MPD diameter is variable. For all BD-IPMN, the *widest* diameter of the MPD should be recorded, even if away from the cyst. A dilated MPD is a suspicious feature with BD-IPMN and should be immediately investigated by EUS and FNA to determine further management.[35,36] MPD may display a localized fusiform dilation at the insertion of the cyst neck in pure BD-IPMN.

Presence of "Worrisome Features" and/or "High-Risk Stigmata"

I encourage radiologists to use the specific terms "worrisome features" or "high-risk stigmata" in their reports, when applicable. These terms are derived from the multiau-thored consensus articles from Sendai,[7] later modified in Fukuoka, Japan,[37] and are universally understood by physicians who treat pancreatic disease and by other refer-ring physicians. *Worrisome features* include a cyst 3 cm or greater; thickened, enhanced cyst walls; and nonenhanced mural nodules. The Fukuoka criteria include MPD dilation to 5 to 9 mm (without other causes of obstruction) as a worrisome feature; we recommend that a simple 7-mm duct threshold be used.[36] *High-risk stig-mata* detected by imaging include extrahepatic biliary obstruction secondary to pancreatic head cyst, an enhanced solid component, and MPD 10 mm or greater without other cause of obstruction.

Growth on Follow-Up Examination

Although an accepted definition of significant "growth" is not established in the litera-ture, we recommend that radiologists report whether growth has occurred on follow-up examinations according to the following criteria: for cysts less than 0.5 cm, growth is represented by a 100% increase in long-axis diameter; for cysts 0.5 to 1.5 cm, growth is represented by a 50% increase in long-axis diameter; and for cysts greater than 1.5 cm, growth is represented by a 20% increase in long-axis diameter.

Although most clinicians, surgeons, and radiologists think that growth indicates a possible progression toward high-grade dysplasia or malignancy, this assumption has been questioned.[25] Even so, growth remains the most widely utilized parameter for long-term surveillance.

When possible, radiologists should also report a cyst's growth rate. Authors have shown that a more rapid growth rate (>2 mm/y) can help separate aggressive from indolent cysts.[38,39]

Multiplicity

Radiologists should report the presence of multiple cysts. The cyst with the longest dimension should be used as the index lesion. However, each cyst must be assessed for growth and for worrisome features and high-risk stigmata on initial and follow-up examinations. Our algorithm applies to patients with single or multiple incidental pancreatic cysts because the literature is not clear about different outcomes for multiple cysts.[40,41]

The importance of multifocal IPMN has been studied by several groups in patients with more than 2 cysts.[8,40–42] Two groups found an increased risk of high-grade dysplasia or malignancy,[40,42] whereas 2 groups did not.[8,41]

INCLUSION/EXCLUSION CRITERIA FOR USE OF THE ALGORITHM

1. All incidental cysts should be presumed mucinous, unless the cyst has definitive features of an alternative histology (eg, SCA) or has been proven by aspiration not to be mucinous. Such presumed mucinous cysts should be followed or considered for surgery.[26,43–46] We generally recommend 9 to 10-year follow-up with varying schedules, based on initial size. If a cyst grows, the frequency of follow-up should increase and/or EUS with FNA should be considered. A study comparing Fukuoka, European evidence-based guidelines, and America Gastroenterological Association (AGA) found that European EBG had the lowest rate of missed malignancy with the highest number of unnecessary resections, Fukuoka had the highest number of missed malignancy, and AGA had the lowest surgical rate with the highest number of missed malignancy.[47]
2. Cyst size directs follow-up or intervention. Although our cyst size thresholds (ie, <1.5, 1.5–2.5, >2.5 cm) differ from the commonly used 3-cm threshold,[11] our choices are sensitive to studies of surgically resected "Sendai-negative" cysts less than 3 cm, which have shown that high-grade dysplasia or frank malignancy may occur.[48–52]
3. Follow-up may "shift" either when a cyst grows from less than 1.5 to 1.5 cm or greater or when a cyst is first discovered in a patient aged close to 80 years, as described above. In general, a new 9 to 10-year follow-up period is not recommended when such a shift occurs; rather, decisions about total follow-up length should be tailored to the patient's circumstance.
4. Development of "worrisome features" or "high-risk stigmata," as described above, should prompt surgical consultation.
5. Comparison to earlier imaging studies is crucial, including those where the pancreas is frequently visualized, such as chest CT, spine CT or MRI, PET/CT, and abdominal ultrasound. Earlier studies should be reviewed for stability and features. The date of an earlier study can be used as a baseline to establish a follow-up schedule.

Surveillance and Follow-Up

Authors have documented delayed growth in small cysts that were unchanged for several years.[53,54] In addition, new knowledge concerning age-related outcomes[55–60] and cysts as a marker for elevated whole-gland PDAC risk[55,61] are important clinical parameters.

For most patients, we advocate 9 to 10 years follow-up terminating at the age of 80 years. For patients aged older than 65 years at the time of initial cyst detection, longer follow-up may be prudent; however, decisions to follow cysts beyond 9 to 10 years should be made at the individual patient level. With our approach, many older patients will not undergo surveillance for the full 9 to 10 years, whereas younger patients may undergo lengthier monitoring. Given the absence of definitive studies to inform optimal follow-up, our recommendations are primarily based on experiential observations.

For patients aged 80 years or older at the time of initial cyst detection, a separate algorithm for follow-up may be instituted. Follow-up beyond 80 years of age, for a cyst first identified at less than 80 years, is generally not advised, as indicated above. The exception is when a cyst is discovered in a patient who is close to—but not yet—80 years of age. When this occurs, case-by-case decisions for ongoing surveillance should be based on patient characteristics (ie, overall health, willingness to undergo treatment, if needed) and accumulated knowledge about the cyst.

We use 3 algorithms for cysts based on the cyst size at presentation and patient age. Cysts less than 1.5 cm in patients aged older than 75 years can be imaged every 2 years; cysts in patients aged between 60 and 74 years are imaged every 2 years for 7 years, or, if growth, the interval is shortened to every year. Patients aged 60 years and younger are imaged every year for 5 years and then every 2 years for 5 years. For cysts between 1.5 and 2.5 cm, imaging follow-up is based on either the presence or absence of MPD communications. If there is MPD communication, the cyst is imaged every 6 months for 2 years, then every year for 2 years, then every 2 years for 5 years. For cysts with no MPD communication, they are imaged every year for 5 years, then every 2 years for 5 years. Any growth warrants EUS/FNA. Alternatively, for cysts near 2.5 cm, EUS/FNA can be immediately used. For cysts greater than 2.5 cm with MPD communication, imaging every 6 months for 2 years followed by every year for 2 years followed by every 2 years for 5 years. For cysts without MPD communication, the cyst can be imaged yearly for 5 years followed by every 2 years for 5 years. Any growth demands EUS/FNA. Alternatively, the cyst can undergo immediate EUS/FNA.

IMAGING PROTOCOL OPTIMIZATION

Follow-up imaging may be performed with *either* MRI with contrast-enhanced sequences *or* "pancreas-protocol" multidetector CT (MDCT). MRI avoids the cumulative radiation exposure of multiple follow-up CT examinations but MRI has not been shown to be superior to pancreatic-protocol CT scanning for detecting worrisome features or PDAC.[62-65]

Regardless of the modality, intravenous contrast, multiphase acquisitions, and thin sections for 3D visualization are needed. Sixteen-slice or greater MDCT scanners acquire submillimeter slices with close to isotropic voxels and allow reformatted thicker slices (3–5 mm). Pancreatic-phase images should begin about 40 seconds after initiating the IV contrast injection. Injection rates of 4 to 5 mL/s may optimally display peripancreatic vasculature and maximize pancreatic enhancement. A second phase is recommended at approximately 80 seconds to evaluate the liver and remainder of the abdomen and pelvis.

MRI studies are best performed at 3T. Fat-suppressed T2-weighted images (single shot or breath hold) and gadolinium-enhanced T1-weighted gradient recalled echo sequences in arterial, early portal, and late portal phases are suggested. MRCP can help to establish if the cyst communicates with the MPD, assisted by 3D analysis of source data (thin slices). Routinely using contrast material for MRI follow-up is controversial. Noncontrast MRI has shorter scan times and lower cost with little difference in detecting evolving dysplastic changes.[66,67] However, contrast-enhanced sequences may help detect enhancement within mural nodules (high-risk stigma), and the pancreatic-phase improves the ability to detect metachronous PDAC elsewhere.

Specifics of pancreatic protocols for CT and MRI are summarized in a joint statement from the American Pancreatic Association and the Society of Abdominal Radiology.[68] These protocols have also been adopted into National Comprehensive Cancer Network guidelines for pancreatic imaging (version 1.2016). Recent studies have shown that deep learning model (DLM) may improve junior interpreter's performance.[69]

SUMMARY

- We propose an updated algorithm for reporting incidental pancreatic cysts, stratified by patient and imaging features.
- Five properties that define our new algorithm include (1) cysts should be managed as mucinous unless proven otherwise, (2) broad use of EUS with FNA for problem solving, (3) more specific definition of cyst measurement and growth criteria, (4) follow-up periods of 9 to 10 years in most patients, and (5) modified management for patients aged 80 years or older.
- We emphasize the importance of shared decision-making between patients and physicians for successfully managing incidental pancreatic cysts.
- We intend our approach to reduce unnecessary variability in care, and provide further insight into the natural history of incidental pancreatic cysts.

CLINICS CARE POINTS

- Identify a cyst as serous cystadenoma
- Measure the length of the cyst as largest dimension on either axial or coronal plane
- Use accompanying table to assess the risk of any individual cyst

---

DISCLOSURE

The authors have nothing to disclose.

REFERENCES

1. Miller FH, Lopes Vendrami C, Recht HS, et al. Pancreatic Cystic Lesions and Malignancy: Assessment, Guidelines, and the Field Defect. Radiographics 2022; 42(1):87–105.
2. Gardner TB, Glass LM, Smith KD, et al. Pancreatic cyst prevalence and the risk of mucin-producing adenocarcinoma in US adults. Am J Gastroenterol 2013; 108(10):1546–50.
3. Zanini N, Giordano M, Smerieri E, et al. Estimation of the prevalence of asymptomatic pancreatic cysts in the population of San Marino. Pancreatology 2015; 15(4):417–22.
4. Stark A, Donahue TR, Reber HA, et al. Pancreatic Cyst Disease: A Review. JAMA 2016;315(17):1882–93.

5. Moris M, Bridges MD, Pooley RA, et al. Association Between Advances in High-Resolution Cross-Section Imaging Technologies and Increase in Prevalence of Pancreatic Cysts From 2005 to 2014. Clin Gastroenterol Hepatol 2016;14(4): 585–593 e3.

6. Sun HY, Kim SH, Kim MA, et al. CT imaging spectrum of pancreatic serous tumors: based on new pathologic classification. Eur J Radiol 2010;75(2):e45–55.

7. Tanaka M, Chari S, Adsay V, et al. International consensus guidelines for management of intraductal papillary mucinous neoplasms and mucinous cystic neoplasms of the pancreas. Pancreatology 2006;6(1–2):17–32.

8. Mori Y, Ohtsuka T, Kono H, et al. Management strategy for multifocal branch duct intraductal papillary mucinous neoplasms of the pancreas. Pancreas 2012;41(7): 1008–12.

9. Canto MI, Hruban RH, Fishman EK, et al. Frequent detection of pancreatic lesions in asymptomatic high-risk individuals. Gastroenterology 2012;142(4):796–804 [quiz: e14-5].

10. Mandai K, Uno K, Yasuda K. Does a family history of pancreatic ductal adenocarcinoma and cyst size influence the follow-up strategy for intraductal papillary mucinous neoplasms of the pancreas? Pancreas 2014;43(6):917–21.

11. Tanaka M, Fernandez-del Castillo C, Adsay V, et al. International consensus guidelines 2012 for the management of IPMN and MCN of the pancreas. Pancreatology 2012;12(3):183–97.

12. Megibow AJ, Baker ME, Morgan DE, et al. Management of Incidental Pancreatic Cysts: A White Paper of the ACR Incidental Findings Committee. J Am Coll Radiol 2017;14(7):911–23.

13. Muraki T, Jang KT, Reid MD, et al. Pancreatic ductal adenocarcinomas associated with intraductal papillary mucinous neoplasms (IPMNs) versus pseudo-IPMNs: relative frequency, clinicopathologic characteristics and differential diagnosis. Mod Pathol 2022;35(1):96–105.

14. Adsay NV. Cystic neoplasia of the pancreas: pathology and biology. J Gastrointest Surg 2008;12(3):401–4.

15. Park JW, Jang JY, Kang MJ, et al. Mucinous cystic neoplasm of the pancreas: is surgical resection recommended for all surgically fit patients? Pancreatology 2014;14(2):131–6.

16. Yamao K, Yanagisawa A, Takahashi K, et al. Clinicopathological features and prognosis of mucinous cystic neoplasm with ovarian-type stroma: a multi-institutional study of the Japan pancreas society. Pancreas 2011;40(1):67–71.

17. Kimura W, Nagai H, Kuroda A, et al. Analysis of small cystic lesions of the pancreas. Int J Pancreatol 1995;18(3):197–206.

18. Brat DJ, Lillemoe KD, Yeo CJ, et al. Progression of pancreatic intraductal neoplasias to infiltrating adenocarcinoma of the pancreas. Am J Surg Pathol 1998;22(2): 163–9.

19. Kobayashi G, Fujita N, Maguchi H, et al. Natural history of branch duct intraductal papillary mucinous neoplasm with mural nodules: a Japan Pancreas Society multicenter study. Pancreas 2014;43(4):532–8.

20. Pérez-Cuadrado-Robles E, Uribarri-González L, Borbath I, et al. Risk of advanced lesions in patients with branch-duct IPMN and relative indications for surgery according to European evidence-based guidelines. Dig Liver Dis 2019; 51(6):882–6.

21. Canto MI, Almario JA, Schulick RD, et al. Risk of Neoplastic Progression in Individuals at High Risk for Pancreatic Cancer Undergoing Long-term Surveillance. Gastroenterology 2018;155(3):740–51.e2.

22. Johansson K, Kaprio T, Nieminen H, et al. A retrospective study of intraductal papillary neoplasia of the pancreas (IPMN) under surveillance. Scand J Surg 2022;111(1). 14574969221076792.
23. Tanno S, Nakano Y, Koizumi K, et al. Pancreatic ductal adenocarcinomas in long-term follow-up patients with branch duct intraductal papillary mucinous neoplasms. Pancreas 2010;39(1):36–40.
24. Law JK, Wolfgang CL, Weiss MJ, et al. Concomitant pancreatic adenocarcinoma in a patient with branch-duct intraductal papillary mucinous neoplasm. World J Gastroenterol 2014;20(27):9200–4.
25. Scheiman JM, Hwang JH, Moayyedi P. American gastroenterological association technical review on the diagnosis and management of asymptomatic neoplastic pancreatic cysts. Gastroenterology 2015;148(4):824–848 e22.
26. Buscarini E, Pezzilli R, Cannizzaro R, et al. Italian consensus guidelines for the diagnostic work-up and follow-up of cystic pancreatic neoplasms. Dig Liver Dis 2014;46(6):479–93.
27. Del Chiaro M, Verbeke C, Salvia R, et al. European experts consensus statement on cystic tumours of the pancreas. Dig Liver Dis 2013;45(9):703–11.
28. Tanaka S, Nakao M, Ioka T, et al. Slight dilatation of the main pancreatic duct and presence of pancreatic cysts as predictive signs of pancreatic cancer: a prospective study. Radiology 2010;254(3):965–72.
29. Luk L, Hecht EM, Kang S, et al. Society of Abdominal Radiology Disease Focused Panel Survey on Clinical Utilization of Incidental Pancreatic Cyst Management Recommendations and Template Reporting. J Am Coll Radiol 2021; 18(9):1324–31.
30. Sahani DV, Kadavigere R, Saokar A, et al. Cystic pancreatic lesions: a simple imaging-based classification system for guiding management. Radiographics 2005;25(6):1471–84.
31. Procacci C, Graziani R, Bicego E, et al. Serous cystadenoma of the pancreas: report of 30 cases with emphasis on the imaging findings. J Comput Assist Tomogr 1997;21(3):373–82.
32. Choi JY, Kim MJ, Lee JY, et al. Typical and atypical manifestations of serous cystadenoma of the pancreas: imaging findings with pathologic correlation. AJR Am J Roentgenol 2009;193(1):136–42.
33. Kim JH, Eun HW, Park HJ, et al. Diagnostic performance of MRI and EUS in the differentiation of benign from malignant pancreatic cyst and cyst communication with the main duct. Eur J Radiol 2012;81(11):2927–35.
34. Jones MJ, Buchanan AS, Neal CP, et al. Imaging of indeterminate pancreatic cystic lesions: a systematic review. Pancreatology 2013;13(4):436–42.
35. Fritz S, Hackert T, Buchler MW. Pancreatic intraductal papillary mucinous neoplasm–where is the challenge? Dig Dis 2015;33(1):99–105.
36. Kang MJ, Jang JY, Lee S, et al. Clinicopathological Meaning of Size of Main-Duct Dilatation in Intraductal Papillary Mucinous Neoplasm of Pancreas: Proposal of a Simplified Morphological Classification Based on the Investigation on the Size of Main Pancreatic Duct. World J Surg 2015;39(8):2006–13.
37. Dbouk M, Brewer Gutierrez OI, Lennon AM, et al. Guidelines on management of pancreatic cysts detected in high-risk individuals: An evaluation of the 2017 Fukuoka guidelines and the 2020 International Cancer of the Pancreas Screening (CAPS) consortium statements. Pancreatology 2021;21(3):613–21.
38. Kang MJ, Jang JY, Kim SJ, et al. Cyst growth rate predicts malignancy in patients with branch duct intraductal papillary mucinous neoplasms. Clin Gastroenterol Hepatol 2011;9(1):87–93.

39. Kwong WT, Lawson RD, Hunt G, et al. Rapid Growth Rates of Suspected Pancreatic Cyst Branch Duct Intraductal Papillary Mucinous Neoplasms Predict Malignancy. Dig Dis Sci 2015;60(9):2800–6.

40. Raman SP, Kawamoto S, Blackford A, et al. Histopathologic findings of multifocal pancreatic intraductal papillary mucinous neoplasms on CT. AJR Am J Roentgenol 2013;200(3):563–9.

41. Castelli F, Bosetti D, Negrelli R, et al. Multifocal branch-duct intraductal papillary mucinous neoplasms (IPMNs) of the pancreas: magnetic resonance (MR) imaging pattern and evolution over time. Radiol Med 2013;118(6):917–29.

42. Fritz S, Schirren M, Klauss M, et al. Clinicopathologic characteristics of patients with resected multifocal intraductal papillary mucinous neoplasm of the pancreas. Surgery 2012;152(3 Suppl 1):S74–80.

43. Tanno S, Nakano Y, Nishikawa T, et al. Natural history of branch duct intraductal papillary-mucinous neoplasms of the pancreas without mural nodules: long-term follow-up results. Gut 2008;57(3):339–43.

44. Maguchi H, Tanno S, Mizuno N, et al. Natural history of branch duct intraductal papillary mucinous neoplasms of the pancreas: a multicenter study in Japan. Pancreas 2011;40(3):364–70.

45. Handrich SJ, Hough DM, Fletcher JG, et al. The natural history of the incidentally discovered small simple pancreatic cyst: long-term follow-up and clinical implications. AJR Am J Roentgenol 2005;184(1):20–3.

46. Arlix A, Bournet B, Otal P, et al. Long-term clinical and imaging follow-up of nonoperated branch duct form of intraductal papillary mucinous neoplasms of the pancreas. Pancreas 2012;41(2):295–301.

47. Vanden Bulcke A, Jaekers J, Topal H, et al. Evaluating the accuracy of three international guidelines in identifying the risk of malignancy in pancreatic cysts: a retrospective analysis of a surgical treated population. Acta Gastroenterol Belg 2021;84(3):443–50.

48. Fritz S, Klauss M, Bergmann F, et al. Small (Sendai negative) branch-duct IPMNs: not harmless. Ann Surg 2012;256(2):313–20.

49. Nakhaei M, Bligh M, Chernyak V, et al. Incidence of pancreatic cancer during long-term follow-up in patients with incidental pancreatic cysts smaller than 2 cm. Eur Radiol 2022;32(5):3369–76.

50. Woo SM, Ryu JK, Lee SH, et al. Branch duct intraductal papillary mucinous neoplasms in a retrospective series of 190 patients. Br J Surg 2009;96(4):405–11.

51. Pelaez-Luna M, Chari ST, Smyrk TC, et al. Do consensus indications for resection in branch duct intraductal papillary mucinous neoplasm predict malignancy? A study of 147 patients. Am J Gastroenterol 2007;102(8):1759–64.

52. Jang JY, Kim SW, Lee SE, et al. Treatment guidelines for branch duct type intraductal papillary mucinous neoplasms of the pancreas: when can we operate or observe? Ann Surg Oncol 2008;15(1):199–205.

53. Brook OR, Beddy P, Pahade J, et al. Delayed Growth in Incidental Pancreatic Cysts: Are the Current American College of Radiology Recommendations for Follow-up Appropriate? Radiology 2016;278(3):752–61.

54. Khannoussi W, Vullierme MP, Rebours V, et al. The long term risk of malignancy in patients with branch duct intraductal papillary mucinous neoplasms of the pancreas. Pancreatology 2012;12(3):198–202.

55. Chernyak V, Flusberg M, Haramati LB, et al. Incidental pancreatic cystic lesions: is there a relationship with the development of pancreatic adenocarcinoma and all-cause mortality? Radiology 2015;274(1):161–9.

56. Morris-Stiff G, Falk GA, Chalikonda S, et al. Natural history of asymptomatic pancreatic cystic neoplasms. HPB (Oxford) 2013;15(3):175–81.
57. Terris B, Ponsot P, Paye F, et al. Intraductal papillary mucinous tumors of the pancreas confined to secondary ducts show less aggressive pathologic features as compared with those involving the main pancreatic duct. Am J Surg Pathol 2000;24(10):1372–7.
58. Udare A, Agarwal M, Alabousi M, et al. Diagnostic Accuracy of MRI for Differentiation of Benign and Malignant Pancreatic Cystic Lesions Compared to CT and Endoscopic Ultrasound: Systematic Review and Meta-analysis. J Magn Reson Imaging 2021;54(4):1126–37.
59. Uehara H, Ishikawa O, Katayama K, et al. Size of mural nodule as an indicator of surgery for branch duct intraductal papillary mucinous neoplasm of the pancreas during follow-up. J Gastroenterol 2011;46(5):657–63.
60. Fritz S, Klauss M, Bergmann F, et al. Pancreatic main-duct involvement in branch-duct IPMNs: an underestimated risk. Ann Surg 2014;260(5):848–55 [discussion: 55-6].
61. Munigala S, Gelrud A, Agarwal B. Risk of pancreatic cancer in patients with pancreatic cyst. Gastrointest Endosc 2016;84(1):81–6.
62. Nougaret S, Reinhold C, Chong J, et al. Incidental pancreatic cysts: natural history and diagnostic accuracy of a limited serial pancreatic cyst MRI protocol. Eur Radiol 2014;24(5):1020–9.
63. Chen FM, Ni JM, Zhang ZY, et al. Presurgical Evaluation of Pancreatic Cancer: A Comprehensive Imaging Comparison of CT Versus MRI. AJR Am J Roentgenol 2016;206(3):526–35.
64. Lee HJ, Kim MJ, Choi JY, et al. Relative accuracy of CT and MRI in the differentiation of benign from malignant pancreatic cystic lesions. Clin Radiol 2011;66(4):315–21.
65. Sainani NI, Saokar A, Deshpande V, et al. Comparative performance of MDCT and MRI with MR cholangiopancreatography in characterizing small pancreatic cysts. AJR Am J Roentgenol 2009;193(3):722–31.
66. Macari M, Lee T, Kim S, et al. Is gadolinium necessary for MRI follow-up evaluation of cystic lesions in the pancreas? Preliminary results. AJR Am J Roentgenol 2009;192(1):159–64.
67. Pozzi-Mucelli RM, Rinta-Kiikka I, Wunsche K, et al. Pancreatic MRI for the surveillance of cystic neoplasms: comparison of a short with a comprehensive imaging protocol. Eur Radiol 2016;27(1):41–50.
68. Al-Hawary MM, Francis IR, Chari ST, et al. Pancreatic ductal adenocarcinoma radiology reporting template: consensus statement of the society of abdominal radiology and the american pancreatic association. Gastroenterology 2014;146(1):291–304 e1.
69. Wang X, Sun Z, Xue H, et al. A deep learning algorithm to improve readers' interpretation and speed of pancreatic cystic lesions on dual-phase enhanced CT. Abdom Radiol (NY) 2022;47(6):2135–47.

Pancreatic Cystic Lesions
Next Generation of Radiologic Assessment

Chenchan Huang, MD[a,*], Sumit Chopra, PhD[b],
Candice W. Bolan, MD[c], Hersh Chandarana, MD[a],
Nassier Harfouch, MD[a], Elizabeth M. Hecht, MD[d],
Grace C. Lo, MD[e], Alec J. Megibow, MD[a]

KEYWORDS

- Pancreatic cystic lesions • Pancreatic cystic neoplasms
- Intraductal papillary mucinous neoplasms (IPMN) • Machine learning • Deep learning
- Radiomics

KEY POINTS

- Current radiology cross-sectional imaging has limited accuracy in subtyping pancreatic cystic lesions and risk stratification of precursor pancreatic cystic lesions
- There is tremendous interest in developing advanced imaging analysis for pancreatic cystic lesions to address the unmet needs of current conventional imaging.
- Radiomics and deep learning are two areas of advanced imaging analysis to potentially serve as the next generation of radiology assessment of pancreatic cystic lesions. However, current publications show limited success and large-scale research is needed to further our understanding of how radiomics and deep learning can truly add value to conventional imaging in pancreatic cystic lesion assessment.

INTRODUCTION

Pancreatic cystic lesions are increasingly detected on imaging with the majority being branch-duct intraductal papillary mucinous neoplasms (BD-IPMN).[1,2] BD-IPMN and the less common, mucinous cystic neoplasms (MCN), are the only macroscopically visible precursor lesions to pancreatic ductal adenocarcinoma (PDAC). Current non-invasive imaging modalities have limited accuracy for accurately subtyping cystic lesions and stratifying risk of malignancy for precursor cystic lesions. This limitation

[a] Department of Radiology, NYU Grossman School of Medicine, 660 1st Avenue, 3F, New York, NY 10016, USA; [b] Department of Radiology, NYU Grossman School of Medicine, 650 First Avenue, 4th Floor, New York, NY 10016, USA; [c] Department of Radiology, Mayo Clinic in Florida, 4500 San Pablo Road South, Jacksonville, FL 32224, USA; [d] Department of Radiology, New York Presbyterian – Weill Cornell Medicine, 520 East 70th Street, Starr 8a, New York, NY 10021, USA; [e] Department of Radiology, New York Presbyterian – Weill Cornell Medicine, 520 East 70th Street, Starr 7a, New York, NY 10021, USA
* Corresponding author.
E-mail address: Chenchan.Huang@nyulangone.org

Gastrointest Endoscopy Clin N Am 33 (2023) 533–546
https://doi.org/10.1016/j.giec.2023.03.004
1052-5157/23/© 2023 Elsevier Inc. All rights reserved.

giendo.theclinics.com

leads to invasive endoscopic ultrasound and fine needle aspiration (EUS/FNA), long-term imaging follow-up, and/or unnecessary pancreatic surgeries for benign pancreatic cystic lesions. Consequently, there is a pressing need for more advanced imaging analysis to improve diagnosis and risk stratification of these precursor cystic lesions to optimize patient management.

Spurred by advances in computing power over the past decade, radiomics, followed by deep learning are two areas of advanced imaging analysis that have ignited tremendous amount of research interest in recent years. These two areas are also rapidly evolving and maturing as the scientific community becomes more familiar with them.

This article will review current imaging modalities for detection and characterization of pancreatic cystic lesion and their limitations, and introduce the use of radiomics and deep learning (DL), current landscape of these techniques, their limitations, as well as future directions pertaining to pancreatic cystic lesions.

CURRENT UNMET NEEDS OF IMAGING PANCREATIC CYSTIC LESION
Characterization of Pancreatic Cystic Lesions

Early studies revealed accuracies of 39.5% to 46% for computed tomography (CT) and MRI in characterizing specific subtypes of pancreatic cystic lesions.[3,4] However, a more recent study demonstrated an overall accuracy of up to 80.5% for combined CT and MRI,[5] although lower for serous cystadenomas at 56.8%. Interestingly, in a 2012 retrospective study that looked at 851 pancreatic resections performed for PCLs, 25% were benign cystic lesions without malignant potential on final pathology, 16.1% of which were serous cystic neoplasms.[6] One of the main reasons for low diagnostic accuracies is the overlapping morphology of these cystic lesions, particularly for serous cystadenomas that have atypical appearances. For example, macrocytic serous cystadenoma can be indistinguishable from the "cluster of grapes" appearance of a BD-IPMN, and when abutting the main pancreatic duct, ductal communication can be challenging to identify. Moreover, BD-IPMNs may not show ductal communication due to small or obstructed cyst necks.

In a multinational study of 2622 patients with serous cystadenomas, 61% of these patients underwent pancreatic surgery, with 60% reporting that the reason for surgery was an uncertain diagnosis.[7] Although most of the incidentally noted PCLs tend to be IPMNs, if imaging could reliably and accurately diagnose benign cystic lesions such as serous cystic neoplasms, this would prevent long-term imaging surveillance, invasive workup with EUS/FNA, and unnecessary surgical resections for a substantial number of patients.

Current Imaging Unable to Accurately Risk Stratify Branch-Duct Intraductal Papillary Mucinous Neoplasms

Currently, there is still limited accuracy for risk stratification of BD-IPMN. Malignancy has been shown to occur at a rate of approximately 24% of BD-IPMNs in surgically resected cases, with surveillance studies showing a much lower malignancy rate of 1% to 2% per year.[8] This is collaborated by a recent Japanese single-center large study of 1404 patients with BD-IPMN undergoing long-term surveillance, which reported a 3.3% risk of malignancy at 5 years and a 15% risk at 15 years.[9] Surgically resected studies tend to overestimate the risk of malignancy (by excluding those under surveillance) while surveillance studies likely underestimate the risk of malignancy (due to lack of pathologic confirmation). To address these selection biases, a recent large retrospective multicenter international study consisted of 292 patients who were initially under imaging surveillance for BD-IPMN but ultimately underwent surgical resection from 2010 to 2019. It is noteworthy that even in these five expert centers with a super-selected patient population, 185 (63%) of the patients who underwent resection due to clinical and radiological "worrisome features" and "high-risk stigmata" had no high-grade dysplasia or invasive carcinoma on pathology.[10]

Diagnostic Performance of Societal Consensus Guidelines

To assist in clinical decision-making of PCL management, societal consensus guidelines based on literature review and expert opinions have been developed, with the intent to stratify cystic lesions into different risk categories with corresponding action plans. There are currently five major societal consensus guidelines: the American Gastrointestinal Association (AGA) guidelines, the American College of Gastroenterology (ACG) guidelines, the American College of Radiology (ACR) recommendations, the European Evidence-Based guidelines, and the International Association of Pancreatology (IAP)/Fukuoka guidelines. Each of these guidelines differs slightly in their intended audiences, target cyst types, and surveillance and management recommendations.[11–15] Detailed review and comparison of these guidelines are out of scope of this article. However, the most important imaging features associated with a perceived elevated risk of malignancy are shared by these guidelines and include main pancreatic duct dilation, presence of mural nodule, cyst size, and interval growth. Depending on local practice preferences, academic institutions may develop their guidelines, which are often a mixture of two or more of the five main societal guidelines.

The overarching goal of these guidelines is to maximize the sensitivity of detecting malignancy, often at the expense of lower specificity and accuracy. A 2017 study compared the diagnostic accuracies of the 2012 International Consensus/Fukuoka (Fukuoka) guideline, 2010 ACR guidelines, and 2015 AGA guideline for preoperative diagnosis of high-grade dysplasia and invasive carcinoma on the pathology of resected cystic lesions. Accuracies were reported as 49.8%, 59.8%, and 75.8%, respectively, with sensitivities of 73.2%, 53.6%, and 7.3%, respectively.[16] A separate study comparing the 2012 Fukuoka, 2015 AGA, and 2013 European guidelines found similar accuracy rates of 54%, 59%, and 53%, respectively. Both studies showed the AGA guidelines as being the most specific, but with the highest risk of missing cases of high-grade dysplasia/invasive carcinoma.

In 2017, updates were made to the Fukuoka and ACR guidelines, which consisted of incorporating additional parameters to the list of criteria. For example, the 2017 Fukuoka guidelines added cyst growth rate of $\geq$ 5 mm/2 years, lymphadenopathy, and elevated Ca 19-9 as worrisome features.[14] Despite these revisions, a 2021 retrospective single-center study[17] comparing the diagnostic performance of the updated 2017 Fukuoka guidelines with the 2018 European guidelines in 137 patients found similar low area under the curve (AUC) values of 0.572 for Fukuoka and 0.621 for European. This study found that more than half of the resections were unnecessary (pathology yielded benign low-grade dysplasia or non-neoplastic cystic lesions), with postoperative 30-day mortality and major morbidity of 0% and 37.5%, respectively. As pancreatic surgery has high morbidity rates, there is a need for better preoperative PCL risk stratification.

NEXT GENERATION OF RADIOLOGY ASSESSMENT
Radiomics

Spurred by advances in computing power over the past decade, and coupled with machine learning, radiomics has garnered tremendous attention as an advancement in imaging analysis. Radiomics is the conversion of standard-of-care images into mineable quantitative data. These quantitative data are also known as radiomics features, and are typically invisible to the human eye.[18] These features include basic parameters, first-order features, and second-order features of a lesion. Basic parameters include data such as size and compactness. First-order features are typically histograms of pixel intensities, and second-order features are sometimes used interchangeably as texture analysis, as these features describe spatial relationships of pixel intensities within a lesion.[18–20]

This type of quantitative imaging data, which is considered more objective than a radiologist's qualitative assessment, can reveal subtle internal heterogeneity that the human eye cannot perceive, and can noninvasively capture whole tumoral heterogeneity beyond what tissue sampling can achieve.[19,21] Radiomics analysis is a multi-step process (**Fig. 1**). Using standard images obtained as part of clinical management, the first step involves segmentation of the 2-dimensional (2D) region of interest or 3D volume of interest, such as the whole pancreas or the PCL. Segmentation is currently the most labor-intensive part of radiomics analysis, as it is mostly done either manually or semi-automated by a radiologist or researcher. DL-based auto-segmentation has emerged in recent years (often a type of U-Net), although currently mostly geared for segmentation of entire organs, and trained algorithm often result in failures when applied to a different dataset.[22] After segmentation, the second step is image processing. The goal here is to homogenize images across datasets to improve reproducibility of radiomics features extracted in the third step. In another word, sequential image processing steps are performed to ensure uniform pixel spacing, gray-level intensities, bins of the gray-level histogram, etc. across segmented images from which

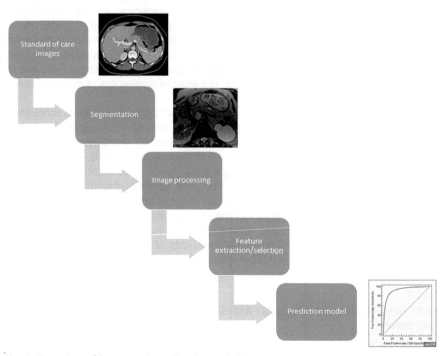

Fig. 1. Overview of key steps in radiomics analysis.

radiomics features will draw from.[23] The third step involves extracting quantitative features of a region of interest, such as volume, shape, histogram, and texture. Usually, far too many radiomics features are extracted initially. However, there are well-established statistical methods for feature reduction, such that only small amount of reproducible and non-redundant radiomics features are selected, which also reduces overfitting. These carefully selected radiomics features can subsequently be chosen as input to develop a multi-parametric machine-learning prediction model, with or without additional clinical variables such as laboratory or pathology data,[24,25] to answer a variety of clinical questions, such as presence of a diagnosis or tumor response to treatment.

RADIOMICS AND SUBTYPING PANCREATIC CYSTIC LESIONS

There has been success and excitement in solid pancreatic cancer detection using radiomics.[26,27] There are fewer publications in the evaluation of cystic lesions using radiomics, likely owing to paucity of cells in cystic lesions compared with that of solid masses. One of the earliest studies on this topic aimed at differentiating IPMN, MCN, SCA, and solid pseudopapillary epithelial neoplasm (SPEN) in a cohort of 74 cases, and found that combining patient demographic information with radiomic features achieved an accuracy of 84% versus that of 60% to 70% for radiologists.[28] A more recent similar but larger study comprised of 214 patients with IPMNs, MCN, SCA, SPEN, or cystic neuroendocrine tumors showed a radiomics-based machine-learning model achieving an AUC of 0.940 for correctly diagnosing the type of cystic lesion compared with an AUC of 0.895 for an expert academic radiologist with more than 25 years of experience.[29] Studies that focus on differentiating serous from mucinous cystic lesions have all reported high AUCs, ranging from 0.89 to 0.96.[30,31]

In day-to-day practice, it is a particularly challenging task for radiologists to distinguish atypical macrocystic serous cystic neoplasm from a branch-duct IPMN or mucinous cystic neoplasm due to overlapping imaging features. As virtually all serous cystic neoplasms are benign, accurate preoperative diagnosis would help avoid unnecessary surgeries and long-term follow-up in asymptomatic patients. Two recent CT-based radiomics studies aimed at differentiating atypical macrocystic serous cystic neoplasm from mucinous cystic neoplasms and achieved AUCs of 0.775 to 0.784.[32,33] However, these studies, which involved 103 MCN and 113 atypical serous cystic neoplasm (SCN) patients, were only marginally better compared with radiologist assessments (radiomics model with AUC of 0.78 vs radiologists AUC of 0.73).[33]

Radiomics and Risk Stratification of Pancreatic Branch-Duct Intraductal Papillary Mucinous Neoplasms

Studies assessing the ability of radiomics to detect malignancy in IPMNs, usually combined with clinical variables, report promising results with AUCs ranging from 0.71 to 0.96.[34–40] However, some of these studies include main duct or mixed type IPMN, neither of which present imaging or management dilemmas. It is more clinically relevant to address the question of how well radiomics perform at risk-stratifying BD-IPMN. Two relatively large studies from the same center consisting of more than 100 patients with BD-IPMNs, showed their models had lower but overall still high diagnostic performance of predicting malignancy when combined with clinical variables, with AUCs ranging from 0.79 to 0.81.[36,37] Charkraborty and colleagues studied a cohort of 103 patients with resected BD-IPMN, including 27 with malignancy (high-grade dysplasia and invasive carcinoma) on pathology, and their model achieved an AUC of 0.77 in identifying malignancy using radiomics features and increased AUC to 0.81 with the addition of clinical variables such as age, gender, and symptoms.[36] Tobaly and colleagues presented the largest multicenter study,[39] consisting of 408 patients with resected IPMNs, including a subgroup of 137 BD-IPMNs (92 benign and 45 malignant). For the BD-IPMN subgroup analysis, their radiomics model achieved AUC of 0.73 in the training cohort, with and without clinical variables, but had a low AUC in the external validation cohort that consisted of a variety of protocols from multiple nearby hospitals, with AUC of 0.55 that slightly improved to 0.57 even when combined with clinical variables. Based on these publications with relatively small sample sizes, and a low AUC on external validation group with the last study, one can conclude that radiomics has not shown adequate success in risk stratification in branch-duct IPMN. Additionally, none of these above studies compared diagnostic performances of their radiomics models with that of radiologists, therefore, it is difficult to truly assess these models' clinical utility.

Artificial Intelligence Overview and Definitions

Artificial intelligence (AI)/machine learning (ML), spurred by advances in the sub-field of DL, has rapidly gained prominence in the scientific communities in the last couple of decades (**Fig. 2**). The term AI refers to the intelligence (perception/reasoning/synthesizing/inference) exhibited by computers and machines as opposed to humans. ML refers to the process of creating a machine (a.k.a., "model") that can "learn" from data to perform tasks in complex environments. The more data the model is exposed to, the better it learns about the environment, which in turn leads to improved performance on the task at hand. The statistical model can be thought of as a parametric function, such as logistic regression, that takes as input a set of "features" describing the environment and produces an output pertaining to the task. Learning (a.k.a., "training") refers to the process of adjusting the parameters of the model to generate the correct output given the input features for every example. The hope is that the features describing every example along with the learned parameters are general enough that if a new (previously unseen) image is passed through this pipeline, it will result in the correct answer. The input features to the model could either be extracted from the

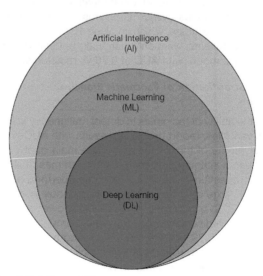

Fig. 2. Relationship of AI, ML, and DL.

raw input using hand-coded rules (such as in radiomics features as described in the above section) or they could themselves be learned (as in the case of DL).

DL is a sub-field of ML where the structure of the "model" in the above-described pipeline is inspired by the mammalian brain's multi-layer architecture and the focus is on "learning" the input features describing the environment in addition to learning the parameters to solve the end task with high accuracy.[41] Specifically, the model is composed of a collection of nodes, called artificial neurons (AN). These nodes are connected so that they can transmit a signal from one AN to another, much like the synapses in a biological brain (**Fig. 3**). "Deep" in DL refers to the number of such layers stacked on top of each other. "Learning" refers to the adjustment of the parameters (weights) of each AN in the network such that for any input example it provides the right answer. The flexibility associated with these "models" enables DL algorithms to learn the features from raw input.

Convolutional Neural Networks (CNNs) are neural networks that can receive a 2D or 3D input, such as 2D images or 3D volumetric images resembling the visual cortex of the brain[41] (**Fig. 4**). Modern DL models (such as CNNs) contain millions of nodes and learnable parameters; as a result, they require large amounts of training examples to train effectively. Because of this, until the 2010s, DL models were generally regarded as too computationally expensive to train on practical tasks. However, advances in computing power over the past decade, along with the availability of large public data sets, such as ImageNet,[42] have accelerated the field's growth.

The use of ML techniques in PCL evaluation can be split into two main categories, namely using handcrafted radiomics features as input for ML models or using raw imaging data as input to the DL models. The radiomics route first involves segmenting and extracting quantitative features from clinical images and then using these features as input to a downstream ML model to solve the task at hand, and has been discussed in an earlier section. In DL, these models can theoretically take the raw pixel values of images as input as opposed to radiomics that need careful segmentations to derive hand-crafted extracted features from images. However, most DL research in radiology at present still requires training an algorithm with large volume of annotated images

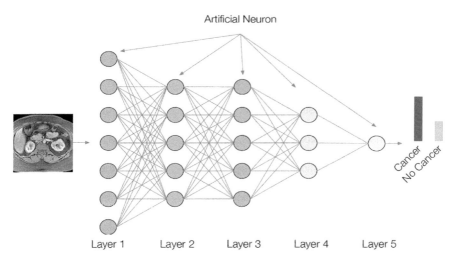

Fig. 3. Neural networks are composed of numerous AN arranged in layers. By incorporating hidden layers and nonlinear operations, neural networks can learn to model intricate patterns and relationships within data.

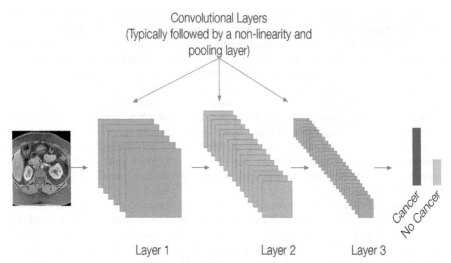

Fig. 4. CNNs are a type of DL model made up of a series of specialized layers that work together to extract features from the input data, such as an image. Convolutional layers use filters to analyze small regions of the image and identify patterns and features, which are subsequently passed through the non-linearity layer to enable CNN to model complex relationships in the data. Pooling layer then aggregates the spatially proximal features to generate high-level features that are robust to small perturbations of the input. It also helps reduce the dimensions of the feature maps.

that have segmented the regions or volumes of interest. One of the main differences between radiomics and DL is the type of features they extract from images. Radiomics extract hand-crafted features, which are predefined, quantifiable, and somewhat interpretable. DL extract features directly from large image datasets via algorithms, and these features are therefore neither predefined nor interpretable. Another difference is that DL usually requires magnitudes of more data and computational resources in comparison to radiomics. Furthermore, DL is newer compared with radiomics. These two latter reasons may contribute to the relative paucity of DL publications on the topic of PCL at present. A few notable papers are discussed below.

Deep Learning and Subtyping Pancreatic Cystic Lesions

When compared with radiomics models, there is a relative void using DL for subtyping PCL. Li and colleagues used densely connected convolutional networks (Dense-Net) on CT images of whole pancreases from 206 patients who had one of four pathologically confirmed cystic lesions (64 IPMN, 35 MCN, 66 SCN, and 41 SPT). Using a stratified 10-fold cross-validation strategy, this DL model achieved an overall accuracy of 72.8% in subtyping cystic lesions, significantly higher than the 48.1% accuracy achieved by radiology interpretation. Interestingly, this DL model also misclassified SCNs as IPMNs, similar to the radiologists in this study and other studies in the literature.[43]

Deep Learning and Risk Stratification of Branch-Duct Intraductal Papillary Mucinous Neoplasms

There is a paucity of DL publications specifically on risk stratification of BD-IPMNs. On the topic of using DL to classify overall IPMNs (including main duct IPMNs), as low risk versus high risk, Corral and colleagues assessed the diagnostic performance of a DL model with MRI from 139 patients (108 patients underwent surgical resection for PCL following MRI, and 31 patients with normal pancreas for MRI performed for non-pancreatic indications). Due to the small sample size, 10-fold cross-validation was used. They used T2-weighted and post-contrast T1-weighted axial images from a standard MRI protocol. A support vector machine classifier assigned pancreases into one of three categories: healthy, low-grade IPMN, or high-grade IPMN with adenocarcinoma. Their DL model achieved similar accuracy when compared with an expert radiologist using AGA or Fukuoka criteria (AUC of 0.783, 0.769, and 0.775, respectively). The DL model had the highest sensitivity and slightly lower specificities (75%, 78%) compared with AGA (25% and 96%) and Fukuoka guidelines (62% and 77%). Notably, the DL model from this study used a fraction of time needed to interpret an MRI (1.82 seconds using this particular study protocol compared with estimated minimum of 5–10 minutes for radiologists to review the pancreas).[44] However, as pointed out earlier, many of the IPMNs from this study were main duct or mixed-type IPMNs, therefore, one cannot ascertain the diagnostic performance of this DL model in the more controversial BD-IPMNs of day-to-day practice.

A more recent study looked into the DL model for differentiating benign versus malignant PCLs.[45] The study included 363 patients' dual-phase CT images from two medical centers. The authors developed a DL model algorithm (3D specially designed densely connected convolutional networks), and compared the diagnostic performances of their DL algorithm versus a traditional radiomics model versus three radiologists. The highest accuracy was among the DL model and senior radiologist, which outperformed the traditional radiomics model and a junior radiologist. The types of PCLs included in this study were diverse and extensive, including IPMN, cystic ductal adenocarcinoma, pseudocyst, and lymphangia. Only 65 of these lesions were IPMNs, and it is not known what percentage were BD-IPMNs. Therefore, it is not known whether this DL model's diagnostic performance will apply to risk stratification of the more controversial and pertinent BD-IPMNs. More studies on DL's ability to stratify BD-IPMNs are needed.

CHALLENGES AND FUTURE DIRECTIONS IN RADIOMICS AND DEEP LEARNING

As seen from these publications, while there are some successes in subtyping cystic lesions with both radiomics and DL, risk stratification of IPMN/PCL still has a long way to go. Many challenges lie ahead before radiomics and DL become part of clinical radiology. For example, most of these studies, particularly the earlier radiomics studies, are comprised of small single-center studies with a few dozen patients. Large cohort studies that contain a sufficient number of pathology-proven malignant BD-IPMNs are needed for robust radiomics and DL projects. Basic challenges include lack of standardization in image acquisition, segmentation, and radiomic features, to name a few. It is not surprising that most of the radiomics studies are CT based despite MRI/MRCP being the modality of choice for PCL evaluation and surveillance, as the MRI has significantly more variations of imaging protocols/acquisitions than CT. Similarly, for DL, there is a need for large cohort multi-institutional studies to develop algorithms that are trained on large-scale diverse data sets.

Inter-reader variability, differences in imaging protocols, and the type of software used for radiomics feature extraction have all been shown to significantly and negatively affect the reproducibility of radiomics features.[46–50] To facilitate large-scale radiomics projects, automated segmentation is essential as manual or semi-automated segmentation methods require significant human effort and are not scalable. This is also a challenge that DL projects face, as currently most of the DL radiology projects are supervised and require a large amount of segmented data to train an algorithm. One of the largest criticism of DL is that it is an extreme example of "black box" nature. As DL models are trained with millions of parameters to extract data patterns correlating with an output (such as presence of a disease), exactly how such a model generates a particular output is impossible for humans to understand. This lack of interpretability and explainability has been termed "black box".[51,52] As "black box" can hinder trust among medical practitioners, interpretable AI is a quickly growing area of interest in the radiology community.[53]

Notable progress and initiatives to counter some of these challenges in radiomics have emerged. For example, the radiomics quality score is a key reference to judge the quality of a research study, thus, elevating the standards for radiomics research and publications. The image biomarker standardization initiative (IBSI)[54] was established with the goal of publishing reference radiomic features that are stable and reproducible.

An area of AI research that largely remains unexplored is multi-modality training. Almost all the previously proposed works focus on training a DL model using a single imaging modality. Combining data from different modalities, including different imaging modalities (EUS/CT/MR) and electronic health records (including patient demographic information, family history, clinical history, cyst fluid, blood test, and genetics) may further increase diagnostic performances. Lastly, all the models proposed thus far take as input data from a single scan of the patient. Development of additional new worrisome features and high-risk stigmata in a surveillance cohort that subsequently underwent surgery have been found to be associated with high-grade dysplasia at final pathology, while patients with a stable worrisome feature on surveillance imaging had the lowest risk of high-grade dysplasia.[10] As this cohort of patients usually undergoes imaging surveillance, changes that occur on serial imaging may contain unmined data that are valuable in further stratifying PCLs and is an area that can be explored.

SUMMARY

As incidental PCLs are increasingly detected and reported, controversy surrounds the management of the highly prevalent BD-IPMNs that have a small chance of progressing into PDAC. Long-term radiology surveillance, invasive EUS/FNA, and unnecessary pancreatic surgeries are some of the expensive costs of catching a small number of high-grade dysplasia/early PDAC. Unmet needs of current radiology imaging have become obvious, including limited accuracy in classifying cystic lesion type and limited accuracy in risk stratification of the highly prevalent BD-IPMN. The presence of multiple societal consensus guidelines likely hinders large multi-institutional and multinational research, and a unified guideline would be helpful. Traditional radiomics coupled with ML and DL are two areas of intense research now. Although some preliminary publications have shown varying degrees of success in PCL diagnosis, data on risk stratification of precursor cystic lesions are still extremely limited. There remains a significant void in large-scale research efforts, particularly in their preferred surveillance imaging modality, which is MRI. As the medical community becomes more familiar with radiomics and AI research, common challenges and roadblocks have emerged and have led to the development of societal initiatives to address some of these challenges. More high-quality research publications are needed before we can confidently proclaim radiomics and DL as the next generation of radiology assessment for PCLs.

CLINICS CARE POINT

- Advanced imaging analysis tools such as radiomics and DL are currently not in clinical use yet.

DISCLOSURE

A.J. Megibow is a consultant for Bracco Diagnostics and Voyager Pharmaceuticals. The remaining authors declare that there are no other disclosures relevant to the subject matter of this article.

REFERENCES

1. Pezzilli R, Buscarini E, Pollini T, et al. Epidemiology, clinical features and diagnostic work-up of cystic neoplasms of the pancreas: Interim analysis of the prospective PANCY survey. Dig Liver Dis 2020;52(5):547–54.
2. Kromrey ML, Bülow R, Hübner J, et al. Prospective study on the incidence, prevalence and 5-year pancreatic-related mortality of pancreatic cysts in a population-based study. Gut 2018;67(1):138–45.
3. Sainani NI, Saokar A, Deshpande V, et al. Comparative Performance of MDCT and MRI With MR Cholangiopancreatography in Characterizing Small Pancreatic Cysts. Am J Roentgenol 2009;193(3):722–31.
4. Visser BC, Yeh BM, Qayyum A, et al. Characterization of Cystic Pancreatic Masses: Relative Accuracy of CT and MRI. Am J Roentgenol 2007;189(3):648–56.
5. Jang DK, Song BJ, Ryu JK, et al. Preoperative Diagnosis of Pancreatic Cystic Lesions: The Accuracy of Endoscopic Ultrasound and Cross-Sectional Imaging. Pancreas 2015;44(8):1329–33.
6. Valsangkar NP, Morales-Oyarvide V, Thayer SP, et al. 851 resected cystic tumors of the pancreas: a 33-year experience at the Massachusetts General Hospital. Surgery 2012;152(3 Suppl 1):S4–12.
7. Jais B, Rebours V, Malleo G, et al. Serous cystic neoplasm of the pancreas: a multinational study of 2622 patients under the auspices of the International Association of Pancreatology and European Pancreatic Club (European Study Group on Cystic Tumors of the Pancreas). Gut 2016;65(2):305–12.
8. Farrell JJ. Prevalence, Diagnosis and Management of Pancreatic Cystic Neoplasms: Current Status and Future Directions. Gut Liver 2015;9(5):571–89.
9. Oyama H, Tada M, Takagi K, et al. Long-term Risk of Malignancy in Branch-Duct Intraductal Papillary Mucinous Neoplasms. Gastroenterology 2020;158(1):226–37.e5.
10. Marchegiani G, Pollini T, Andrianello S, et al. Progression vs Cyst Stability of Branch-Duct Intraductal Papillary Mucinous Neoplasms After Observation and Surgery. JAMA Surg 2021;156(7):654–61.
11. European evidence-based guidelines on pancreatic cystic neoplasms. Gut 2018;67(5):789–804.
12. Elta GH, Enestvedt BK, Sauer BG, et al. ACG Clinical Guideline: Diagnosis and Management of Pancreatic Cysts. Am J Gastroenterol 2018;113(4):464–79.
13. Megibow AJ, Baker ME, Morgan DE, et al. Management of Incidental Pancreatic Cysts: A White Paper of the ACR Incidental Findings Committee. J Am Coll Radiol 2017;14(7):911–23.

14. Tanaka M, Fernández-Del Castillo C, Kamisawa T, et al. Revisions of international consensus Fukuoka guidelines for the management of IPMN of the pancreas. Pancreatology 2017;17(5):738–53.

15. Vege SS, Ziring B, Jain R, et al. American gastroenterological association institute guideline on the diagnosis and management of asymptomatic neoplastic pancreatic cysts. Gastroenterology 2015;148(4):819–22 [quize:12-3].

16. Xu MM, Yin S, Siddiqui AA, et al. Comparison of the diagnostic accuracy of three current guidelines for the evaluation of asymptomatic pancreatic cystic neoplasms. Medicine (Baltimore) 2017;96(35):e7900.

17. Kovacevic B, Hansen MC, Kristensen TS, et al. Diagnostic performance of current guidelines and postoperative outcome following surgical treatment of cystic pancreatic lesions - a 10-year single center experience. Scand J Gastroenterol 2020;55(12):1447–53.

18. Gillies RJ, Kinahan PE, Hricak H. Radiomics: Images Are More than Pictures. They Are Data 2016;278(2):563–77.

19. Davnall F, Yip CSP, Ljungqvist G, et al. Assessment of tumor heterogeneity: an emerging imaging tool for clinical practice? Insights into Imaging 2012;3(6): 573–89.

20. Lambin P, Rios-Velazquez E, Leijenaar R, et al. Radiomics: extracting more information from medical images using advanced feature analysis. European journal of cancer 2012;48(4):441–6.

21. Lubner MG, Smith AD, Sandrasegaran K, et al. CT Texture Analysis: Definitions, Applications, Biologic Correlates, and Challenges. Radiographics 2017;37(5): 1483–503.

22. van Timmeren JE, Cester D, Tanadini-Lang S, et al. Radiomics in medical imaging-"how-to" guide and critical reflection. Insights Imaging 2020;11(1):91.

23. Lafata KJ, Wang Y, Konkel B, et al. Radiomics: a primer on high-throughput image phenotyping. Abdominal radiology (New York) 2022;47(9):2986–3002.

24. Scapicchio C, Gabelloni M, Barucci A, et al. A deep look into radiomics. La radiologia medica 2021;126(10):1296–311.

25. Horvat N, Miranda J, El Homsi M, et al. A primer on texture analysis in abdominal radiology. Abdom Radiol 2022;47(9):2972–85.

26. Chu LC, Park S, Kawamoto S, et al. Utility of CT Radiomics Features in Differentiation of Pancreatic Ductal Adenocarcinoma From Normal Pancreatic Tissue. AJR Am J Roentgenol 2019;213(2):349–57.

27. Mukherjee S, Patra A, Khasawneh H, et al. Radiomics-Based Machine-Learning Models Can Detect Pancreatic Cancer on Prediagnostic CTs at a Substantial Lead Time Prior to Clinical Diagnosis. Gastroenterology 2022. https://doi.org/10.1053/j.gastro.2022.06.066.

28. Dmitriev K, Kaufman AE, Javed AA, et al. Classification of Pancreatic Cysts in Computed Tomography Images Using a Random Forest and Convolutional Neural Network Ensemble. Medical image computing and computer-assisted intervention 2017;10435:150–8.

29. Chu LC, Park S, Soleimani S, et al. Classification of pancreatic cystic neoplasms using radiomic feature analysis is equivalent to an experienced academic radiologist: a step toward computer-augmented diagnostics for radiologists. Abdominal radiology (New York) 2022. https://doi.org/10.1007/s00261-022-03663-6.

30. Chen HY, Deng XY, Pan Y, et al. Pancreatic Serous Cystic Neoplasms and Mucinous Cystic Neoplasms: Differential Diagnosis by Combining Imaging Features and Enhanced CT Texture Analysis. Frontiers in oncology 2021;11:745001.

31. Yang R, Chen Y, Sa G, et al. CT classification model of pancreatic serous cystic neoplasms and mucinous cystic neoplasms based on a deep neural network. Abdominal radiology (New York) 2022;47(1):232–41.
32. Xie H, Ma S, Guo X, et al. Preoperative differentiation of pancreatic mucinous cystic neoplasm from macrocystic serous cystic adenoma using radiomics: Preliminary findings and comparison with radiological model. Eur J Radiol 2020;122: 108747.
33. Xie T, Wang X, Zhang Z, et al. CT-Based Radiomics Analysis for Preoperative Diagnosis of Pancreatic Mucinous Cystic Neoplasm and Atypical Serous Cystadenomas. Frontiers in oncology 2021;11:621520.
34. Hanania AN, Bantis LE, Feng Z, et al. Quantitative imaging to evaluate malignant potential of IPMNs. Oncotarget 2016;7(52):85776.
35. Permuth JB, Choi J, Balarunathan Y, et al. Combining radiomic features with a miRNA classifier may improve prediction of malignant pathology for pancreatic intraductal papillary mucinous neoplasms. Oncotarget 2016;7(52):85785.
36. Chakraborty J, Midya A, Gazit L, et al. CT radiomics to predict high-risk intraductal papillary mucinous neoplasms of the pancreas. Med Phys 2018;45(11): 5019–29.
37. Attiyeh MA, Chakraborty J, Gazit L, et al. Preoperative risk prediction for intraductal papillary mucinous neoplasms by quantitative CT image analysis. HPB Oxford 2019;21(2):212–8.
38. Polk SL, Choi JW, McGettigan MJ, et al. Multiphase computed tomography radiomics of pancreatic intraductal papillary mucinous neoplasms to predict malignancy. World J Gasteroenterol 2020;26(24):3458.
39. Tobaly D, Santinha J, Sartoris R, et al. CT-Based Radiomics Analysis to Predict Malignancy in Patients with Intraductal Papillary Mucinous Neoplasm (IPMN) of the Pancreas. Cancers 2020;(11):12. https://doi.org/10.3390/cancers12113089.
40. Jeon SK, Kim JH, Yoo J, et al. Assessment of malignant potential in intraductal papillary mucinous neoplasms of the pancreas using MR findings and texture analysis. Eur Radiol 2021;31(5):3394–404.
41. LeCun Y, Bengio Y, Hinton G. Deep learning. Nature 2015;521(7553):436–44.
42. Deng J., Dong W., Socher R., et al., "ImageNet: A large-scale hierarchical image database," 2009 IEEE Conference on Computer Vision and Pattern Recognition, Miami, FL, USA, 2009, pp. 248-255, https://doi.org/10.1109/CVPR.2009.5206848.
43. Li H, Shi K, Reichert M, et al. Differential Diagnosis for Pancreatic Cysts in CT Scans Using Densely-Connected Convolutional Networks. Annu Int Conf IEEE Eng Med Biol Soc 2019;2019:2095–8. https://doi.org/10.1109/EMBC.2019. 8856745.
44. Corral JE, Hussein S, Kandel P, et al. Deep learning to classify intraductal papillary mucinous neoplasms using magnetic resonance imaging. Pancreas 2019; 48(6):805–10.
45. Wang X, Sun Z, Xue H, et al. A deep learning algorithm to improve readers' interpretation and speed of pancreatic cystic lesions on dual-phase enhanced CT. Abdominal radiology (New York) 2022;47(6):2135–47.
46. Doshi AM, Tong A, Davonport MS, et al. Assessment of Renal Cell Carcinoma by Texture Analysis in Clinical Practice: A Six-Site, Six-Platform Analysis of Reliability. AJR Am J Roentgenol 2021;217(5):1132–40.
47. Dreyfuss LD, Abel EJ, Nystrom J, et al. Comparison of CT Texture Analysis Software Platforms in Renal Cell Carcinoma: Reproducibility of Numerical Values and Association With Histologic Subtype Across Platforms. AJR Am J Roentgenol 2021;216(6):1549–57.

48. Yamashita R, Perrin T, Chakraborty J, et al. Radiomic feature reproducibility in contrast-enhanced CT of the pancreas is affected by variabilities in scan parameters and manual segmentation. Eur Radiol 2020;30(1):195–205.
49. Prabhu V, Gillingham N, Babb JS, et al. Repeatability, robustness, and reproducibility of texture features on 3 Tesla liver MRI. Clin Imaging 2022;83:177–83.
50. Kocak B, Durmaz ES, Kaya OK, et al. Reliability of Single-Slice-Based 2D CT Texture Analysis of Renal Masses: Influence of Intra- and Interobserver Manual Segmentation Variability on Radiomic Feature Reproducibility. AJR Am J Roentgenol 2019;213(2):377–83.
51. Baselli G, Codari M, Sardanelli F. Opening the black box of machine learning in radiology: can the proximity of annotated cases be a way? European Radiology Experimental 2020;4(1):1–7.
52. Vellido A. The importance of interpretability and visualization in machine learning for applications in medicine and health care. Neural Comput Appl 2020;32(24): 18069–83.
53. Reyes M, Meier R, Pereira S, et al. On the Interpretability of Artificial Intelligence in Radiology: Challenges and Opportunities. Radiology 2020;2(3):e190043.
54. Zwanenburg A, Vallières M, Abdalah MA, et al. The Image Biomarker Standardization Initiative: Standardized Quantitative Radiomics for High-Throughput Image-based Phenotyping. Radiology 2020;295(2):328–38.

Are All Cysts Created Equal?
Pancreatic Cystic Neoplasms in Patients with Familial or Genetic Risk Factors for Pancreatic Cancer

Ido Haimi, MD[a,1], Shenin Dettwyler, MS, CGC[b,1],
Jessica Everett, MS, CGC[b], Diane M. Simeone, MD[a,b,c,*]

KEYWORDS

- Pancreatic cysts • Familial • Adenocarcinoma • Pathogenic germline variant

KEY POINTS

- The recognition of pancreatic cystic lesions in the general population continues to increase over time. Ongoing surveillance of pancreatic cysts is required, due to malignant potential.
- Relative to the general population, high-risk individuals (HRI) with familial and/or genetic pancreatic cancer risk factors may have a greater prevalence of pancreatic cysts.
- Currently available data regarding pancreatic cysts in HRI are limited, with inconclusive evidence regarding the behavior and natural history of cysts in this population compared to the general population.
- Larger datasets with standardized imaging spanning longer timeframes are needed to elucidate connections between pancreatic cysts incidence and subsequent pancreatic cancer risk in HRI.
- These larger datasets will determine whether current HRI pancreatic surveillance guidelines should be updated to include more nuanced management for HRI with pancreatic cysts.

The number of pancreatic cystic lesions in the United States population between the ages of 40 and 89 is estimated to be 3.5 million. This translates to a prevalence of 2.5%.[1] Over the past two decades, there has been a steady rise in the prevalence of pancreatic cysts, with many diagnosed in asymptomatic individuals. This rise is attributed to the increased utilization of cross-sectional imaging, improved quality and

[a] Department of Surgery, NYU Langone Health, 240 East 38th Street, 20th Floor, New York, NY 10016, USA; [b] Perlmutter Cancer Center, NYU Langone Health, 240 East 38th Street, 20th Floor, New York, NY 10016, USA; [c] Pancreatic Cancer Center, 240 East 38th Street, 20th Floor, New York, NY 10016, USA
[1] These two authors contributed equally to the work.
* Corresponding author. Pancreatic Cancer Center, 240 East 38th Street, 20th Floor, New York, NY 10016, USA.
E-mail address: diane.simeone@nyulangone.org

Gastrointest Endoscopy Clin N Am 33 (2023) 547–557
https://doi.org/10.1016/j.giec.2023.03.002
1052-5157/23/© 2023 Elsevier Inc. All rights reserved.

availability of advanced imaging modalities, and an expanding elderly population, as these lesions are known to increase with age.[2–4] The frequency of incidental pancreatic cysts among patients undergoing cross-sectional imaging for unrelated indications may be as high as 49% to 71%.[2,5,6] Data suggest that 2.2% of abdominal computed tomography (CT) scans and 19.6% of MRIs detect the presence of a pancreatic cyst.[7–9] Furthermore, the prevalence of pancreatic cysts is thought to be even higher in patients classified as high-risk individuals (HRI) with an increased likelihood to develop pancreatic cancer (PDAC) due to pathogenic germline variants (PGV) in PDAC susceptibility genes and/or a family history of familial pancreatic cancer (FPC).[10] The criteria defining HRIs established by the American College of Gastroenterology (ACG),[11] the International Cancer of the Pancreas Screening (CAPS) Consortium,[12] and the National Comprehensive Cancer Network (NCCN),[13] are summarized in **Table 1**.

Historically, pancreatic cysts were considered the result of inflammatory processes.[14,15] However, over the past two decades, research and clinical experience have demonstrated that a large majority of these lesions are neoplastic—a significant proportion of which have malignant potential or harbor cancer,[15,16] in particular mucin-producing cystic lesions such as intraductal papillary mucinous neoplasms (IPMNs, the most common), and mucinous cystic neoplasms (MCN). Although most of these lesions do not transform into cancer, to the best of our current knowledge, IPMNs and MCNs all have malignant PDAC potential. Until better biomarkers are developed to define those at high risk for progression or cancer development, all patients with these lesions require surveillance; in some instances, surgical resection is warranted if the cyst becomes large (>3 cm) or possesses worrisome features. Of all PDACs that are diagnosed in the United States, 10% are from malignant degeneration

Table 1
Definitions of high-risk individuals for the development of pancreatic adenocarcinoma

	Personal and/or Family History Criteria	Age to Initiate Pancreatic Screening
PGV-HRI	• Carrier of a PGV in a gene with increased PDAC risks (*ATM, BRCA1, BRCA2, MLH1, MSH2, MSH6, EPCAM, PALB2*), and • ≥1 FDR or SDR with PDAC (known or presumed to be on the same side of the family as the PGV)	• Age 50, or 10 y younger than earliest PDAC diagnosis in family
	• *STK11* PGV carrier	• Age 30–35, or 10 y younger than earliest PDAC diagnosis in family
	• *CDKN2A* PGV carrier	• Age 40, or 10 y younger than earliest PDAC diagnosis in family
	• *PRSS1* PGV carrier	• Age 40, or 20 y after onset of pancreatitis

FPC-HRI	• No identifiable PGV, and a family history meeting one of the following FPC designations:
	  ○ ≥2 individuals with PDAC on same side of the family; ≥2 affected are FDRs to each other; and ≥1 is an FDR to the HRI considering surveillance, or
	  ○ ≥3 FDRs and/or SDRs with PDAC on the same side of the family
		• Age 50, or 10 y younger than earliest PDAC diagnosis in family

Abbreviations: FDR, first-degree relative; FPC, familial pancreatic cancer; HRI, high-risk individual; PDAC, pancreatic cancer; PGV, pathogenic germline variant; SDR, second-degree relative; y, years.

of a pancreatic cystic neoplasm.[17] Diagnosis of PDAC at an advanced stage portends a 5-year survival of less than 5%; hence, significant effort has been placed on screening patients with pancreatic cysts to prevent the development of advanced PDAC in this cohort.[18–20] As more patients are diagnosed with pancreatic cysts, a challenging clinical lacuna arises: how to accurately assess the risk associated with pancreatic cysts. In practical terms, clinicians need data-driven guidance to strike a balance between the risks of less frequent screenings (missed precursor lesions) versus overtreatment (unnecessary surgery).

Screening guidelines for incidentally detected pancreatic cysts in the general population have been issued by several societies, including the American Gastrointestinal Association (2015), the American College of Radiology (2017), the International Association of Pancreatology (Fukuoka guidelines, 2019), the American College of Gastroenterology (2018), and a group of European expert societies (European guidelines, 2018).[21–25] Although varying in scope, these guidelines offer a unified approach to imaging and surgical procedures for pancreatic cysts based on a combination of "worrisome features" such as cyst size, pancreatic duct abnormalities, mural nodules, as well as cyst location and type. For low-risk pancreatic cysts, these guidelines generally recommend surveillance with MRI/magnetic resonance cholangiopancreatography (MRCP) at regular intervals, with the use of endoscopic ultrasound (EUS) and/or CT if the pancreatic cyst increases in size or develops high-risk features.[26] The guidelines do not address the potential need for a more nuanced and cautious approach in the management of pancreatic cysts in HRI.

In clinical practice, especially in high-volume pancreatic centers, HRI are often found to have pancreatic cysts and vice versa.[27,28] These patients are either targeted for surveillance at regular intervals (typically annually) or considered for surgical resection due to a presumed increased PDAC risk in the cystic lesion. However, consistent, large-scale evidence to substantiate these practices has not been generated to date. This lack of evidence is also highlighted in the Fukuoka guidelines,[21] which support "more aggressive" surveillance of individuals with IPMN and two or more first-degree relatives with PDAC, but provide only a general approach to screening without stratification of different HRI. Instead, a host of smaller, isolated studies with conflicting and anecdotal results provide limited and incomplete guidance. Consequently, the question of whether having both a pancreatic cystic neoplasm (especially IPMNs) and a family history of PDAC carries a higher risk than either factor alone remains unanswered.

Generally, two approaches have been utilized to explore the relationship between HRI status and the presence of pancreatic cysts. In the first approach, studies have focused on individuals presenting with pancreatic cysts, and may also report on the presence and impact of HRI criteria. For example, a study of 300 patients with mixed-type and branch-duct IPMN by Mandai and colleagues[28] showed an increased risk of PDAC in 17 patients meeting FPC criteria compared with 283 patients without a family history (17% vs 2%). However, after risk stratification by age, the difference between groups disappeared. Data from Nehra and colleagues[29] focused on a retrospective analysis of 324 patients with resected IPMNs; of these, 13% were from FPC families. Here, PDAC risk did not differ between IPMN patients with and without FPC. Further stratification based on Fukuoka criteria also did not reveal a difference between these two groups. Del Chiaro and colleagues[30] conducted a prospective observational study of 40 HRI, 35% of whom had pancreatic cysts. Of these, 5% developed PDAC and 2.5% had an IPMN-associated invasive malignancy.

A second approach involves calculating the percentage of HRI who have pancreatic cysts detected during pancreatic surveillance, and subsequent impact on the development of PDAC. Numerous studies since 1999 have reported on pancreatic abnormalities detected during the screening of HRI (including pancreatic cysts). However, the majority are single-institution studies published over a decade ago, or with cohort sizes of fewer than 100 patients.[5,10,31–49] Additionally, many studies published sequentially contain overlapping data from the same clinical site[31,32,49] and/or HRI screening study, including the National Familial Pancreas Tumor Registry/CAPS,[5,47,48,50–52] the Dutch Familial Pancreatic Cancer Study,[36–38,46,53,54] and the National German Familial Pancreatic Cancer Registry.[36,39–41] This makes it difficult to ascertain the true incidence of pancreatic cysts in HRI since some patients are "double-counted" across publications.[38–41]

Several of the largest and most recent studies are summarized in **Table 2**. Canto and colleagues[52] followed 354 HRI enrolled in the CAPS 1 through 4 studies across multiple US sites. The overall incidence of pancreatic cysts in HRI was not described. Rather, the study endpoints focused on IPMNs with high-grade dysplasia (IPMN-HGD) and/or PDAC. Of the 4% of HRI diagnosed with PDAC, two had IPMNs and FPC. An additional 2% had IPMN-HGDs, including four FPC and two STK11 PGV carriers. Dbouk and colleagues[51] reported 732 HRI enrolled in the CAPS 1 through 5 study at one hospital, and found pancreatic cysts in nearly half of the cohort (356/732, 49%). Ultimately, 3% of HRI with pancreatic cysts were diagnosed with PDAC, with at least two PDACs arising from a pancreatic cyst. Eight of these HRI met FPC criteria, while the remainder were BRCA1 or BRCA2 PGV carriers. Of note, a portion of these HRI were previously described by Canto and colleagues[52] Finally, Overbeek and colleagues[54] assessed 366 HRI (FPC and PGV) and noted pancreatic cysts in 53%, with 10 patients diagnosed with PDAC. Half of the PDAC diagnoses occurred in HRI with no pancreatic cysts, while the other five occurred in PGV carriers with pancreatic cysts (one BRCA2, two CKDN2A, and two STK11). Ardeshna and colleagues[55] recently performed an extensive literature review on pancreatic cyst incidence in PGV carriers. Interestingly, while most single-institution studies report no difference in pancreatic cyst rates between HRI and non-HRI, their comprehensive overview of available data suggests that intraductal papillary mucinous neoplasms (IPMNs) may be more prevalent in HRI with PGV relative to non-HRI.

Clearly, larger datasets with standardized imaging and reporting spanning longer timeframes are needed to elucidate connections between pancreatic cyst incidence and subsequent PDAC risks in HRI. Furthermore, the lack of consistency regarding inclusion of cases (PDAC diagnoses) and controls (non-HRI with pancreatic cysts) for comparison also needs to be corrected. Among past surveillance studies (including those in **Table 2**), few PDAC diagnoses have been documented in HRI with pancreatic cysts overall. This is partially due to short study durations.[5,10,31–49] However, even in HRI with screen-detected PDACs, studies have not consistently noted whether the malignancy arose from a pancreatic cyst or as a separate solid mass.[38,51,54] Regarding comparison groups, only Shin and colleagues[34] included non-HRI controls in their analysis of MRI/MRCP pancreatic findings, and found pancreatic cysts in 17% of both the FPC and non-HRI control groups.

The currently available data also contain a knowledge gap regarding "HRI-like" patients with pancreatic cysts who have genetic or family history risk factors, but do not meet current HRI criteria. According to the current ACG, CAPS, and NCCN recommendations,[11–13] annual surveillance is not routinely offered to either (1) individuals with ATM, BRCA1, BRCA2, PALB2, or Lynch syndrome PGVs without a family history of PDAC, or (2) PGV-negative individuals with a single affected first- or second-degree relative. Recent guidelines from the American Society of Gastrointestinal Endoscopy (ASGE) include conditional recommendations for annual pancreatic surveillance in all BRCA1, BRCA2, and PALB2 PGV carriers, regardless of family PDAC history,

Table 2
Summary of pancreatic cystic lesions previously reported in high-risk individuals undergoing pancreatic surveillance

Publication	Institution/Location	Study Population	Study Timeframe	Genetic Testing Done?	Surveillance Imaging	Cysts Identified
Canto et al,[52] 2018	Multiple US sites (CAPS 1–4)	354 HRI • 344 FPC FHx • 57 PGV carriers[a]: ○ 4 CDKN2A ○ 39 BRCA1/BRCA2/PALB2 + ≥1 FDR/SDR ○ 1 unspecified Lynch + ≥1 FDR/SDR ○ 1 PRSS1 + ≥1 FDR/SDR ○ 8 STK11	1998–2014	Known PGVs noted, but testing not required for study inclusion	Baseline EUS; then EUS, MRI/MRCP, or CT	14/354 (4%) HRI developed PDAC • 2/14 (14%) had IPMNs; both FPC-HRI, PGV status not specified 7/354 (2%) HRI had IPMNs + HGD • 4 FPC-HRI, PGV status not specified • 2 STK11 PGV carriers
Overbeek et al,[54] 2022[b]	Dutch Familial Pancreatic Cancer study: • Erasmus MC Cancer Institute • University of Amsterdam • University Medical Center Utrecht	366 HRI • 201 FPC FHx • 96 CDKN2A PGV • 7 BRCA1 PGV • 45 BRCA2 PGV • 1 ATM PGV • 2 PALB2 PGV • 9 STK11 PGV • 5 TP53 PGV	10/2006–2019	Yes, for 302/266 (82.5%) HRI. Analysis of ATM, BRCA1, BRCA2, CDKN2A, MLH1, MSH2, MSH6, PALB2, STK11, TP53 genes	MRI/MRCP and EUS	10/366 (3%) HRI developed PDAC 5/10 (50%) with PDAC had cyst(s) • 1 BRCA2 PGV • 2 CDKN2A PGV • 2 STK11 PGV 188/356 (53%) HRI without PDAC had cyst(s) Subgroups not specified • At least 1 BRCA2 PGV • At least 2 FPC FHx

(continued on next page)

Table 2
(continued)

Publication	Institution/Location	Study Population	Study Timeframe	Genetic Testing Done?	Surveillance Imaging	Cysts Identified

Dbouk et al,[51] 2021[c]	Johns Hopkins Hospital, MD, United States (CAPS 1–5)	732 HRI
		• No information provided on stratification into FPC vs PGV subgroups
			1998–5/2018	Yes: *ATM, BRCA1, BRCA2, CDKN2A, PRSS1, STK11*, all Lynch syndrome gene analysis	MRI/MRCP, EUS, or CT	*356/732 (49%) HRI with cysts*
						• 24/356 (7%) pancreatic cysts resected; 1 with PDAC (FPC)
						• *12/356 (3%) pancreatic cysts developed separate solid mass; 10/12 dx PDAC*
						  ○ 1 each *BRCA1* and *BRCA2* PGV + ≥1 FDR/SDR
						  ○ 8 FPC
						• 320/356 (90%) with pancreatic cysts did not develop mass/require resection; no information on FPC vs PGV status

Abbreviations: Dx, diagnosed; EUS, endoscopic ultrasound; FDR, first-degree relative; FHx, family history; FPC, familial pancreatic cancer; HGD, high-grade dysplasia; HRI, high-risk individual; MRI/MRCP, magnetic resonance imaging cholangiopancreatography; PDAC, pancreatic ductal adenocarcinoma; PGV, pathogenic germline variant; SDR, second-degree relative.

[a] Total n = 397 rather than 354; some FPC-HRI must also have PGVs, but no information is provided regarding which PGVs were observed in FPC-HRI.

[b] Includes overlapping data from HRI described in Poley et al, 2009, Potjer et al, 2013, and Harinck et al, 2015 (Dutch Familial Pancreatic Cancer Study).

[c] Includes overlapping data from HRI described in Canto et al, 2004 and Canto et al, 2006 (Johns Hopkins National Familial Pancreas Tumor Registry; later, CAPS) as well as Canto et al, 2012, Canto et al, 2018, and Abe et al, 2019 (CAPS 1–5 Studies).

acknowledging the low quality of evidence behind this suggestion.[56] As noted above, neither family history nor PGV status are presently included in the prevailing pancreatic cyst guidelines.[21–23,25] Thus, HRI-like patients with incidentally detected pancreatic cysts receive the same screening as the general population. No information is currently available regarding the appropriateness of this strategy, or if the presence of any genetics/familial PDAC risk factor should influence surveillance.

Considered collectively, several key insights are gleaned from the literature on pancreatic cysts in HRI. First, few comprehensive studies on pancreatic surveillance in HRI have been performed in recent decades, and the existing data do not focus on elucidating connections between HRI, pancreatic cysts, and PDAC risk. Notably, all completed studies were limited by small sample sizes, and the majority represented heterogeneous patient cohorts, such that no strict definition of either FPC or PGV was consistently adopted. Several studies lacked genetic testing entirely; this omission confounds the reported findings, since an HRI from an untested FPC family may actually harbor an unrecognized PGV. Others included analyses of only select genes relevant to PDAC risk, skewed toward *BRCA1*, *BRCA2*, and *CDKN2A*. Finally, much of the data were derived from retrospective reviews of relatively short timelines, making the observations susceptible to lead-time bias. It is important to note that these observations are not an indictment of any individual study, or the field. Rather, they emphasize the significant need and difficulty of collecting standardized, longitudinal data at a large scale in this diverse and complicated patient population.

To address this gap, several groups are working on collecting standardized, longitudinal data on subjects with personal or familial PDAC risk factors. One such effort is the Pancreatic Cancer Early Detection (PRECEDE) Consortium. PRECEDE is the first international partnership designed to collect uniform data via a federated learning approach. The study seeks to enroll 10,000 individuals over a 5-year period for a planned 10-year study, and opened in May 2020.[57,58] Over 3700 HRI have enrolled to date, with 40 sites across North America, Europe, Asia, and South America using standardized genetic testing, clinical and laboratory data acquisition, and imaging (MRI/MRCP and EUS). The overarching purpose of PRECEDE is to establish a multi-site cohort of HRI to research PDAC early detection and prevention, with data shared between all collaborating institutions. Through this effort, data will be consolidated and shared between new locations and single centers with a robust history of HRI surveillance (including sites from CAPS, the Dutch Familial Pancreatic Cancer Study, and the European Registry of Hereditary Pancreatitis and Familial Pancreatic Cancer [EUROPAC]).[11,45,51,54] Furthermore, the widespread geographic distribution of PRECEDE sites is intended to facilitate data collection outside of previously characterized American and Western European populations, toward the goal of remedying the lack of diversity in PDAC early detection research. This effort should help better define the contribution of pancreatic cysts to PDAC development in both HRI and non-HRI populations. In addition, it represents an example of how the field can address long-standing, challenging questions in the era of big data and global hyperconnectivity.

The rapid rise in the detection of pancreatic cysts and the improved ability to both identify and characterize HRI requires more nuanced guidelines. Efforts such as PRECEDE and others represent a paradigm shift that is focused on stratifying, analyzing, and enriching screened populations, such that screening and management recommendations are more accurate and sophisticated. This approach to more accurately determine risk stratification of pancreatic cysts with a high level of curated and comprehensive data should add substantially to current cyst management guidelines. These, in turn, will help tackle questions such as which patients should be screened and how, and who warrants surgical resection. In the future, these answers will not be based on topographic and historical commonalities between patients, but rather on a personalized approach built on novel modalities such as radiogenomics, biomarkers, and advanced genetic analysis. In other words, not all cysts in HRI were created equal.

CLINICS CARE POINTS

- Limited information is available regarding the optimal surveillance strategy for HRI with familial and/or genetic PDAC risk factors who also have pancreatic cysts.
- To distinguish HRI from the general population, health care providers should collect information regarding any family history of PDAC and other cancers for patients presenting with an incidentally detected pancreatic cyst or worrisome finding.
- Patients with ≥1 close relatives with PDAC need germline genetic testing to clarify whether they meet HRI criteria. At a minimum, testing should include analysis of the *ATM, BRCA1, BRCA2, CDKN2A, EPCAM, MLH1, MSH2, MSH6, PALB2, PMS2, STK11,* and *PRSS1* genes.
- Providers are encouraged to refer HRI to pancreatic cancer screening studies, especially those with (1) germline pathogenic variants and ≥1 close relatives with pancreatic cancer, or (2) a family history meeting FPC Criteria.
- Until further data are available, HRI (with or without pancreatic cysts) should continue to undergo pancreatic screening as outlined by the American College of Gastroenterology, the International Cancer of the Pancreas Consortium, and/or the NCCN.

REFERENCES

1. Gardner TB, Glass LM, Smith KD, et al. Pancreatic cyst prevalence and the risk of mucin-producing adenocarcinoma in US adults. Am J Gastroenterol 2013;108: 1546–50.
2. de Jong K, Nio CY, Hermans JJ, et al. High prevalence of pancreatic cysts detected by screening magnetic resonance imaging examinations. Clin Gastroenterol Hepatol 2010;8:806–11.
3. Sohn TA, Yeo CJ, Cameron JL, et al. Intraductal papillary mucinous neoplasms of the pancreas: an updated experience. Ann Surg 2004;239:788–99.
4. Laffan TA, Horton KM, Klein AP, et al. Prevalence of unsuspected pancreatic cysts on MDCT. AJR Am J Roentgenol 2008;191:802–7.
5. Canto MI, Hruban RH, Fishman EK, et al. Frequent detection of pancreatic lesions in asymptomatic high-risk individuals. Gastroenterology 2012;142:796–804.
6. Ferrone CR, Correa-Gallego C, Warshaw AL, et al. Current Trends in Pancreatic Cystic Neoplasms. Arch Surg 2009;144:448–54.
7. Zanini N, Giordano M, Smerieri E, et al. Estimation of the prevalence of asymptomatic pancreatic cysts in the population of San Marino. Pancreatology 2015; 15:417–22.
8. Moris M, Bridges MD, Pooley RA, et al. Association Between Advances in High-Resolution Cross-Section Imaging Technologies and Increase in Prevalence of Pancreatic Cysts From 2005 to 2014. Clin Gastroenterol Hepatol 2016;14: 585–93.e3.
9. Stark A, Donahue TR, Reber HA, et al. Pancreatic cyst disease a review. JAMA, J Am Med Assoc 2016;315:1882–93.
10. Verna EC, Hwang C, Stevens PD, et al. Pancreatic cancer screening in a prospective cohort of high-risk patients: A comprehensive strategy of imaging and genetics. Clin Cancer Res 2010;16:5028–37.

11. Syngal S, Brand RE, Church JM, et al. ACG clinical guideline: Genetic testing and management of hereditary gastrointestinal cancer syndromes. Am J Gastroenterol 2015;110:223–62.

12. Goggins M, Overbeek KA, Brand RE, et al. Management of patients with increased risk for familial pancreatic cancer: updated recommendations from the International Cancer of the Pancreas Screening (CAPS) Consortium. Gut 2020;69:7–17.

13. National Comprehensive Cancer Network. NCCN Clinical Practice Guidelines in Oncology (NCCN Guidelines ®) Genetic/Familial High-Risk Assessment: Breast, Ovarian, and Pancreatic. Available at: https://www.nccn.org/home/member- (2023).

14. Warshaw AL, Rutledge PL. Cystic tumors mistaken for pancreatic pseudocysts. Ann Surg 1987;205:393.

15. Fernández-Del Castillo C, Targarona J, Thayer SP, et al. Incidental pancreatic cysts: clinicopathologic characteristics and comparison with symptomatic patients. Arch Surg 2003;138:427–34.

16. Allen PJ, D'Angelica M, Gonen M, et al. A selective approach to the resection of cystic lesions of the pancreas: results from 539 consecutive patients. Ann Surg 2006;244:572–9.

17. Singhi A, Koay E, Chari S, et al. Early Detection of Pancreatic Cancer: Opportunities and Challenges. Gastroenterology 2019;156:2024–40.

18. Rahib L, Wehner MR, Matrisian LM, et al. Estimated Projection of US Cancer Incidence and Death to 2040. JAMA Netw Open 2021;4.

19. Balaban EP, Mangu PB, Khorana AA, et al. Locally Advanced, Unresectable Pancreatic Cancer: American Society of Clinical Oncology Clinical Practice Guideline. J Clin Oncol 2016;34:2654–67.

20. Surveillance Epidemiology and End Results (SEER) Program. Pancreatic Cancer — Cancer Stat Facts. Available at: https://seer.cancer.gov/statfacts/html/pancreas. html. (2022).

21. Tanaka M, Fernández-del Castillo C, Kamisawa T, et al. Revisions of international consensus Fukuoka guidelines for the management of IPMN of the pancreas. Pancreatology 2017;17:738–53.

22. Vege SS, Ziring B, Jain R, et al. American gastroenterological association institute guideline on the diagnosis and management of asymptomatic neoplastic pancreatic cysts. Gastroenterology 2015;148:819–22.

23. Elta GH, Enestvedt BK, Sauer BG, et al. ACG Clinical Guideline: Diagnosis and Management of Pancreatic Cysts. Am J Gastroenterol 2018;113:464–79.

24. van Huijgevoort NCM, del Chiaro M, Wolfgang CL, et al. Diagnosis and management of pancreatic cystic neoplasms: current evidence and guidelines. Nat Rev Gastroenterol Hepatol 2019;16:676–89.

25. Megibow AJ, Baker ME, Morgan DE, et al. Management of Incidental Pancreatic Cysts: A White Paper of the ACR Incidental Findings Committee. J Am Coll Radiol 2017;14:911–23.

26. Aziz H, Acher AW, Krishna SG, et al. Comparison of Society Guidelines for the Management and Surveillance of Pancreatic Cysts: A Review. JAMA Surg 2022;157:723–30.

27. Mukewar S, de Pretis N, Aryal-Khanal A, et al. Fukuoka criteria accurately predict risk for adverse outcomes during follow-up of pancreatic cysts presumed to be intraductal papillary mucinous neoplasms. Gut 2017;66:1811–7.

28. Mandai K, Uno K, Yasuda K. Does a family history of pancreatic ductal adenocarcinoma and cyst size influence the follow-up strategy for intraductal papillary mucinous neoplasms of the pancreas? Pancreas 2014;43:917–21.

29. Nehra D, Oyarvide VM, Mino-Kenudson M, et al. Intraductal papillary mucinous neoplasms: Does a family history of pancreatic cancer matter? Pancreatology 2012;12:358.

30. del Chiaro M, Verbeke CS, Kartalis N, et al. Short-term Results of a Magnetic Resonance Imaging–Based Swedish Screening Program for Individuals at Risk for Pancreatic Cancer. JAMA Surg 2015;150:512–8.

31. Kimmey MB, Bronner MP, Byrd DR, et al. Screening and surveillance for hereditary pancreatic cancer. Gastrointest Endosc 2002;56:S82–6.

32. Brentnall TA, Bronner MP, Byrd DR, et al. Early diagnosis and treatment of pancreatic dysplasia in patients with a family history of pancreatic cancer. Ann Intern Med 1999;131:247–55.

33. Ludwig E, Olson SH, Bayuga S, et al. Feasibility and yield of screening in relatives from familial pancreatic cancer families. Am J Gastroenterol 2011;106:946.

34. Shin SS, Armao DM, Burke LMB, et al. Comparison of the incidence of pancreatic abnormalities between high risk and control patients: prospective pilot study with 3 Tesla MR imaging. J Magn Reson Imaging 2011;33:1080–5.

35. Al-Sukhni W, Borgida A, Rothenmund H, et al. Screening for Pancreatic Cancer in a High-Risk Cohort: An Eight-Year Experience. J Gastrointest Surg 2012;16: 771–83.

36. Potjer TP, Schot I, Langer P, et al. Variation in precursor lesions of pancreatic cancer among high-risk groups. Clin Cancer Res 2013;19:442–9.

37. Klatte DCF, Boekestijn B, Wasser MNJM, et al. Pancreatic Cancer Surveillance in Carriers of a Germline CDKN2A Pathogenic Variant: Yield and Outcomes of a 20-Year Prospective Follow-Up. J Clin Oncol 2022;4.

38. Vasen H, Ibrahim I, Guillen Ponce C, et al. Benefit of Surveillance for Pancreatic Cancer in High-Risk Individuals: Outcome of Long-Term Prospective Follow-Up Studies From Three European Expert Centers. J Clin Oncol 2016;34:2010–9.

39. Schneider R, Slater EP, Sina M, et al. German national case collection for familial pancreatic cancer (FaPaCa): Ten years experience. Fam Cancer 2011;10: 323–30.

40. Langer P, Kann PH, Fendrich V, et al. Five years of prospective screening of high-risk individuals from families with familial pancreatic cancer. Gut 2009;58:1410–8.

41. Bartsch DK, Slater EP, Carrato A, et al. Refinement of screening for familial pancreatic cancer. Gut 2016;65:1314–21.

42. Joergensen MT, Gerdes AM, Sorensen J, et al. Is screening for pancreatic cancer in high-risk groups cost-effective? - Experience from a Danish national screening program. Pancreatology 2016;16:584–92.

43. Lachter J, Rosenberg C, Hananiya T, et al. Screening to Detect Precursor Lesions of Pancreatic Adenocarcinoma in High-risk Individuals: A Single-center Experience. Rambam Maimonides Med J 2018;9:e0029.

44. Gangi A, Malafa M, Klapman J. Endoscopic Ultrasound-Based Pancreatic Cancer Screening of High-Risk Individuals A Prospective Observational Trial. Pancreas 2018;47:586–91.

45. Sheel ARG, Harrison S, Sarantitis I, et al. Identification of Cystic Lesions by Secondary Screening of Familial Pancreatic Cancer (FPC) Kindreds Is Not Associated with the Stratified Risk of Cancer. Am J Gastroenterol 2019;114:155–64.

46. Poley JW, Kluijt I, Gouma DJ, et al. The yield of first-time endoscopic ultrasonography in screening individuals at a high risk of developing pancreatic cancer. Am J Gastroenterol 2009;104:2175–81.
47. Canto MI, Goggins M, Yeo CJ, et al. Screening for pancreatic neoplasia in high-risk individuals: an EUS-based approach. Clin Gastroenterol Hepatol 2004;2: 606–21.
48. Canto MI, Goggins M, Hruban RH, et al. Screening for Early Pancreatic Neoplasia in High-Risk Individuals: A Prospective Controlled Study. Clin Gastroenterol Hepatol 2006;4:766–81.
49. Rulyak SJ, Brentnall TA. Inherited pancreatic cancer: surveillance and treatment strategies for affected families. Pancreatology 2001;1:477–85.
50. Abe T, Blackford AL, Tamura K, et al. Deleterious germline mutations are a risk factor for neoplastic progression among high-risk individuals undergoing pancreatic surveillance. J Clin Oncol 2019;37:1070–80.
51. Dbouk M, Brewer Gutierrez OI, Lennon AM, et al. Guidelines on management of pancreatic cysts detected in high-risk individuals: An evaluation of the 2017 Fukuoka guidelines and the 2020 International Cancer of the Pancreas Screening (CAPS) consortium statements. Pancreatology 2021;21:613–21.
52. Canto M.I., Almario J.A., Schulick R.D., et al., Risk of Neoplastic Progression in Individuals at High Risk for Pancreatic Cancer Undergoing Long-term Surveillance, Gastroenterology, 155, 2018, 740–751.e2.
53. Harinck F, Konings ICAW, Kluijt I, et al. A multicentre comparative prospective blinded analysis of EUS and MRI for screening of pancreatic cancer in high-risk individuals. Gut 2016;65:1505–13.
54. Overbeek KA, Levink IJM, Koopmann BDM, et al. Long-term yield of pancreatic cancer surveillance in high-risk individuals. Gut 2022;71:1152–60.
55. Ardeshna DR, Rangwani S, Cao T, et al. Intraductal Papillary Mucinous Neoplasms in Hereditary Cancer Syndromes. Biomedicines 2022;10.
56. Sawhney MS, Calderwood AH, Thosani NC, et al. ASGE guideline on screening for pancreatic cancer in individuals with genetic susceptibility: summary and recommendations. Gastrointest Endosc 2022;95:817–26.
57. Gonda TA, Everett JN, Wallace M, et al. Recommendations for a More Organized and Effective Approach to the Early Detection of Pancreatic Cancer From the PRECEDE (Pancreatic Cancer Early Detection) Consortium. Gastroenterology 2021;161:1751–7.
58. Gonda T.A., Farrell J., Wallace M., et al., Standardization of EUS imaging and reporting in high-risk individuals of pancreatic adenocarcinoma: consensus statement of the Pancreatic Cancer Early Detection Consortium, *Gastrointest Endosc*, 95, 2022, 723–732.e7.

Blood-Based Biomarkers in the Diagnosis and Risk Stratification of Pancreatic Cysts

Matthew T. Peller, MD, Koushik K. Das, MD*

KEYWORDS

- Pancreatic cystic lesion • Intraductal papillary mucinous neoplasm • Biomarkers
- Blood based • Pancreatic ductal adenocarcinoma • Tumor marker

KEY POINTS

- Blood-based biomarkers offer significant potential for the noninvasive assessment of pancreatic cystic lesions.
- CA 19-9 remains the only blood-based marker in routine clinical practice with limited utility in terms of diagnosis and risk stratification.
- Novel biomarkers show early promise in the fields of proteomics, metabolomics, cell-free DNA/circulating tumor DNA, extracellular vesicles, and microRNA.
- Barriers to successful biomarker development include confounding variables, a lack of longitudinal cohort data on pancreatic cystic lesions, and variations in technique and reproducibility for biomarker isolation and measurement.
- The combination of multiple biomarkers along with clinical factors, radiomics, and machine learning will likely lead to improved performance over individual biomarkers.

INTRODUCTION

Pancreatic cystic lesions (PCLs) are common incidental findings, the vast majority of which never require intervention or develop overt malignancy. An estimated 7.9% of patients under the age of 70 years have pancreatic cysts.[1] Several types of PCLs, most notably serous cyst adenoma and pseudocysts, are definitively benign or harbor negligible risk of malignancy and do not require surveillance or resection unless symptomatic because of a mass effect on surrounding organs. However, pancreatic ductal adenocarcinoma (PDAC) arises from several unique precursor lesions within the pancreas: a noncystic precursor (pancreatic intraepithelial neoplasia) and mucinous

Disclosure
The authors have nothing to disclose.
Division of Gastroenterology, Washington University School of Medicine, 660 South Euclid Avenue Campus Box 8124, Saint Louis, MO 63110, USA
* Corresponding author.
E-mail address: k.das@wustl.edu

cystic lesions (MCLs), specifically mucinous cystic neoplasm (MCN) and intraductal papillary mucinous neoplasm (IPMN). While there have been multiple reports published on cohorts establishing a continued, although highly variable, risk of pancreatic cancer development from PCL followed up beyond 5 years,[2,3] it is well established that the vast majority of these lesions are indolent with an estimated risk of malignant transformation of 0.72% per year (or 2.8% overall).[4–6] Even though pancreatic resection remains potentially curative, it continues to carry a 1% to 2% mortality and 30% to 60% morbidity rate.[7] As such, there remains an unmet need for molecular tools to stratify high-risk/malignant lesions from low-risk ones.

The diagnosis of PCL can often be made by radiographic evaluation using ultrasound, computed tomography, and magnetic resonance imaging, and they are safely evaluated by endoscopic ultrasound (EUS) with diagnostic sampling by fine needle aspiration (FNA). MCL can often be distinguished by their radiographic or endosonographic appearance (ie, the presence of pancreatic duct communication, presence of a characteristic central scar, and so forth), but there remains a majority of cases where the identity or subtype of the cyst is not definitively assessed.[8] There have been considerable advances in molecular cyst fluid analysis that can help in the determination of the subtype of PCL. For example, the identification of VHL mutations is ~70% sensitive and 100% specific for SCA, and MEN1 alterations are ~70% sensitive and 98% specific for pancreatic neuroendocrine tumors.[9,10] The current standard approach in most centers remains for cyst fluid biochemical analysis (traditionally with carcinoembryonic antigen [CEA] and amylase) augmented with cytology. Overall, FNA is safe, but the diagnostic yield with cytology alone for assessing advanced neoplasia is limited with poor sensitivity but high specificity (sensitivity 27%–48%, specificity 83%–100%).[11–13] Radiographic and sonographic characteristics such as size, nodularity, and involvement of the main pancreatic duct help identify MCL at higher risk of harboring or progressing to malignancy that may benefit from surgical resection.[8,14] Even so, 25% of resected cystic lesions are found to represent benign cysts rather than MCL, and 77% of resected MCL have no evidence of high-grade dysplasia or malignancy.[15,16] In the past decade, however, considerable progress has been made in the discovery and validation of molecular cyst fluid analyses, with multiple biomarkers achieving near-90% sensitivity and near-100% specificity including panels of next-generation sequencing (NGS),[9,17] methylation panels,[18] and unique glycosylation epitopes.[19–21] In addition to ever-improving cyst fluid molecular analysis panels and well-established radiographic characteristics, there are now a myriad of tools being developed to aid in the process of PCL risk stratification including radiomics, applications of machine learning, and a wide array of laboratory-based tests on both cyst fluid and blood. Indeed, we may reach a limit of sensitivity in PCL cyst fluid analysis alone because of both biological factors (ie, divergent clonal behavior of progenitor lesions developing into PCL) and technical factors (ie, limitations in dominant cyst sampling, acellular specimens, and degraded DNA). The hope and goal of many researchers, including ourselves, would be to assess a new generation of noninvasive biomarkers (ie, serologic, other body fluids) together in concert with clinical parameters and periodic imaging to inform future guidelines. Such biomarkers would allow for broad, population screening/surveillance for a condition that is extremely common and provide an economical means to serially survey a condition that has generally been limited to assessments with costly and invasive radiologic and endoscopic interventions.

The current chapter will focus on the emerging evidence and future directions of blood-based biomarkers in the diagnosis and risk stratification of pancreatic cysts. While the majority of the literature reviewed here is more broadly evaluated as efforts to improve the early detection of PDAC and its precursor lesions, we will highlight those studies that pertain more specifically to PCL.

BIOMARKERS

Unsurprisingly, the blood-based biomarkers currently under investigation for PCL often mirror those explored in cyst fluid. Overall, blood-based biomarkers offer several important advantages over cyst fluid analysis. Cyst fluid procurement generally requires an EUS with FNA that implies access to appropriate expertise and consultation with gastroenterology/interventional endoscopy. In addition, the procedure itself, while generally safe, carries a risk of bleeding, perforation, and pancreatitis with overall estimated incidence of 1.7%.[22] Cyst fluid sampling is not always feasible based on cyst size and location in relation to intervening vascular structures and may not be complete/fully representative as acellular specimens are frequent and clonal divergence in PCL development has now been demonstrated by several groups.[23–25] Aside from these technical issues and limitations of access, the procedure itself has considerable financial burden to individuals and health systems and likely only represents a single "snapshot in time" of what is ultimately an ever-evolving process. In comparison, despite their limitations in overall sensitivity, blood-based biomarkers potentially hold the promise of a safe and widely available means to globally assess the pancreas (in cases of multifocal PCL), relatively inexpensively, accessibly, and serially over time in patients with PCL.

One challenge in risk stratification of PCL and early detection of PDAC is the heterogeneous nature of these lesions, which have variable biosignatures.[26] Consequently, it is unlikely that any singular biomarker will ever be adequate for assessing the identity and potential risk of a PCL. A common theme then is the combination of multiple biomarkers and the inclusion of radiographic or clinical factors such as the presence of new-onset diabetes (NOD) (which itself carries a 5.4-fold increased risk of PDAC within 1 year of diagnosis[27]) to boost the pretest probability of the sample population of patients in which a putative biomarker panel is being assessed. For example, the computer learning algorithm CompCyst combined cyst fluid markers, clinical features, and radiographic features in a large cohort of 862 patients with surgically resected PCL to significantly predict those individuals who did not require surgical management.[28]

In addition to the heterogeneous nature of PCL and PDAC, there are several other challenges that researchers face when attempting to identify novel biomarkers. Known confounders for detecting PDAC include chronic pancreatitis (CP), obstructive jaundice, and the coexistence of diabetes.[29] Numerous biomarkers including CA 19-9 have been identified as potential predictors of PDAC but have reduced sensitivity and performance when controlling for obstructive jaundice and CP.[30–32] The finding that NOD is a risk factor for the development of PDAC can be advantageous in identifying patients that may benefit from additional testing; however, it also serves as a confounder when searching for novel biomarkers. To help control for these variables, there has been a call for improved prediagnostic cohorts to better understand baseline characteristics leading up to a diagnosis of PDAC in sporadic patients, those with NOD, those with increased risk due to germline gene mutations, and those under surveillance for PCL.[33]

ESTABLISHED TUMOR MARKERS
CA 19-9

Certainly, the most well-known biomarker for PDAC is CA 19-9. This tumor-associated glycoprotein has a clear association with PDAC but is limited first and foremost by its sensitivity. In fact, approximately 10% of individuals carry a genotype (Lewis-negative) that results in undetectable levels of CA 19-9 in 94% of cases.[34] Reported sensitivities for PDAC vary widely from as low as 34.2% and up to 85% and tend to increase with more advanced cancer, with only 65% of resectable disease demonstrating elevated serum levels of CA 19-9.[35–40] The specificity of CA 19-9 is generally more favorable, consistently demonstrating performance greater than 85%,[36,38–40] although nonspecific elevations of CA 19-9 have been well documented in patients with and without pancreaticobiliary disease.[41] Several studies have evaluated the utility of CA 19-9 for risk stratifying IPMNs. Fritz and colleagues obtained preoperative serum levels in 142 patients undergoing resection of IPMNs. CA 19-9 levels greater than 37 u/ml identified invasive disease with a sensitivity and specificity of 74% and 85.9%, respectively, but was unable to distinguish between those cases with noninvasive disease including low-, moderate-, or high-grade dysplasia.[38] A meta-analysis of 9 studies on the diagnostic performance of CA 19-9 for predicting benign versus invasive IPMN found a pooled sensitivity of 52% and specificity of 88% using a CA 19-9 greater than 35 u/ml.[36] As with many biomarkers, CA 19-9 is prone to confounding variables such as CP and obstructive jaundice, as well as the selection bias of several of these studies recruiting patients from surgical cohorts.[31,37,40] In current practice, CA 19-9 is generally limited in use for surveillance after an established tissue diagnosis of malignancy, especially in patients undergoing treatment. CA 19-9 may offer some ability to risk stratify PCL, increasing the preoperative clinical concern for underlying advanced neoplasia in patients who are secretors; however, its use as a screening tool is not widely accepted because of its low sensitivity and unacceptable level of false positivity.

Carcinoembryonic Antigen

While CEA is an established tool in the diagnostic evaluation of cyst fluid, its utility as a serum marker in PCL and PDAC is less clear. Multiple studies have evaluated its performance in predicting invasive IPMN. Serum CEA greater than 5 ng/mL demonstrates poor sensitivity ranging from 18% to 40% but a high specificity of 92% to 95%.[36,38] Its performance is less accurate than that of CA 19-9 and similarly is unsuitable for screening but may offer some ability to rule in invasive disease or improve the performance of biomarker panels.[42,43]

PROTEOMICS
Amylase

In addition to its common use in diagnosing acute pancreatitis, amylase is another valuable tool in cyst fluid diagnosis. Its potential use as a serum marker for IPMN was demonstrated in a single study that showed low levels of amylase were associated with a higher incidence of invasive IPMN (odds ratio 9.6) in a series of 146 patients undergoing surgical resection of IPMN.[44]

Novel Proteomics

With advances in the study of proteomics using techniques including microarray and tandem mass spectrometry, it has become possible to identify a myriad of potential novel biomarkers for the detection of any number of disease processes including malignancy. Within the study of PCL-associated PDAC, large panels of proteins have been identified in discovery cohorts that have either a positive or negative association with PDAC. These proteins have then generally been tested and validated in subsequent cohorts, oftentimes resulting in the elimination of many of the initial candidate proteins due to poor performance or issues with confounding variables. Examples of such proteins include TSP-1, TSP-2, haptoglobin, alpha-1-antichymotrypsin, and CEMIP among many others.[32,45–47] Two studies investigated the performance of TSP-1 (THSB1) in panels of additional biomarkers for detecting PDAC with area under the curve (AUC) of 0.85 and 0.92, with the latter study including both IPMN and MCN in the control population. CEMIP has been implicated in other malignancies including breast cancer. In 1 study, it improved the detection of PDAC versus healthy controls when combined with CA 19-9 yielding a high sensitivity of 96.6%, but lower specificity of 59.2%.[47] Individual studies pertaining to these proteins and others are listed in **Table 1** and **Table 2**. As mentioned previously, none of these biomarkers provide sufficient sensitivity and specificity to be independently clinically applicable and, therefore, are often combined with other novel biomarkers and frequently combined with CA 19-9 to improve diagnostic performance.

A proprietary biomarker panel and algorithm that falls into this category is that of the IMMray PanCan-d test.[48] This is currently one of the only blood tests that are commercially available for early detection of pancreatic cancer. It is not yet Food and Drug Administration (FDA) approved and is listed as a laboratory-developed test by the FDA. In their original proteomic investigation, Mellby and colleagues used a large Scandinavian discovery cohort with various stages of pancreatic cancer and healthy controls and validated in a smaller cohort of US patients with controls and pancreatic cancer.[49] In this group, they identified 25 optimal targets that were enhanced to include 29 consensus biomarkers with an AUC of 0.97 in the discovery and 0.84 in the validation cohort, corresponding to a sensitivity and specificity of 93% and 95%, respectively, for detecting early PDAC (stage I and II) compared to healthy controls. Notably, in the limited cases available, the assay showed promise in distinguishing malignant IPMNs from benign or borderline IPMNs. A final, commercial iteration of the test was recently introduced with a simplified panel of 8 biomarkers in combination with CA 19-9 and a proprietary algorithm. In a cohort of 167 PDAC patients, 203 high-risk patients (without known PDAC) and 221 normal controls, CA 19-9 alone/ PanCan-D demonstrated a sensitivity and specificity of 75.8%/85% and 97.6%/ 98%, respectively.[48,50] Importantly, CA 19-9 nonsecretors in this cohort were found in 26% of African Americans, 24% of Hispanics, and 8% to 14% of Caucasians, which may limit the application especially in certain populations. The specific application of this assay to PCL risk stratification and clinical follow-up remains unknown but an area of ongoing exploration.

METABOLOMICS

In a similar approach to that of proteomics, there are various metabolites under investigation as potential biomarkers of invasive PDAC. Two separate studies examining large panels of metabolites for detection of PDAC developed final models each containing 4 and 9 metabolites, respectively; the latter with the addition of CA 19-9. These two studies detected PDAC with sensitivities of 71.4% and 89.9% and specificities of 78.1% and 91.3%, respectively. Neither of these studies included subjects with PCL specifically, and the only overlapping metabolite within the final models was histidine.[51,52]

CIRCULATING DNA-BASED BIOMARKERS

DNA-based markers are a promising method for risk stratifying PCL and for the early detection of PDAC. The field of study has expanded rapidly with the development of massively parallel sequencing, which allows for the detection of DNA mutations

Table 1
Summary of studies on blood-based biomarkers for the risk stratification and assessment of pancreatic cystic lesions

Biomarker	Detected Outcome	Study, Year	Sample Details	AUC	Sensitivity	Specificity	Other
Established tumor markers							
CA 19–9	Invasive IPMN (PDAC)	Fritz et al,[38] 2010	N = 142 IPMNs undergoing resection		74%	85.9%	CA 19–9 was unable to differentiate between IPMN with high-grade dysplasia and those with low- or moderate-grade dysplasia.
CA 19–9	Invasive IPMN (histology)	Wang et al,[36] 2015	Meta-analysis including 9 studies		52%	88%	
CA 19–9	High-grade dysplasia and invasive IPMN	Kim et al,[39] 2015	N = 367 IPMNs undergoing resection		34.2%	92.4%	
CEA	Invasive IPMN (PDAC)	Fritz et al,[38] 2010	N = 142 IPMNs undergoing resection		40%	92.4%	CA 19–9 was unable to differentiate between IPMN with high-grade dysplasia and those with low- or moderate-grade dysplasia.
CEA	Invasive IPMN (histology)	Wang et al,[36] 2015	Meta-analysis including 9 studies		18%	95%	
Proteomics							
Amylase	Invasive IPMN	Yagi et al,[44] 2016	N = 146 IPMNs undergoing surgical resection				Patients with low serum amylase were more likely to have invasive IPMN with odds ratio 9.6.

Marker	Comparison	Study	Cohort	AUC	Sensitivity	Specificity	Notes
Biomarker signature (29 biomarkers)	Benign/borderline IPMN vs malignant IPMN (not primary outcome of study)	Mellby et al,[49] 2018	Validation cohort: N = 658 including PDAC stage I-IV, CP, IPMN, and healthy controls.	0.96	93%	95%	Of the 20 IPMNs included in the validation cohort, the assay correctly distinguished malignant from benign/borderline IPMNs.
DNA-based markers							
cfDNA	IPMN (vs PDAC vs serous cystadenoma vs healthy control)	Berger et al,[60] 2016	N = 125 including IPMN (active surveillance as well as resected with borderline histology), PDAC stage IV, serous cystadenoma, and healthy controls.		IPMN vs control: 81% PDAC vs IPMN: 75%	IPMN vs control: 84%, PDAC vs IPMN: 71%	Results based on cfDNA quantification. The detection of KRAS and GNAS mutations was specific for IPMN vs serous cystadenomas.
Miscellaneous							
Circulating epithelial cells (Pdx-1 staining)	PDAC (vs PCL vs healthy controls)	Rhim et al,[83] 2014	N = 51 including PDAC, IPMN, MCN, and healthy controls				Pancreas-specific circulating epithelial cells were detected in 78% of PDAC, 33% of PCL, and 0% of healthy controls
Circulating epithelial cells (cytokeratin and Pdx-1 staining)	IPMN vs other PCL	Poruk et al,[89] 2017	N = 26 undergoing surgical resection of IPMN, solid pseudopapillary neoplasm, MCN, or lobular pancreatic proliferation		58%	100%	Circulating epithelial cells were more likely to be found in patients with IPMN with high-grade dysplasia.

(continued on next page)

Table 1
(continued)

Biomarker	Detected Outcome	Study, Year	Sample Details	AUC	Sensitivity	Specificity	Other
NLR >4 and radiographic and clinical features	Invasive IPMN	Gemenetzis et al,[94] 2017	N = 272 including invasive IPMN, IPMN with high-grade dysplasia, and benign IPMN	0.89			Other features included in the model were main duct dilation >5 mm, enhancing solid component, jaundice, and cyst size >3 cm.
NLR >2.074	Invasive IPMN	Arima et al,[93] 2015	N = 76 undergoing surgical resection of IPMN		73.1%	58%	
NLR >3.1	IPMN with high-grade dysplasia or invasive carcinoma (vs low-grade dysplasia)	Sugimachi et al,[92] 2021	N = 50 undergoing surgical resection of IPMN	0.75	56%	87%	NLR was followed during surveillance up to 5 y before resection and demonstrated a significant rise immediately before resection in those with high-grade dysplasia or invasive carcinoma compared to those with low-grade dysplasia.
NLR and CEA and CA 19-9	IPMN with high-grade dysplasia or invasive carcinoma (vs low-grade dysplasia)	Hata et al,[95] 2019	N = 205 undergoing surgical resection of IPMN		58.8%	76.8%	

Abbreviations: cfDNA, cell-free DNA; NLR, neutrophil-to-lymphocyte ratio.

Table 2
Summary of studies on blood-based biomarkers for the detection of pancreatic ductal adenocarcinoma

Biomarker	Study, Year	Sample Details	Detected Outcome	AUC	Sensitivity	Specificity	Other
Established tumor markers							
CA 19–9 >37 u/ml	O'brien et al,[40] 2015	N = 458 including PDAC and noncancer controls. Samples obtained before cancer diagnosis	PDAC		68%	95%	Diagnostic performance at 1 y before cancer diagnosis
Proteomics							
TSP-1 and CA 19-9	Jenkinson et al,[46] 2016	N = 472 including PDAC, CP, benign biliary obstruction, DM II, and healthy controls	PDAC	0.85			Serum TSP-1 levels were lower up to 24 mo before diagnosis of PDAC. TSP-1 levels were lower in PDAC with diabetes.
TSP-1 (THBS1), haptoglobin, alpha-1-antichymotrypsin and CA 19-9	Nie et al,[32] 2014	N = 179 including PDAC, CP, IPMN, MCN, DM, and healthy controls	PDAC grade 1A-4	0.92			Obstructive jaundice affected performance of all biomarkers in the study. AUC excluding obstructive jaundice increased to 0.95.
TSP-2 (THBS2) and CA 19–9	Kim et al,[45] 2017	N = 312 including PDAC and noninvasive IPMN	PDAC	0.95			
CEMIP and CA 19-9	Lee et al,[47] 2018	N = 324 including PDAC and healthy controls	PDAC	0.94	96.6%	59.2%	CEMIP identified 86.1% of CA 19-9 negative PDAC.
8-Plex biomarker signature and CA 19-9	Delfani et al,[48] (IMMray PanCan-D) 2021	N = 1113 including PDAC, DM, CP, and healthy controls	PDAC stage 1 & II (vs all controls)	0.95			
8-Plex biomarker signature and CA 19-9	Brand et al,[50] 2022	203 High risk, 167 PDAC I-IV	Stage I and II (vs high-risk patients)		85%	98%	Sensitivity improved to 89% when excluding Lewis-null
cfDNA and 8 proteins (CA 19–9, CEA, CA-125, prolactin, hepatocyte growth factor, osteopontin, myeloperoxidase, and tissue inhibitor of metalloproteinases 1	Cohen et al,[43] (CancerSEEK) 2018	1005	8 Different cancers (ovary, liver, stomach, pancreas, esophagus, colorectum, lung, or breast)		69%–98% for all cancer types	99%	See DNA-based markers for cfDNA description.

(continued on next page)

Table 2
(continued)

Biomarker	Study, Year	Sample Details	Detected Outcome	AUC	Sensitivity	Specificity	Other
Glypican-1 (GPC-1) detected on circulating exosomes	Melo et al,[61] 2015	N = 335 including PDAC, breast cancer, CP, serous cystadenomas, IPMN, and healthy controls	PDAC (vs benign disease and healthy controls)	1.0	100%	100%	No direct comparison between PDAC and IPMN
GPC-1 detected on circulating exosomes	Lai et al,[64] 2017	N = 46 including PDAC, CP, and healthy controls	PDAC (vs CP and healthy controls)	0.75			See performance of miRNA signature from same study under "RNA-based markers"
Metabolomics							
Xylitol, 1,5-anhydro-D-glucitol, histidine, inositol	Kobayashi et al,[51] 2013	N = 191 including PDAC, CP, and healthy controls	PDAC		71.4%	78.1%	Metabolites selected from a panel of 45 candidate biomarkers.
Proline, sphingomyelin (d18:2,C17:0), phosphatidylcholine (C18:0,C22:6), isocitrate, sphinganine 1-phosphate (d18:0), histidine, pyruvate, ceramide (d18:1,C24:0). sphingomyelin (d17:1,C18:0), and CA 19-9	Mayerle et al,[52] 2018	N = 914 including PDAC, CP, cirrhosis, nonpancreatic disease controls, and healthy controls	PDAC	0.94	89.9%	91.3%	Metabolites were selected specifically with the intention of differentiating between CP and PDAC. NPV 99.8%
DNA-based markers							
cfDNA	Pietrasz et al,[58] 2017	N = 135 with resectable, locally advanced, or metastatic PDAC	Overall survival and disease-free survival				Circulating tumor DNA was associated with shorter overall survival. In patients with resectable disease, the presence of circulating tumor DNA was associated with shorter overall survival (19.3 vs 32.3 mo, P = .027).
cfDNA	Sausen et al,[57] 2015	N = 51 PDAC stage II	Presence of circulating tumor DNA				Circulating tumor DNA was found in 43% of patients. Detection ctDNA after resection was associated with relapse.

Marker/Genes	Study	N	Cancer Type	AUC	Sensitivity	Specificity	Findings
8 Proteins and cfDNA from 16 genes (CTNNB1, PIK3CA, FBXW7, APC, EGFR, BRAF, CDKN2A, PTEN, FGFR2, HRAS, KRAS, AKT1, TP53, PPP2R1A, GNAS)	Cohen et al,[43] (CancerSEEK) 2018	1005	8 Different cancers (ovary, liver, stomach, pancreas, esophagus, colorectum, lung, or breast)		72%		Sensitivity and specificity for all cancer types were 69%–98% and 99%, respectively.
Exosomal DNA mutations (KRAS)	Allenson et al,[65] 2017	N = 142 including PDAC and healthy controls	PDAC (vs healthy controls)				KRAS mutations were found in 66.7% of localized, 80% of locally advanced, and 85% of metastatic PDAC.
Exosomal DNA mutations ($KRAS^{G12D}$, $TP53^{R273H}$)	Yang et al,[66] 2017	N = 171 undergoing pancreatic resection including PDAC, IPMN, CP, autoimmune pancreatitis, pancreatic neuroendocrine tumor, duodenal adenoma, pancreatic cystadenoma, common bile duct cancer, and uterine sarcoma.	PDAC				$KRAS^{G12D}$ mutation was found in 39.6% of PDAC, 28.5% of IPMN, 55.6% CP, and 2.6% healthy controls. $TP53^{R273H}$ mutation was found in 4.2% of PDAC, 14.2% IPMN, and no healthy controls.
cfDNA Methylation (BMP3, RASSF1A, BNC1, MESTv2, TFPI2, APC, SFRP1, and SFRP2)	Henriksen et al,[69] 2016	N = 278 including PDAC, CP, acute pancreatitis, and patients with negative screen for PDAC	PDAC	0.86	76%	83%	
cfDNA	Liu et al,[71] 2020	N = 6689 including cancer and noncancer controls	50 Different cancer types stage I-III including PDAC		43.9%	99.3%	Cancer localization was predicted in 96% of cases with an accuracy of 93%.
RNA-based biomarkers							
GPC-1 mRNA from extracellular vesicles	Hu et al,[62] 2017	N = 193 including PDAC I-IV, pancreatitis, and healthy controls	PDAC (vs. benign disease and healthy controls)	1.0	100%	100%	
miRNA-10b, 21, 30c, 181a, let7a	Lai et al,[64] 2017	N = 46 including PDAC, CP, and healthy controls	PDAC (vs healthy controls)	1.0	100%	100%	See GLP-1 performance from same study under "proteomics"
miRNA-21, 196a, 155	Kong et al,[75] 2011	N = 65 including PDAC, CP, and healthy controls	PDAC				Levels of expression were significantly different between PDAC and

(continued on next page)

Table 2
(continued)

Biomarker	Study, Year	Sample Details	Detected Outcome	AUC	Sensitivity	Specificity	Other
							controls for each of the individual miRNAs in the study. miRNA-196a expression was correlated with median survival in PDAC.
miRNA-21, 34a	Alemar et al,[74] 2016	N = 34 including PDAC and healthy controls	PDAC	0.89 (miRNA-21) 0.87 (miRNA-34a)			
miRNA-27a-3p and CA 19–9	Wang et al,[78] 2013	N = 352 including preoperative PDAC, benign disease, and healthy controls	PDAC (vs benign disease)	0.89	85.3%	81.6%	Benign disease included chronic pancreatitis, serous cystadenoma, pseudocyst, autoimmune pancreatitis, biliary calculus disease, and "other benign pancreas cysts."
miRNA-938	Xu et al,[79] 2016	N = 363 including PDAC, CP, pancreatic neuroendocrine tumor, healthy controls, and other pancreas tumors (serous cystadenomas, mucinous cystadenomas, IPMNs, pseudopapillary tumors, epithelial cysts)	PDAC (vs other pancreas tumors)	0.62			
miRNA-486	Xu et al,[79] 2016	N = 363 including PDAC, CP, pancreatic neuroendocrine tumor, healthy controls, and other pancreas tumors (serous cystadenomas, mucinous cystadenomas, IPMNs, pseudopapillary tumors, epithelial cysts)	PDAC (vs health controls)	0.86			

miRNA-16, 24, 27a, 30a.5p, 323.3p, 20a, 25, 29c, 483.5p and CA 19-9	Johansen et al,[73] 2016	N = 417 including PDAC, CP, and healthy controls	PDAC (vs CP and healthy controls)	0.90	0.85	0.76	
miRNA-20a, 21, 24, 25, 99a, 185, 191	Liu et al,[72] 2012	N = 437 including PDAC, CP, and cancer-free controls	PDAC	0.99	94%	93%	The panel had an accuracy of 83.6% in a subsequent prospective cohort of 55 patients suspected of having PDAC and eventually had histologic diagnosis.
Miscellaneous							
Circulating tumor cells	Allard et al,[86] 2004	N = 21 PDAC	Presence of circulating tumor cells				Circulating tumors cells were found in 19% of patients with PDAC.
Circulating tumor cells	Kurihara et al,[84] 2008	N = 47 including PDAC, CP, and healthy controls	PDAC (vs CP and healthy controls)				Circulating tumor cells were found in 42% of patients with PDAC and none of the controls.
Circulating tumor cells	Bidard et al,[87] 2013	N = 79 patients with nonresectable, nonmetastatic PDAC	Presence of circulating tumor cells				Circulating tumor cells were found in 11% of patients and were associated with shorter overall survival (RR 2.5, $P = .01$).
Circulating tumor cells	Kulemann et al,[88] 2017	N = 68 (including PDAC and healthy controls)	Presence of circulating tumor cells				Circulating tumor cells were found in 67.3% of PDAC and none of the controls. Circulating tumor cells and corresponding tumor cells had discordant KRAS mutation profiles in 42% of patients.

Abbreviation: CEMIP, cell migration-inducing hyaluronan binding protein; ctDNA, circulating tumor DNA; DM II, diabetes mellitus type II; NPV, negative predictive value; RR, relative risk.

occurring even at very low frequencies. Early studies applying this method to cyst fluid analysis have been very promising[17,53,54] although blood-based testing introduces unique challenges in translation. While circulating tumor DNA (ctDNA)/liquid biopsy technology has taken a leading role in the treatment direction of epithelial malignancies like colorectal cancer,[55] its application and adoption into the clinical management of pancreatic cancer has been much more limited. A considerable amount of work has been published on a variety of platforms for capturing tumor-associated components including ctDNA and extracellular vesicles (EVs) although both technical and biological factors have limited their expansion and clinical utilization.[56] Given the low prevalence of pancreatic cancer even in enriched populations of patients with PCL or germline genetic mutations, sensitivity of liquid biopsy for screening purposes would have to be greater than 95% for broad application.

Cell-Free DNA/Cell-Tumor DNA

Cell-free DNA (cfDNA)/ctDNA represents fragments of DNA shed by cells into the blood stream. By sequencing these fragments of DNA, it is possible to identify and quantify mutations that may indicate tumorigenesis. Several studies have shown the feasibility of identifying ctDNA with droplet digital PCR (ddPCR) and NGS, correlating its presence with poorer overall survival, although sensitivity (especially in early-stage patients) was moderate (40%–60%).[57,58] Using molecular barcodes and the "safe-sequencing" approach, investigators found the presence of ctDNA before surgical resection correlated to median recurrence-free survival.[58,59] However, adoption of this into clinical practice for screening and surveillance has been low because of the modest sensitivity and the low abundance of ctDNA, respectively. Specifically, among patients with PCL, Berger and colleagues found that the quantity of isolated cfDNA could distinguish patients with IPMN from those with PDAC or healthy controls, while detection of GNAS and KRAS mutations could discriminate between IPMN and serous cystadenomas.[60] CancerSEEK is an example of a multicancer early detection test that uses a combination of cfDNA and 8 proteins to detect 8 different cancers at stages I-III, including pancreatic cancer. The cfDNA portion of the test measures 61 amplicons originating from 16 different genes (see **Table 2**). This test is not yet approved by the FDA but demonstrated promising sensitivities; it has not yet been specifically evaluated for segregating high-risk PCL patients.[43]

Extracellular Vesicles

EVs, including exosomes and microvesicles, may be isolated via density-based separation, size-based separation, or affinity-based separation, each of which may introduce technical hurdles in clinical application in PDAC. Ultracentrifugation are time-consuming procedures in clinical practice, and the high speed may damage exosomes. Chromatography and filtration may generate contaminated solutions with low specificity and concentration of exosomes. Affinity purification relies on antibodies against specific exosomal surface proteins that have limited their general use. For example, Melo and colleagues used mass spectrometry to identify glypican 1 to have 100% sensitivity/specificity in identifying early- and late-stage PDAC from healthy tissue/benign disease.[61] However, while this was confirmed by some investigators,[62] others found that it had poor performance in larger cohorts, underscoring the need for large, unbiased, validation in this field.[63,64] A pooled approach with antibodies to multiple surface proteins (CLDN4, EpCAM, CD151, LGALS3BP, HIST2H2BF, and HIST2H2BE) was found to have improved performance, in 73% of cases.[63] Exosomal DNA has been evaluated via ddPCR for mutant KRAS, and while enriched versus ctDNA, sensitivity was still moderate in early PDAC (67% vs 46%).[65] This study and another identified a low level of circulating KRAS/TP53 mutations in an apparently healthy population, suggesting a baseline rate of these mutations in an aging population.[66] Using exosomal DNA, KRAS and TP53 mutations were found in 28.5% and 14.2% of patients with IPMNs versus 2.6% and 0% of healthy controls, respectively.[66] These findings suggest exosomal DNA could be leveraged to risk stratify these patients and detect early malignancy.

cfDNA Methylation

Methylation and posttranslational modifications have been well studied in the context of tumor regulation and oncogenesis; however, it remains understudied specifically in the field of PCL. There are some data derived primarily from the analysis of cyst fluid, pancreatic juice, or tissue samples.[67] Blood-based cfDNA methylation studies do exist for the early detection of PDAC but are prone to confounding by CP and, for the most part, are small and lack validation.[68] In one study examining 28 promoter regions for 8 genes, a predictive model including age over 65 years predicted PDAC at any stage with a sensitivity of 76% and specificity of 83%.[69] While not specific to PDAC, Galleri is a commercially available test that is not yet approved by the FDA but is based on cfDNA methylation. The test is designed to detect variations in greater than 100,000 methylation regions for the detection of 50 different cancers, including PDAC. In early testing and validation sets, the test was 67.3% sensitive and 99.3% specific for detection of 12 cancers including PDAC. Sensitivity decreased to 43.9% when including all cancer types of stage I-III.[70,71] This method shows great promise in early cancer detection; however, data relating to the diagnosis and risk stratification in PCL populations specifically are lacking.

RNA-BASED BIOMARKERS

MicroRNAs (miRNA) refer to small noncoding RNA molecules that alter posttranscriptional gene regulation at an epigenetic level and have been implicated in tumorigenesis and progression to malignancy.[72,73] There are many promising studies evaluating miRNA as a biomarker isolated from cyst fluid, but like cfDNA, these molecules can also be found in the circulation and serve as potential biomarkers for differentiating PCL from PDAC. miRNA-21 and miRNA-196a have been studied in both cyst fluid and blood as markers of invasive disease as well as prognostic tools for PDAC.[74–77] In an early study on serum-based miRNA, Kong and colleagues found that miRNA-21 and miRNA-196a were expressed differently between patients with PDAC, those with CP, and healthy controls and that miRNA-196a was correlated with median survival of patients with PDAC.[75] When combined with CA 19-9, miRNA-27a-3p isolated from peripheral mononuclear cells could discriminate preoperative PDAC samples from benign disease (including benign cysts and CP among others) with an AUC of 0.89 with similar performance in PDAC I, II, and III.[78] miRNA-938 had a modest AUC of 0.62 for differentiating PDAC from other pancreatic tumors (serous cystadenomas, epithelial cysts, MCN, IPMNs, and pseudopapillary tumor).[79] Other studies have used panels consisting of multiple miRNAs to improve detection of PDAC with an AUC of 0.9 (including CA 19–9) and 0.99.[72,73] Limitations remain with miRNA as a blood-based biomarker including a lack of standardization of quantification techniques, small sample sizes, and variable performance of individual miRNAs across validation cohorts.[80]

OTHER BIOMARKERS
Circulating Epithelial/Tumor Cells

Previous studies have suggested that metastatic seeding of pancreatic cancer can occur before a clinically evident tumor exists.[81–83] In a prospective study by Rhim and colleagues, pancreatic circulating epithelial cells (CECs) confirmed by Pdx-1 (pancreas-specific transcription factor) staining were detected in 8 of 11 patients with PDAC (78%), 7 of 21 patients with IPMN or MCN (33%), and 0 of 19 patients of healthy controls (0%). This suggests that CEC could become a tool for risk stratification of PCL.[83] While circulating tumor cell (CTC) capture technology varies considerably in approach and implementation, studies with CellSearch have demonstrated detectable CTCs in a varying number of PDAC patients (19%–92%).[84–86] When present, CTCs do appear to correlate to poorer clinical outcomes.[87] Interestingly, however, in a single study that used ScreenCell filtration to isolate CTCs from PDAC patients and ddPCR to identify KRAS mutations, 11 of 26 of the solid tissues and matched CTCs had a discordant KRAS mutation status, with interesting potential implications for tumor seeding, dissemination, and heterogeneity.[88] In a separate study, cytokeratin-positive CECs had a sensitivity of 58% and specificity of 100% for identifying IPMNs versus other PCLs in patients undergoing surgical resection.[89] The quantity of isolated CECs was correlated with progression toward invasive pathology in both these studies, and while analysis of the genetic composition of these CECs is technically challenging, it may also help identify early cancers before early seeding events.[83,89] In a study of a mouse model of pancreatic cancer, RNA sequencing of CECs demonstrated upregulation of WNT genes in CEC tumor cells.[90] There are no large studies investigating this technique on a clinical level for PCL although it potentially shows promise as CTC/CEC capture technologies continue to progress.

Neutrophil-to-Lymphocyte Ratio

Tumor-associated neutrophils are thought to create a protumor environment through the release of cytokines and chemokines that ultimately shift the local immune response in favor of tumorigenesis and failure of immunosurveillance.[91] On a systemic level, this may be observed as an increased neutrophil-to-lymphocyte ratio (NLR).[42] A higher preoperative NLR has been shown to be associated with IPMN harboring higher-grade dysplasia and invasive disease versus low-grade dysplasia and healthy controls, and it decreases after curative resection.[92–95] A predictive model combining NLR with radiologic and clinical features had an AUC of 0.893 for predicting an invasive disease.[94] Sugimachi and colleagues demonstrated a significant rise in NLR immediately before surgical resection in those ultimately diagnosed with high-grade dysplasia or invasive carcinoma when compared to those with low-grade dysplasia.[92] A threshold NLR has not been agreed upon, and in general, NLR has modest sensitivity and specificity on its own but can improve the performance of other clinical predictors or blood-based biomarkers.[95]

FUTURE DIRECTIONS

As the discovery of blood-based novel biomarkers continues, the success of producing clinically applicable tools will depend on several key factors. As mentioned throughout this article, there is no (and likely will not be) a single biomarker capable of diagnosing and risk stratifying PCL or detecting PDAC. Successful tests will most likely combine multiple biomarkers and clinical/radiographic factors to improve sensitivity and specificity. The few commercially available tests for early detection of malignancy are in fact panels of multiple biomarkers themselves, sometimes combining various types of biomarkers (eg, cfDNA and proteomics).[28,43,48] Another limitation of novel biomarkers is reproducibility. As with most new technologies, methods and values must also be established, and standardized reporting methods must be followed to allow for adequate reproducibility and external validation of findings.[29]

Control of confounding factors is also a significant challenge. CP, jaundice, and NOD are among the most commonly cited confounding variables, and these must be addressed in larger validation studies before being applied to a clinical population. Skaro and colleagues identified germline mutations associated with increased risk of pancreatic cancer in 2.9% of patients undergoing surgical resection of IPMNs.[96] Those with germline mutations were more likely to have PDAC than those without.[96] One important approach to addressing this issue is collecting data from prediagnostic cohorts. The ECOG ACRIN EA2185 prospective study following up patients over 5 years with incidental cysts, randomized to high- and low-intensity surveillance programs and biospecimen banking, will hopefully create an ideal repository for putative biomarker panel validation.[97] Owing to the relatively low incidence of pancreas cancer, specific panels/thresholds/approaches may be required for risk stratification of PCL in sporadic patients, those with NOD, those with increased risk due to germline gene mutations, and those with concerning family histories without germline mutations for example. Ultimately, however, focusing on high-risk patient populations would not only improve test performance but also provide the greatest clinical impact.[60] Identifying those patients with PCL at the highest risk of PDAC will be an important step in applying noninvasive biomarkers in a clinical setting.

SUMMARY

Blood-based biomarkers hold incredible potential for the noninvasive assessment of PCLs and early detection of PDAC. CA 19-9 remains the only blood-based marker in current, common clinical practice, and its use remains primarily limited to postresection surveillance, with significant uncertainty regarding its proper use as a diagnostic test or preoperative risk stratification tool. Many novel biomarkers show promising results in early phases of investigation in the fields of proteomics, metabolomics, cfDNA/ctDNA, EV, and miRNA. Combinations of these novel biomarkers and integration with clinicoradiographic data will improve diagnostic accuracy. Future work will need to account for confounding variables and develop a longitudinal understanding of which patients with PCL go on to develop PDAC.

CLINICS CARE POINTS

- CA 19-9 remains the only blood-based marker in routine clinical practice with limited utility in terms of diagnosis and risk stratification.
- IMMray PanCan-d is a proprietary test based on proteomics that is commercially available for use in screening for pancreatic cancer and has been evaluated in high-risk cohorts although not specifically evaluated in patients with PCL.
- Novel biomarkers show promise in the fields of proteomics, metabolomics, cfDNA/ctDNA, extracellular vesicles, and miRNA but are early in the phases of development and validation.

REFERENCES

1. Lee KS, Sekhar A, Rofsky NM, et al. Prevalence of incidental pancreatic cysts in the adult population on MR imaging. Am J Gastroenterol 2010;105(9):2079–84.
2. Oyama H, Tada M, Takagi K, et al. Long-term Risk of Malignancy in Branch-Duct Intraductal Papillary Mucinous Neoplasms. Gastroenterology 2020;158(1):226–37.e5.

3. Pergolini I, Sahora K, Ferrone CR, et al. Long-term Risk of Pancreatic Malignancy in Patients With Branch Duct Intraductal Papillary Mucinous Neoplasm in a Referral Center. Gastroenterology 2017;153(5):1284–94.e1.
4. Scheiman JM, Hwang JH, Moayyedi P. American gastroenterological association technical review on the diagnosis and management of asymptomatic neoplastic pancreatic cysts. Gastroenterology 2015;148(4):824–48.e22.
5. Crippa S, Bassi C, Salvia R, et al. Low progression of intraductal papillary mucinous neoplasms with worrisome features and high-risk stigmata undergoing non-operative management: a mid-term follow-up analysis. Gut 2017;66(3): 495–506.
6. Vege SS, Ziring B, Jain R, et al. American gastroenterological association institute guideline on the diagnosis and management of asymptomatic neoplastic pancreatic cysts. Gastroenterology 2015;148(4):819–22.
7. Ho CK, Kleeff J, Friess H, et al. Complications of pancreatic surgery. HPB 2005; 7(2):99–108.
8. Masica DL, Molin MD, Wolfgang CL, et al. A novel approach for selecting combination clinical markers of pathology applied to a large retrospective cohort of surgically resected pancreatic cysts. J Am Med Inform Assoc 2017;24(1): 145–52.
9. Paniccia A, Polanco PM, Boone BA, et al. Prospective, Multi-Institutional, Real-Time Next-Generation Sequencing of Pancreatic Cyst Fluid Reveals Diverse Genomic Alterations That Improve the Clinical Management of Pancreatic Cysts. Gastroenterology 2022. https://doi.org/10.1053/J.GASTRO.2022.09.028.
10. Springer S, Wang Y, Dal Molin M, et al. A combination of molecular markers and clinical features improve the classification of pancreatic cysts. Gastroenterology 2015;149(6):1501–10.
11. Thornton GD, McPhail MJW, Nayagam S, et al. Endoscopic ultrasound guided fine needle aspiration for the diagnosis of pancreatic cystic neoplasms: a meta-analysis. Pancreatology 2013;13(1):48–57.
12. Wang KX, Ben QW, Jin ZD, et al. Assessment of morbidity and mortality associated with EUS-guided FNA: a systematic review. Gastrointest Endosc 2011;73(2): 283–90.
13. del Chiaro M, Besselink MG, Scholten L, et al. European evidence-based guidelines on pancreatic cystic neoplasms. Gut 2018;67(5):789–804.
14. Canto MI, Almario JA, Schulick RD, et al. Risk of Neoplastic Progression in Individuals at High Risk for Pancreatic Cancer Undergoing Long-term Surveillance. Gastroenterology 2018;155(3):740–51.e2.
15. Valsangkar NP, Morales-Oyarvide V, Thayer SP, et al. 851 resected cystic tumors of the pancreas: A 33-year experience at the Massachusetts General Hospital. Surgery 2012;152(3):S4–12.
16. Sahora K, Mino-Kenudson M, Brugge W, et al. Branch duct intraductal papillary mucinous neoplasms: Does cyst size change the tip of the scale? A critical analysis of the revised international consensus guidelines in a large single-institutional series. Ann Surg 2013;258(3):466–74.
17. Singhi AD, McGrath K, Brand RE, et al. Preoperative next-generation sequencing of pancreatic cyst fluid is highly accurate in cyst classification and detection of advanced neoplasia. Gut 2018;67(12). https://doi.org/10.1136/GUTJNL-2016-313586.
18. Majumder S, Taylor WR, Yab TC, et al. Novel Methylated DNA Markers Discriminate Advanced Neoplasia in Pancreatic Cysts: Marker Discovery, Tissue Validation, and Cyst Fluid Testing. Am J Gastroenterol 2019;114(9):1539–49.

19. Brown JW, Das KK, Kalas V, et al. mAb Das-1 recognizes 3'-Sulfated Lewis A/C, which is aberrantly expressed during metaplastic and oncogenic transformation of several gastrointestinal Epithelia. PLoS One 2021;16(12). https://doi.org/10.1371/JOURNAL.PONE.0261082.
20. Das KK, Geng X, Brown JW, et al. Cross Validation of the Monoclonal Antibody Das-1 in Identification of High-Risk Mucinous Pancreatic Cystic Lesions. Gastroenterology 2019;157(3):720–30.e2.
21. Das KK, Xiao H, Geng X, et al. mAb Das-1 is specific for high-risk and malignant intraductal papillary mucinous neoplasm (IPMN). Gut 2014;63(10):1626–34.
22. Kanno A, Yasuda I, Irisawa A, et al. Adverse events of endoscopic ultrasound-guided fine-needle aspiration for histologic diagnosis in Japanese tertiary centers: Multicenter retrospective study. Dig Endosc 2021;33(7):1146–57.
23. Omori Y, Ono Y, Tanino M, et al. Pathways of Progression From Intraductal Papillary Mucinous Neoplasm to Pancreatic Ductal Adenocarcinoma Based on Molecular Features. Gastroenterology 2019;156(3):647–61.e2.
24. Fischer CG, Beleva Guthrie V, Braxton AM, et al. Intraductal Papillary Mucinous Neoplasms Arise From Multiple Independent Clones, Each With Distinct Mutations. Gastroenterology 2019;157(4):1123–37.e22.
25. Felsenstein M, Noë M, Masica DL, et al. IPMNs with co-occurring invasive cancers: neighbours but not always relatives. Gut 2018;67(9):1652–62.
26. Campbell PJ, Yachida S, Mudie LJ, et al. The patterns and dynamics of genomic instability in metastatic pancreatic cancer. Nature 2010;467(7319):1109–13.
27. Ben Q, Xu M, Ning X, et al. Diabetes mellitus and risk of pancreatic cancer: A meta-analysis of cohort studies. Eur J Cancer 2011;47(13):1928–37.
28. Springer S, Masica DL, Molin MD, et al. A multimodality test to guide the management of patients with a pancreatic cyst. Sci Transl Med 2019;11(501):4772.
29. Jenkinson C, Earl J, Ghaneh P, et al. Biomarkers for early diagnosis of pancreatic cancer. Expert Rev Gastroenterol Hepatol 2015;9(3):305–15.
30. Yan L, Tonack S, Smith R, et al. Confounding effect of obstructive jaundice in the interpretation of proteomic plasma profiling data for pancreatic cancer. J Proteome Res 2009;8(1):142–8.
31. Tonack S, Jenkinson C, Cox T, et al. iTRAQ reveals candidate pancreatic cancer serum biomarkers: influence of obstructive jaundice on their performance. Br J Cancer 2013;108(9):1846–53.
32. Nie S, Lo A, Wu J, et al. Glycoprotein biomarker panel for pancreatic cancer discovered by quantitative proteomics analysis. J Proteome Res 2014;13(4):1873–84.
33. Pereira SP, Oldfield L, Ney A, et al. Early detection of pancreatic cancer. Lancet Gastroenterol Hepatol 2020;5(7):698–710.
34. Parra-Robert M, Santos VícM, Canis SM, et al. Relationship Between CA 19.9 and the Lewis Phenotype: Options to Improve Diagnostic Efficiency. Anticancer Res 2018;38(10):5883–8.
35. Safi F, Schlosser W, Falkenreck S, et al. CA 19-9 serum course and prognosis of pancreatic cancer. Int J Pancreatol 1996;20(3):155–61.
36. WANG W, ZHANG L, CHEN L, et al. Serum carcinoembryonic antigen and carbohydrate antigen 19-9 for prediction of malignancy and invasiveness in intraductal papillary mucinous neoplasms of the pancreas: A meta-analysis. Biomed Rep 2015;3(1):43–50.
37. Goggins M. Molecular markers of early pancreatic cancer. J Clin Oncol 2005;23(20):4524–31.

38. Fritz S, Hackert T, Hinz U, et al. Role of serum carbohydrate antigen 19-9 and carcinoembryonic antigen in distinguishing between benign and invasive intraductal papillary mucinous neoplasm of the pancreas. Br J Surg 2010;98(1):104–10.
39. Kim JR, Jang JY, Kang MJ, et al. Clinical implication of serum carcinoembryonic antigen and carbohydrate antigen 19-9 for the prediction of malignancy in intraductal papillary mucinous neoplasm of pancreas. J Hepatobiliary Pancreat Sci 2015;22(9):699–707.
40. O'Brien DP, Sandanayake NS, Jenkinson C, et al. Serum CA19-9 is significantly upregulated up to 2 years before diagnosis with pancreatic cancer: Implications for early disease detection. Clin Cancer Res 2015;21(3):622–31.
41. Kim S, Park BK, Seo JH, et al. Carbohydrate antigen 19-9 elevation without evidence of malignant or pancreatobiliary diseases. Sci Rep 2020;10(1). https://doi.org/10.1038/S41598-020-65720-8.
42. Moris D, Damaskos C, Spartalis E, et al. Updates and Critical Evaluation on Novel Biomarkers for the Malignant Progression of Intraductal Papillary Mucinous Neoplasms of the Pancreas. Anticancer Res 2017;37(5):2185–94.
43. Cohen JD, Li L, Wang Y, et al. Detection and localization of surgically resectable cancers with a multi-analyte blood test. Science 2018;359(6378):926.
44. Yagi Y, Masuda A, Zen Y, et al. Predictive value of low serum pancreatic enzymes in invasive intraductal papillary mucinous neoplasms. Pancreatology 2016;16(5):893–9.
45. Kim J, Bamlet WR, Oberg AL, et al. Detection of early pancreatic ductal adenocarcinoma using thrombospondin-2 and CA19-9 blood markers. Sci Transl Med 2017;9(398). https://doi.org/10.1126/SCITRANSLMED.AAH5583.
46. Jenkinson C, Elliott VL, Evans A, et al. Decreased serum thrombospondin-1 levels in pancreatic cancer patients up to 24 months prior to clinical diagnosis: Association with diabetes mellitus. Clin Cancer Res 2016;22(7):1734–43.
47. Lee HS, Jang CY, Kim SA, et al. Combined use of CEMIP and CA 19-9 enhances diagnostic accuracy for pancreatic cancer. Sci Rep 2018;8(1):1–7.
48. Delfani P, Carlsson A, King T, et al. Commercial Test Model Study-A multicenter survey. Published online 2021. Available at: www.immunovia.com. Accessed November 24, 2022.
49. Mellby LD, Nyberg AP, Johansen JS, et al. Serum biomarker signature-based liquid biopsy for diagnosis of early-stage pancreatic cancer. J Clin Oncol 2018;36(28):2887–94.
50. Brand RE, Persson J, Bratlie SO, et al. Detection of Early-Stage Pancreatic Ductal Adenocarcinoma From Blood Samples: Results of a Multiplex Biomarker Signature Validation Study. Clin Transl Gastroenterol 2022;13(3):E00468.
51. Kobayashi T, Nishiumi S, Ikeda A, et al. Anovel serum metabolomics-based diagnostic approach to pancreatic cancer. Cancer Epidemiology Biomarkers and Prevention 2013;22(4):571–9.
52. Mayerle J, Kalthoff H, Reszka R, et al. Original article: Metabolic biomarker signature to differentiate pancreatic ductal adenocarcinoma from chronic pancreatitis. Gut 2018;67(1):128.
53. Amato E, Molin MD, Mafficini A, et al. Targeted next-generation sequencing of cancer genes dissects the molecular profiles of intraductal papillary neoplasms of the pancreas. J Pathol 2014;233(3):217–27.
54. Tsiatis AC, Norris-Kirby A, Rich RG, et al. Comparison of Sanger sequencing, pyrosequencing, and melting curve analysis for the detection of KRAS mutations: diagnostic and clinical implications. J Mol Diagn 2010;12(4):425–32.

55. Tie J, Cohen JD, Lahouel K, et al. Circulating Tumor DNA Analysis Guiding Adjuvant Therapy in Stage II Colon Cancer. N Engl J Med 2022;386(24):2261–72.
56. Kamyabi N, Bernard V, Maitra A. Liquid biopsies in pancreatic cancer. Expert Rev Anticancer Ther 2019;19(10):869–78.
57. Sausen M, Phallen J, Adleff V, et al. Clinical implications of genomic alterations in the tumour and circulation of pancreatic cancer patients. Nat Commun 2015;6. https://doi.org/10.1038/NCOMMS8686.
58. Pietrasz D, Pécuchet N, Garlan F, et al. Plasma Circulating Tumor DNA in Pancreatic Cancer Patients Is a Prognostic Marker. Clin Cancer Res 2017;23(1):116–23.
59. Lee JS, Rhee TM, Pietrasz D, et al. Circulating tumor DNA as a prognostic indicator in resectable pancreatic ductal adenocarcinoma: A systematic review and meta-analysis. Sci Rep 2019;9(1). https://doi.org/10.1038/S41598-019-53271-6.
60. Berger AW, Schwerdel D, Costa IG, et al. Detection of Hot-Spot Mutations in Circulating Cell-Free DNA From Patients With Intraductal Papillary Mucinous Neoplasms of the Pancreas. Gastroenterology 2016;151(2):267–70.
61. Melo SA, Luecke LB, Kahlert C, et al. Glypican-1 identifies cancer exosomes and detects early pancreatic cancer. Nature 2015;523(7559):177–82.
62. Hu J, Sheng Y, Kwak KJ, et al. A signal-amplifiable biochip quantifies extracellular vesicle-associated RNAs for early cancer detection. Nat Commun 2017;8(1).
63. Castillo J, Bernard V, San Lucas FA, et al. Surfaceome profiling enables isolation of cancer-specific exosomal cargo in liquid biopsies from pancreatic cancer patients. Ann Oncol 2018;29(1):223–9.
64. Lai X, Wang M, McElyea SD, et al. A microRNA signature in circulating exosomes is superior to exosomal glypican-1 levels for diagnosing pancreatic cancer. Cancer Lett 2017;393:86–93.
65. Allenson K, Castillo J, San Lucas FA, et al. High prevalence of mutant KRAS in circulating exosome-derived DNA from early-stage pancreatic cancer patients. Ann Oncol 2017;28(4):741–7.
66. Yang S, Che SPY, Kurywchak P, et al. Detection of mutant KRAS and TP53 DNA in circulating exosomes from healthy individuals and patients with pancreatic cancer. Cancer Biol Ther 2017;18(3):158.
67. Sato N, Ueki T, Fukushima N, et al. Aberrant methylation of CpG islands in intraductal papillary mucinous neoplasms of the pancreas. Gastroenterology 2002;123(1):365–72.
68. Henriksen SD, Thorlacius-Ussing O. Cell-Free DNA Methylation as Blood-Based Biomarkers for Pancreatic Adenocarcinoma—A Literature Update. Epigenomes 2021;5(2):8.
69. Henriksen SD, Madsen PH, Larsen AC, et al. Cell-free DNA promoter hypermethylation in plasma as a diagnostic marker for pancreatic adenocarcinoma. Clin Epigenetics 2016;8(1). https://doi.org/10.1186/S13148-016-0286-2.
70. Nadauld LD, McDonnell CH, Beer TM, et al. The PATHFINDER Study: Assessment of the Implementation of an Investigational Multi-Cancer Early Detection Test into Clinical Practice. Cancers 2021;13(14). https://doi.org/10.3390/CANCERS13143501.
71. Liu MC, Oxnard GR, Klein EA, et al. Sensitive and specific multi-cancer detection and localization using methylation signatures in cell-free DNA. Ann Oncol 2020;31(6):745–59.
72. Liu R, Chen X, Du Y, et al. Serum MicroRNA Expression Profile as a Biomarker in the Diagnosis and Prognosis of Pancreatic Cancer. Clin Chem 2012;58(3):610–8.

73. Johansen JS, Calatayud D, Albieri V, et al. The potential diagnostic value of serum microRNA signature in patients with pancreatic cancer. Int J Cancer 2016; 139(10):2312–24.
74. Alemar B, Izetti P, Gregório C, et al. MiRNA-21 and miRNA-34a Are Potential Minimally Invasive Biomarkers for the Diagnosis of Pancreatic Ductal Adenocarcinoma. Pancreas 2016;45(1):84–92.
75. Kong X, Du Y, Wang G, et al. Detection of differentially expressed microRNAs in serum of pancreatic ductal adenocarcinoma patients: miR-196a could be a potential marker for poor prognosis. Dig Dis Sci 2011;56(2):602–9.
76. Farrell JJ, Toste P, Wu N, et al. Endoscopically acquired pancreatic cyst fluid microRNA 21 and 221 are associated with invasive cancer. Am J Gastroenterol 2013;108(8):1352–9.
77. Ryu JK, Matthaei H, Dal Molin M, et al. Elevated microRNA miR-21 levels in pancreatic cyst fluid are predictive of mucinous precursor lesions of ductal adenocarcinoma. Pancreatology 2011;11(3):343–50.
78. Wang WS, Liu LX, Li GP, et al. Combined serum CA19-9 and miR-27a-3p in peripheral blood mononuclear cells to diagnose pancreatic cancer. Cancer Prev Res 2013;6(4):331–8.
79. Xu J, Cao Z, Liu W, et al. Plasma miRNAs effectively distinguish patients with pancreatic cancer from controls a multicenter study. Ann Surg 2016;263(6): 1173–9.
80. le Large TYS, Meijer LL, Mato Prado M, et al. Circulating microRNAs as diagnostic biomarkers for pancreatic cancer. Expert Rev Mol Diagn 2015;15(12): 1525–9.
81. Agarwal B, Correa AM, Ho L. Survival in pancreatic carcinoma based on tumor size. Pancreas 2008;36(1). https://doi.org/10.1097/MPA.0B013E31814DE421.
82. Rhim AD, Mirek ET, Aiello NM, et al. EMT and dissemination precede pancreatic tumor formation. Cell 2012;148(1–2):349.
83. Rhim AD, Thege FI, Santana SM, et al. Detection of Circulating Pancreas Epithelial Cells in Patients with Pancreatic Cystic Lesions. Gastroenterology 2014; 146(3):647.
84. Kurihara T, Itoi T, Sofuni A, et al. Detection of circulating tumor cells in patients with pancreatic cancer: a preliminary result. J Hepatobiliary Pancreat Surg 2008;15(2):189–95.
85. Gall TMH, Jacob J, Frampton AE, et al. Reduced dissemination of circulating tumor cells with no-touch isolation surgical technique in patients with pancreatic cancer. JAMA Surg 2014;149(5):482–5.
86. Allard WJ, Matera J, Miller MC, et al. Tumor cells circulate in the peripheral blood of all major carcinomas but not in healthy subjects or patients with nonmalignant diseases. Clin Cancer Res 2004;10(20):6897–904.
87. Bidard FC, Huguet F, Louvet C, et al. Circulating tumor cells in locally advanced pancreatic adenocarcinoma: the ancillary CirCe 07 study to the LAP 07 trial. Ann Oncol 2013;24(8):2057–61.
88. Kulemann B, Rösch S, Seifert S, et al. Pancreatic cancer: Circulating Tumor Cells and Primary Tumors show Heterogeneous KRAS Mutations. Sci Rep 2017;7(1). https://doi.org/10.1038/S41598-017-04601-Z.
89. Poruk KE, Valero V, He J, et al. Circulating Epithelial Cells in Intraductal Papillary Mucinous Neoplasms and Cystic Pancreatic Lesions. Pancreas 2017;46(7): 943–7.
90. Yu M, Ting DT, Stott SL, et al. RNA sequencing of pancreatic circulating tumour cells implicates WNT signaling in metastasis. Nature 2012;487(7408):510.

91. Gregory AD, Houghton AMG. Tumor-associated neutrophils: New targets for cancer therapy. Cancer Res 2011;71(7):2411–6.
92. Sugimachi K, Mano Y, Matsumoto Y, et al. Neutrophil-to-lymphocyte Ratio as a Predictor of Malignancy of Intraductal Papillary Mucinous Neoplasms. Anticancer Res 2021;41(3):1663–9.
93. Arima K, Okabe H, Hashimoto D, et al. The Neutrophil-to-Lymphocyte Ratio Predicts Malignant Potential in Intraductal Papillary Mucinous Neoplasms. J Gastrointest Surg 2015;19(12):2171–7.
94. Gemenetzis G, Bagante F, Griffin JF, et al. Neutrophil-to-lymphocyte Ratio is a Predictive Marker for Invasive Malignancy in Intraductal Papillary Mucinous Neoplasms of the Pancreas. Ann Surg 2017;266(2):339–45.
95. Hata T, Mizuma M, Motoi F, et al. Diagnostic and Prognostic Impact of Neutrophil-to-Lymphocyte Ratio for Intraductal Papillary Mucinous Neoplasms of the Pancreas With High-Grade Dysplasia and Associated Invasive Carcinoma. Pancreas 2019;48(1):99–106.
96. Skaro M, Nanda N, Gauthier C, et al. Prevalence of Germline Mutations Associated with Cancer Risk in Patients With Intraductal Papillary Mucinous Neoplasms. Gastroenterology 2019;156(6):1905.
97. Weinberg DS, Gatsonis C, Zeh HJ, et al. Comparing the clinical impact of pancreatic cyst surveillance programs: A trial of the ECOG-ACRIN cancer research group (EA2185). Contemp Clin Trials 2020;97:106144.

Endoscopic Imaging of Pancreatic Cysts

Ahmad M. Al-Taee, MD[a],*, Jason R. Taylor, MD[b]

KEYWORDS

- Pancreatic cysts • Pancreatic cystic lesions • Pancreatic cystic neoplasms
- Intraductal papillary mucinous neoplasm (IPMN) • Mucinous cystic neoplasm (MCN)
- Serous cystic neoplasm (SCN) • Endoscopic ultrasound (EUS)
- Contrast-enhanced EUS

KEY POINTS

- Pancreatic cystic lesions (PCLs) are increasingly diagnosed due to the widespread use of cross-sectional imaging.
- Cross-sectional imaging alone is often inadequate to determine the type of PCL.
- Endoscopic ultrasound (EUS) especially when combined with fine needle aspiration provides valuable information that help determine the type of PCL. The cyst is examined for the presence of high-risk or worrisome features and the sampled pancreatic cyst fluid can be tested for cytology, glucose, carcinoembryonic antigen (CEA), amylase, and molecular markers.
- A low cyst fluid glucose seems to be associated with improved diagnostic accuracy compared with CEA alone for the diagnosis of mucinous cysts.
- Adjunct techniques such as microforceps, contrast-enhanced EUS, pancreatoscopy, and confocal laser endomicroscopy can be helpful in the evaluation of PCLs.

INTRODUCTION

During the past few decades, pancreatic cystic lesions (PCLs) have been diagnosed with an increasing frequency. One potential explanation is the increasing and widespread use of cross-sectional imaging such as computed tomography and MRI. Most of these cysts are discovered incidentally on cross-sectional imaging performed for nonpancreatic indications. The reported prevalence of PCLs in imaging-based studies ranges from 1.2% to 49.1% with increasing incidence with age.[1–4]

A precise diagnosis of the PCL is important because it helps identify patients in need of surgical resection and those who can undergo surveillance with cross-sectional

[a] Carle Illinois College of Medicine, University of Illinois Urbana-Champaign, Digestive Health Institute, 611 West Park Street, Urbana, IL 61801, USA; [b] St Luke's Hospital, 224 South Woods Mill Road, Suite 410, Chesterfield, MO 63017, USA
* Corresponding author.
E-mail address: aal@illinois.edu

Gastrointest Endoscopy Clin N Am 33 (2023) 583–598
https://doi.org/10.1016/j.giec.2023.03.005
1052-5157/23/© 2023 Elsevier Inc. All rights reserved.

imaging. A combination of clinical and imaging findings in addition to cyst fluid markers can help classify PCLs appropriately and guide management. Although some lesions require surgical resection, the majority of PCLs can be surveyed safely by imaging over the long run.

This review focuses on endoscopic imaging of PCLs. We start with discussing endoscopic diagnosis of PCLs including endoscopic and endosonographic features as well as the role of fine needle aspiration. We then review the role of adjunct techniques, such as microforceps, contrast-enhanced endoscopic ultrasound (EUS), pancreatoscopy, and confocal laser endomicroscopy, in the diagnosis of PCLs.

ENDOSCOPIC EVALUATION OF PANCREATIC CYSTIC LESIONS

Most patients with PCLs have already undergone cross-sectional imaging before referral for EUS. Despite advances in cross-sectional imaging, the ability of computed tomography and MRI to identify the exact type of the PCL remains limited. Therefore, EUS is indicated when the diagnosis is not clear or when the patient has worrisome features. When classic radiological and EUS features are inconclusive, EUS-fine needle aspiration (FNA) is indicated to obtain a sample of the cyst fluid for cytological, chemical, and molecular analysis.

ENDOSCOPIC EXAMINATION

The presence of mucin extruding from a patulous major or minor papilla, described as fish-mouth appearance of papilla, is pathognomonic for main duct intraductal papillary mucinous neoplasm of the pancreas (**Fig. 1**). Although only present in about 50% of cases, this finding has a specificity of 91% for a diagnosis of main duct-intraductal papillary mucinous neoplasm (IPMN).[5] A pancreaticoduodenal fistula extruding mucous is seen in up to 2% of IPMNs and this finding suggests malignant invasion.[6]

Larger PCLs, especially those located in the pancreatic head and uncinate process, may cause extrinsic compression of the duodenum and/or the bile duct and result in gastric outlet and/or biliary obstruction. Rarely, larger pseudocysts may spontaneously fistulize into the stomach, small bowel, or colon, and the luminal side of the fistula can be identified endoscopically.[7]

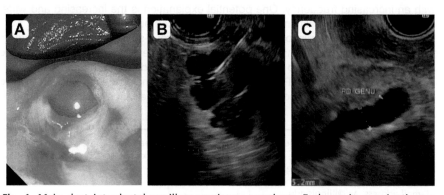

Fig. 1. Main duct intraductal papillary mucinous neoplasm. Endoscopic examination revealed a patulous major papilla, also known as fish mouth papilla (A). Endoscopic ultrasound examination revealed a 35-mm head of pancreas cystic lesion (B) with a dilated main pancreatic duct (C). Patient was referred for surgical resection.

ENDOSCOPIC IMAGING
Endoscopic Ultrasound

EUS serves 2 main functions when evaluating PCLs. First, evaluating morphologic features of the cyst and identifying high-risk or worrisome features. Second, allowing FNA as discussed below. Adjunctive techniques such as contrast-enhanced EUS and confocal laser endomicroscopy are discussed below.

EUS examination can provide a wealth of data on the morphologic features of PCLs. A linear echoendoscope is usually used but a radial echoendoscope can also be used. It important to note the number of the cysts as well as the size and location of each cyst. Each cyst should also be evaluated for the presence of septations (and thickness of each septation), a mural nodule, or an associated mass. The cyst wall thickness should also be noted. The size of the pancreatic duct and whether it connects to the cyst is also important to note. Furthermore, it is important to inspect the entire pancreatic parenchyma as some PCLs such as IPMN tend to be multifocal and can develop concomitant pancreatic adenocarcinoma in a region separate from the cyst. Certain endosonographic features can help classify PCLs into one of the following types. These features are also summarized in **Table 1**.

1. IPMNs are usually macrocystic and are more likely to be found in the pancreatic head than the body or tail. They usually communicate with pancreatic duct and can be associated with a dilated main pancreatic duct or its side branches (see **Fig. 1**; **Fig. 2**). These can be multifocal and pancreatic parenchymal atrophy may also be seen. A mucin ball, mural nodule, or an associated mass may also be visualized.
2. Mucinous cystic neoplasms (MCNs) are most commonly found in the body and tail of the pancreas. They usually have a macrocystic appearance and typically do not communicate with main pancreatic duct. Septations, nodularity, or papillary projections can also be seen. Peripheral calcification, which is seen in 10%–25% of MCNs, is a classic feature of MCNs.
3. Serous cystic neoplasms (SCNs) can be found anywhere in the pancreas and are usually described as having a microcystic or honeycomb appearance. Multiple small (<3 mm) compartments within a cystic lesion suggest a SCN with an accuracy of 92% to 96%, and this feature is not seen in MCNs.[8,9] A central scar or calcification can also be seen. They typically do not communicate with pancreatic duct. Macrocystic and solid variants have also been reported also possible. Microcystic and solids variants of SCN can be mistaken for solid tumors on cross-sectional imaging. The presence of any intramural nodules, cyst wall thickening, floating debris, mucin, or associated pancreatic duct dilation or communication should raise the suspicion for a mucinous lesion.
4. Pseudocysts are usually unilocular, have a thick wall, and may contain echogenic material. They typically communicate with the pancreatic duct. Depending on the clinical context, concomitant features of acute or chronic pancreatitis may be seen. A PCL without septations or solid components along with parenchymal features suggestive of acute or chronic pancreatitis indicate a pseudocyst with a sensitivity of 94% and a specificity of 85%.10 It is also important to evaluate the pseudocyst for feasibility of endoscopic drainage in symptomatic patients.
5. Cystic pancreatic neuroendocrine tumors (PaNETs) usually seem as unilocular or multilocular lesions that can be anechoic or mixed solid and cystic (**Fig. 3**). Wall thickening and intramural nodule may also be seen.
6. Solid pseudopapillary neoplasms (SPNs) seem as well-defined lesions that can have solid, mixed solid and cystic, or cystic appearance. Peripheral or central

Table 1
Endoscopic and endosonographic characteristics of pancreatic cystic lesions

	IPMNs	MCNs	SCNs	Pseudocysts	SPTs	Cystic PaNET
Age	60s–70s	50s–70s	60s–70s	Variable	20s–30s	50s–60s
Gender	Male > female	Female > male	Female > male	Variable	Female > male	Male = female
Endoscopic features	Fish mouth papilla is pathognomonic	No specific features	No specific features	Larger pseudocysts may cause luminal compression or fistulization	No specific features	No specific features
Location	Head > body and tail	Body and tail > head	Body and tail > head	Variable	Body and tail > head	Variable
Endosonographic features	Unilocular or septated cyst. Dilated main (and/or side branch) pancreatic duct ± parenchymal atrophy Solid component may suggest malignancy	Unilocular or septated cyst ± wall calcifications Solid component may suggest malignancy	Microcystic "honeycomb" appearance ± central scar or calcification Oligocystic or macrocystic less common	Anechoic with thick wall and rare septations	Solid and cystic mass ± calcifications	Solid and cystic mass
Communication with the pancreatic duct	Yes	No	No	Yes	No	No
Cyst fluid viscosity and color	Viscous and clear	Viscous and clear	Thin and often bloody	Thin and muddy-brown	Bloody	Variable
Cyst fluid cytology (or cell block)	Mucin-producing columnar cells	Mucin-producing columnar cells supported by ovarian-type stroma	Cuboidal cells that stain positive for glycogen	Neutrophils, macrophages, and histiocytes	Branching papillae with myxoid stroma on cell block	Small homogenous cells with round nuclei that stain positive for chromogranin and synaptophysin on cell block

Cyst fluid amylase	>250 U/L	Variable	<250 U/L	>250 U/L	Insufficient data	Insufficient data
Cyst fluid CEA	>200 ng/mL	>200 ng/mL	<20 ng/mL	<20 ng/mL	Insufficient data	Insufficient data
Cyst fluid glucose	<50 mg/dL	<50 mg/dL	>50 mg/dL	>50 mg/dL	Insufficient data	Insufficient data
Molecular markers	Kras and GNAS mutations	Kras mutation	VHL mutation	None	CTNNB1 mutation	No specific mutations

Abbreviations: CEA, carcinoembryonic antigen; IPMN, intraductal papillary mucinous neoplasm; MCN, mucinous cystic neoplasm; SCN, serous cystic neoplasm; SPT, solid pseudopapillary tumor; PaNET, pancreatic neuroendocrine tumor.

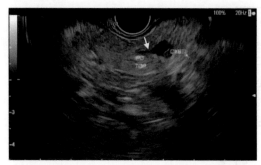

Fig. 2. Side branch intraductal papillary mucinous neoplasm. Endoscopic ultrasound examination showed an 8-mm cystic lesion in the tail of the pancreas with communication with the pancreatic duct (*yellow arrow*).

calcifications may also be seen resulting in acoustic shadowing during EUS examination.

A number of studies have evaluated the role of EUS imaging alone in distinguishing neoplastic from nonneoplastic PCLs. When surgical pathology was used as a reference, the diagnostic accuracy of EUS imaging alone ranged between 40% and 96%.[10] One prospective study investigated the role EUS imaging alone for differentiating mucinous (MCN and IPMN) from nonmucinous cysts showed a low sensitivity, specificity, and accuracy at 45%, 45%, and 51%, respectively.[10] Moreover, using EUS morphologic criteria, the agreement among experienced endosonographers on whether a cyst is neoplastic or not was fair.[11] In the same study, moderate agreement was noted for solid components and SCNs.

In the absence of advanced disease, predicting malignant transformation in IPMNs and MCNs based on EUS imaging alone remains challenging. Multiple studies have demonstrated that EUS imaging alone cannot reliably distinguish benign from malignant IPMNs.[12–15] A meta-analysis of 23 studies found that cyst size greater than 3 cm, main pancreatic duct dilation, presence of a mural nodule, and thickened septal walls were independent predictors of malignant transformation in branch duct-IPMN.[16]

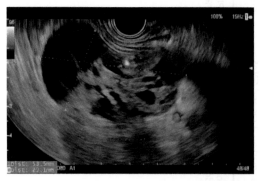

Fig. 3. Cystic pancreatic neuroendocrine tumor. Endoscopic ultrasound examination revealed a 54-mm pancreatic tail cystic lesion that contained large and thick septations. Fine needle aspiration revealed neuroendocrine tumor. Patient was referred to for surgical resection.

Similarly, an international consensus guideline document identified the following features as *high-risk* features for malignancy: obstructive jaundice in a patient with a cystic lesion of head of the pancreas, the presence of an enhancing mural nodule 5 mm or greater on imaging (**Fig. 4**), or main pancreatic duct diameter 10 mm or greater. *Lower risk*, or *worrisome*, features, included clinical evidence of acute pancreatitis, cyst size of 3 cm or greater, rapid cyst growth of greater than 5 mm during 2 years, enhancing mural nodule less than 5 mm, thick enhancing cyst walls, main pancreatic duct diameter between 5 and 9 mm, an abrupt change in the main pancreatic duct caliber with upstream pancreatic parenchymal atrophy, the presence of peripancreatic lymphadenopathy, or an elevated serum CA 19 to 9 level.[17] It is important to note that small cyst size does not exclude malignancy. One surgical series of 212 patients reported that 20% of lesions 2 cm or lesser were malignant, and an additional 45% of lesions had malignant potential.[18]

Another challenging task during EUS evaluation of PCLs is distinguishing a mural nodule from a mucin ball. Several features can aid in distinguishing the 2 lesions. A mucin ball typically has a hypoechoic center surrounded by a well-demarcated hyperechoic rim. Furthermore, a mucin ball can move inside the cysts either by changing the patient's position or by targeting it during fine needle aspiration. However, a mural nodule usually has an isoechoic or hyperechoic center and an irregular (not hyperechoic) rim. PCLs with a large or ill-defined mural nodule are concerning for high-grade dysplasia or cancer. Evaluation with contrast-enhanced EUS, as discussed below, may also aid in distinguishing the two. Moreover, a mural nodule can also be targeted for sampling using a microforceps (Steris, Mentor, OH) that is introduced through a 19G needle during FNA.

Endoscopic Ultrasound Fine-Needle Aspiration

EUS-FNA serves 2 functions: identifying the type of the cyst as well as the presence of high-grade dysplasia or malignancy. The addition of EUS-FNA to cross-sectional imaging has been shown to significantly increase the overall accuracy for diagnosing PCLs.[19] The utility of FNA appears greatest in patients with cysts demonstrating the imaging features most associated with malignancy at surgical resection: cyst size greater than 3 cm, main pancreatic duct dilation, and the presence of a mural nodule or mass lesion.[20–22]

In addition to the international consensus guideline document mentioned above, several guideline documents have been published on the evaluation of PCLs during

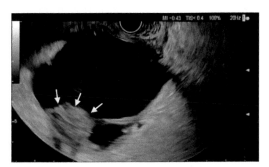

Fig. 4. Mural nodule. Endoscopic ultrasound showed a 65-mm cystic lesion in the pancreatic head with an associated 10-mm intramural nodule (*yellow arrows*). Fine needle aspiration of the cyst and biopsy of the nodule revealed adenocarcinoma.

the past decade. The 2015 American Gastroenterological Association (AGA) guideline recommends patients undergo EUS-FNA if the PCL has 2 or more of the high-risk features that were defined as cyst size 3 cm or greater, presence of a solid component, or a dilated main pancreatic duct.[23] Compared with the AGA guidelines, the American Society of Gastrointestinal Endoscopy (ASGE) had a lower threshold for EUS-FNA, which was recommended for PCLs with any of the following features: cyst size greater than 3 cm, presence of an epithelial nodule, a dilated main pancreatic duct, or the presence of a suspicious mass lesion.[24] For cysts less than 3 cm in size without other indications for performing EUS-FNA, the ASGE suggested EUS-FNA as an optional test.

The American College of Gastroenterology guidelines published in 2018 recommended EUS-FNA for high-risk features that were defined as cyst size 3 cm or greater, main pancreatic duct diameter greater than 5 mm, and change in main duct caliber with upstream atrophy.[25] For PCLs with associated obstructive jaundice or solid mass, discussion with a multidisciplinary group with consideration for EUS-FNA was recommended. For cysts that are 2 to 3 cm in size without classic imaging features on cross-sectional imaging, EUS-FNA is recommended. If the cyst is determined to be a mucinous cyst (IPMN or MCN) by EUS-FNA, surveillance utilizing either MRI or EUS is recommended every 6 to 12 months for the first 3 years. If the cyst is stable, then the ACG recommends annual MRI for an additional 4 years, followed by a lengthened surveillance interval if the cyst remains stable. PCLs that are 1 to 2 cm in size are followed with an MRI/MRCP in 12 months while PCLs less than 1 cm are surveyed with an MRI/MRCP in 2 years.

FNA typically follows a careful EUS examination of the morphologic features of the target cyst as well as the rest of the pancreas. EUS-FNA is usually reserved for cysts that are more than 1 to 1.5 cm in size. If more than one PCL is visualized, the largest lesion is usually targeted for sampling, unless high-risk or worrisome features are noted in more than 1 lesion. For multiseptated PCLs, the largest compartment is usually targeted. Several FNA needles with different needle tip designs are available such as EchoTip Ultra (Cook Medical, Bloomington, IN), Sharkcore (Medtronic, Minneapolis, MN), Expect (Boston Scientific, Marlborough, MA), and EZ Shot (Olympus America, Center Valley, PA). No single needle type or size has shown superiority over another in terms of diagnostic yield and accuracy. Color Doppler imaging is usually used before needle puncture to confirm a lack of significant vascular structures within the needle path. When the needle has entered the lesion of interest, the stylet is withdrawn, and a suction syringe is attached to the needle apparatus. The amount, color, and viscosity of the sampled fluid is noted. Viscous mucinous fluid may be difficult to aspirate with smaller needles. Any solid component associated with a cystic lesion or regional lymph nodes can be aspirated for cytology or histology.[26] FNA of the cyst wall may provide additional cytologic material and can increase the diagnostic yield for mucinous lesions by as much as 37%.[27] A dilated pancreatic duct also can be safely targeted for FNA when IPMN is suspected.[28,29] The string sign is an on-site test that can be performed by measuring the maximal length of sample without being disrupted when stretched between the examiner fingers. It has been shown to be highly specific for the diagnosis of mucinous pancreatic cysts and improves the overall diagnostic accuracy of pancreatic cyst fluid analysis.[30]

Overall, the diagnostic accuracy of cytology from EUS-FNA for cystic lesions ranges between 54% and 97% and may be lower in smaller cysts.[31] Malignancy within a cystic neoplasm can be identified by cytology with 83% to 99% specificity, although reported sensitivities vary from 25% to 88%.[28,29,31,32] Two systematic reviews have evaluated the performance characteristics of EUS-FNA to differentiate between mucinous and nonmucinous cysts.[33,34] The reported sensitivities were 54% and 63% and reported specificities were 93% and 88%, respectively.

Because of the limited sensitivity of cytology, cyst fluid may be analyzed for levels of amylase, tumor markers such as carcinoembryonic antigen (CEA), and molecular markers.

Cyst fluid amylase is typically elevated when the lesion communicates with pancreatic duct (ie, IPMNs and pseudocysts). In a pooled analysis from 12 studies, a cyst fluid amylase of less than 250 U/L virtually excluded pseudocysts.[35]

CEA is typically elevated in mucinous cysts. A meta-analysis found that pancreatic cyst fluid CEA level had a sensitivity of 63% (95% CI, 59%–67%) and specificity of 88% (95% CI, 83%–91%) for the identification of mucinous cystic tumors.[33] A CEA level greater than 192 ng/mL is seen in more than 75% of IPMNs and MCNs.[10] Higher CEA levels increase the specificity for the diagnosis of a mucinous cyst but do not correlate with the risk of malignancy.[10,35] However, a CEA level of less than 5 ng/mL virtually excludes mucinous cysts.[36] In one study, a CEA level less than 5 ng/mL was seen in only 7% of mucinous cysts and all SCNs.[9]

More recently, a low cyst fluid glucose was found to be associated with an improved diagnostic accuracy compared with CEA alone for the diagnosis of mucinous cysts.[37] An intracystic glucose level cutoff of 50 mg/dL had a pooled sensitivity of 90% and a pooled specificity of 88% in differentiating mucinous and nonmucinous pancreatic cysts.[38]

Analysis of molecular markers in PCLs has been proposed to improve on the diagnostic accuracy limitations of cytology and tumor markers. The combination of CEA and DNA molecular analysis has been shown to improve the diagnostic accuracy compared with either test alone.[39,40] Analysis of molecular markers requires only 0.2 mL of cyst fluid and therefore may be most useful in small cysts with nondiagnostic cytology, equivocal cyst fluid CEA results, or when insufficient fluid is present for CEA testing.[39]

Cyst fluid analysis results can help classify PCLs into one of the following types. These findings are also summarized in **Table 1**.

1. IPMNs: The cyst aspirate is typically clear and viscous with elevated amylase and CEA levels and low glucose level. Cytology, which has a yield of less than 50%, might show columnar cells that stain positive for mucin. Although K-ras mutation can be seen in both IPMNs and MCNs, GNAS mutation is seen exclusively in IPMNs. The finding of mutations in both K-ras and GNAS is highly specific for IPMNs but is only seen in less than 50% of cases.
2. MCNs: The cyst aspirate is typically clear and thick with a low amylase and glucose levels and an elevated CEA level. Cytology, which has a yield of less than 50%, might show columnar cells that stain positive for mucin. Mutations in K-ras gene are highly specific for MCNs but are only seen in about one-third of patients.[41] Unlike IPMNs, GNAS is typically negative.
3. SCNs: The characteristic endosonographic appearance of microcystic SCA can obviate cyst sampling. Moreover, the cyst aspirate is usually scant and bloody due to its microcystic nature and the relatively vascular septa. The cyst aspirate is typically thin appearing and is often bloody with a low cyst fluid amylase and CEA levels. Cyst fluid is usually hypocellular or acellular but cuboidal cells that stain positive for glycogen may be seen in less than 50% of cases. Von Hippel-Lindau (VHL) gene mutations have been reported to be present in 22% to 50% of SCNs.[42,43]
4. Pseudocysts lack a true epithelial lining and cytology typically shows inflammatory cells such as neutrophils, macrophages, and histiocytes.

5. PaNETs: Cytology shows small homogenous cells with round nuclei that stain positive for chromogranin and synaptophysin. Targeting the solid component, if present, for cell block preparation is recommended.

6. SPNs: Histologic examination shows monomorphic cells forming pseudopapillary structures. Microscopically, SPTPs are composed of solid nests of uniform neuroendocrine-appearing epithelial cells around delicate fibrovascular stalks. FNA usually shows branching papillae with myxoid stroma. Catenin beta 1 (CTNNB1) mutation is highly sensitive and specific for SPNs.[44] Targeting the solid component, if present, for cell block preparation is recommended.

EUS is considered an overall safe procedure and the risk of major adverse events is rare. Bleeding has a rate between 0.13% and 0.69%, especially when FNA or FNB is performed. Perforation has an overall rate ranging between 0.02% and 0.08%. Acute pancreatitis is a risk after sampling of pancreatic lesions with overall rate of 0.44% to 0.92%.

Infection has an overall reported rate of 1.7%, most of the cases are not clinically significant.[45] Current ASGE guidelines suggest administration of antibiotics for 3 to 5 days after EUS-FNA of a PCL. Routine administration of antibiotics has come into question with a growing body of literature showing this practice do not seem to substantially reduce the risk of infections after EUS-FNA of PCLs.[46]

Microbiopsy Forceps

Given the relatively low yield of cyst fluid cytology, cyst wall sampling using through-the-needle forceps (Moray Micro Forceps, Steris, Mentor, OH) has gained interest during the past few years. This device must be used with a 19G needle and allows for tissue sampling of the cyst wall or mural nodule. Several studies have showed a high technical success and tissue acquisition rates.[47,48] Technical failures are usually related to unfavorable echoendoscope position such as in the second portion of duodenum. A systematic review showed an overall diagnostic yield of 68.6%.[47] Compared with conventional cyst fluid analysis, though-the-needle forceps biopsy resulted in a significant increase in diagnostic yield and improved ability to distinguish neoplastic from nonneoplastic PCLs.[49,50] The overall adverse events rate ranged between 0% and 22.9%.[51,52] Although intracystic bleeding was one of the most commonly reported adverse events, patients are typically asymptomatic and no intervention is required in the vast majority of cases. Acute pancreatitis, which can be potentially severe, has been reported in 3% to 7% of cases.[53,54]

Pancreatoscopy

Pancreatoscopy involves direct visual examination of the main pancreatic duct and is used as an adjunct tool in the evaluation of IPMNs. Pancreatoscopy is helpful to confirm the diagnosis of IPMN in equivocal cases and can guide biopsy specimens to assess for the presence of high-grade dysplasia or malignancy. Moreover, pancreatoscopy can guide surgical resection margins by identifying the extent of IPMN and presence of skip lesions. A systematic review reported a high technical success rate.[55] Cannulation is usually facilitated by the presence of fish mouth papilla as well as a dilated pancreatic duct. A study of 44 patients suspected to have IPMN based on cross-sectional imaging found that pancreatoscopy identified 76% and 78% of surgically resected main duct and side-branch IPMNs, respectively. Furthermore, findings on pancreatoscopy affected clinical decision-making in 76% of cases[56] and altered the surgical approach in up 62% of cases.[55] The most common adverse

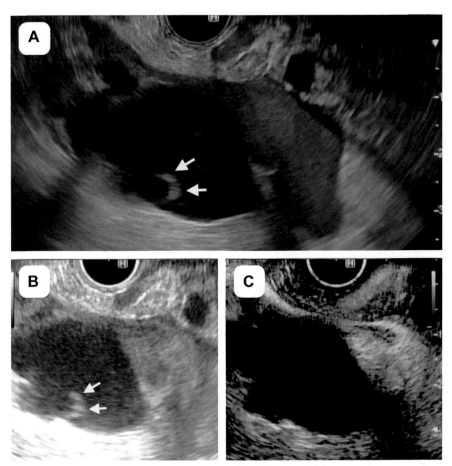

Fig. 5. Mucin ball. A 30-mm cystic lesion was seen in the pancreatic head with an associated 8-mm intramural lesion (*yellow arrows, A*) originating from the wall of the cyst. The lesion had a hypoechoic center surrounded by a well-demarcated hyperechoic rim. Furthermore, the lesion did *not* enhance on contrast-enhanced EUS (*B, C*). These findings were consistent with a mucin ball.

event is postpancreatoscopy pancreatitis with a reported rate ranging between 7% and 20%, with most cases being mild to moderate in severity.[57,58]

Contrast-Enhanced Endoscopic Ultrasound

Contrast-enhanced EUS uses a contrast agent to assess the microcirculation of lesions and nodules. It can aid in distinguishing pseudocysts from pancreatic cystic neoplasms and mural nodules from mucin balls in IPMN. The contrast agent utilized is sulfur hexafluoride lipid-type A microspheres (Lumason, Bracco diagnostics, Milan, Italy). Contraindications include patients with a history of sulfa allergy or chronic kidney disease. After intravenous injection, the arterial phase occurs within 15 to 30 seconds before a venous phase starts about 30 to 45 seconds after injection.[59] The cyst wall of PCNs would typically enhance in the vast majority of cases while the wall of most pseudocysts will be nonenhancing.[60,61] In mucinous cysts, mural nodules will appear enhancing whereas the mucin plugs will be nonenhancing (**Fig. 5**).[60,62] Current evidence suggests that contrast-enhanced EUS is highly accurate for distinguishing nonneoplastic cysts from neoplastic cysts and mural nodules from mucin balls.

Confocal Laser Endomicroscopy

Needle-based confocal laser endomicroscopy (nCLE) is an emerging technology that allows real time in vivo microscopic examination of the cyst epithelium during EUS. After intravenous injection of fluorescein, which highlights tissue architecture and blood vessels, the CLE probe illuminates the target area with a low-power laser and a small aperture in the probe captures the emitted fluorescent light, and real-time images of the target area are generated.[63]

One study that involved 66 patients who underwent nCLE found that the presence of epithelial villous structures had a sensitivity of 59% and a specificity of 100% for mucinous cysts or adenocarcinoma.[64] Another study demonstrated that a superficial vascular network pattern was only seen in SCNs.[65] Moderate-to-high rates of interobserver agreement were demonstrated.[63] nCLE can be helpful in challenging cases where imaging and cyst fluid analysis failed to reach a diagnosis.

SUMMARY

The combination of clinical and imaging findings in addition to cyst fluid analysis can help classify PCLs appropriately and guide management. A precise diagnosis is important because it helps identify patients in need for surgical resection and risk stratify those who can undergo surveillance with cross-sectional imaging.

CLINICS CARE POINTS

- MRI/magnetic resonance cholangiopancreatography) is the cross-sectional imaging modality of choice in the initial evaluation of PCLs.

- EUS serves 2 main functions when evaluating PCLs. First, evaluating morphologic features of the cyst and identifying high-risk or worrisome feature. Second, it allows fine needle aspiration to obtain cyst fluid for analysis.

- In equivocal cases, adjunct techniques contrast-enhanced EUS, confocal laser endomicroscopy, microforceps biopsy, and pancreatoscopy can be helpful in the evaluation of PCLs.

CONFLICTS OF INTEREST

The authors have no commercial or financial conflicts of interest.

FUNDING

None.

REFERENCES

1. Kromrey ML, Bulow R, Hubner J, et al. Prospective study on the incidence, prevalence and 5-year pancreatic-related mortality of pancreatic cysts in a population-based study. Gut 2018;67(1):138–45.
2. Moris M, Bridges MD, Pooley RA, et al. Association Between Advances in High-Resolution Cross-Section Imaging Technologies and Increase in Prevalence of

Pancreatic Cysts From 2005 to 2014. Clin Gastroenterol Hepatol 2016;14(4): 585–93, e3.

3. Schweber AB, Agarunov E, Brooks C, et al. Prevalence, Incidence, and Risk of Progression of Asymptomatic Pancreatic Cysts in Large Sample Real-world Data. Pancreas 2021;50(9):1287–92.

4. Lee KS, Sekhar A, Rofsky NM, et al. Prevalence of incidental pancreatic cysts in the adult population on MR imaging. Am J Gastroenterol 2010;105(9):2079–84.

5. Azar C, Van de Stadt J, Rickaert F, et al. Intraductal papillary mucinous tumours of the pancreas. Clinical and therapeutic issues in 32 patients. Gut 1996;39(3): 457–64.

6. Telford JJ, Carr-Locke DL. The role of ERCP and pancreatoscopy in cystic and intraductal tumors. Gastrointest Endosc Clin N Am 2002;12(4):747–57.

7. Al-Taee A, Taylor J, Chittajallu V, et al. 3524199 Practice patterns in management of walled-off pancreatic necrosis with spontaneous enteral fistulization: a multi-center study. Gastrointest Endosc 2021;93(6):AB250–1.

8. Koito K, Namieno T, Nagakawa T, et al. Solitary cystic tumor of the pancreas: EUS-pathologic correlation. Gastrointest Endosc 1997;45(3):268–76.

9. O'Toole D, Palazzo L, Hammel P, et al. Macrocystic pancreatic cystadenoma: The role of EUS and cyst fluid analysis in distinguishing mucinous and serous lesions. Gastrointest Endosc 2004;59(7):823–9.

10. Brugge WR, Lewandrowski K, Lee-Lewandrowski E, et al. Diagnosis of pancreatic cystic neoplasms: a report of the cooperative pancreatic cyst study. Gastroenterology 2004;126(5):1330–6.

11. Ahmad NA, Kochman ML, Brensinger C, et al. Interobserver agreement among endosonographers for the diagnosis of neoplastic versus non-neoplastic pancreatic cystic lesions. Gastrointest Endosc 2003;58(1):59–64.

12. Song MH, Lee SK, Kim MH, et al. EUS in the evaluation of pancreatic cystic lesions. Gastrointest Endosc 2003;57(7):891–6.

13. Cellier C, Cuillerier E, Palazzo L, et al. Intraductal papillary and mucinous tumors of the pancreas: accuracy of preoperative computed tomography, endoscopic retrograde pancreatography and endoscopic ultrasonography, and long-term outcome in a large surgical series. Gastrointest Endosc 1998;47(1):42–9.

14. Sugiyama M, Atomi Y, Saito M. Intraductal papillary tumors of the pancreas: evaluation with endoscopic ultrasonography. Gastrointest Endosc 1998;48(2): 164–71.

15. Kubo H, Chijiiwa Y, Akahoshi K, et al. Intraductal papillary-mucinous tumors of the pancreas: differential diagnosis between benign and malignant tumors by endoscopic ultrasonography. Am J Gastroenterol 2001;96(5):1429–34.

16. Kim KW, Park SH, Pyo J, et al. Imaging features to distinguish malignant and benign branch-duct type intraductal papillary mucinous neoplasms of the pancreas: a meta-analysis. Ann Surg 2014;259(1):72–81.

17. Tanaka M, Fernandez-Del Castillo C, Kamisawa T, et al. Revisions of international consensus Fukuoka guidelines for the management of IPMN of the pancreas. Pancreatology 2017;17(5):738–53.

18. Fernandez-del Castillo C, Targarona J, Thayer SP, et al. Incidental pancreatic cysts: clinicopathologic characteristics and comparison with symptomatic patients. Arch Surg 2003;138(4):427–33, discussion 433-4.

19. Khashab MA, Kim K, Lennon AM, et al. Should we do EUS/FNA on patients with pancreatic cysts? The incremental diagnostic yield of EUS over CT/MRI for prediction of cystic neoplasms. Pancreas 2013;42(4):717–21.

20. Donahue TR, Hines OJ, Farrell JJ, et al. Cystic neoplasms of the pancreas: results of 114 cases. Pancreas. Nov 2010;39(8):1271–6.
21. Atef E, El Nakeeb A, El Hanafy E, et al. Pancreatic cystic neoplasms: predictors of malignant behavior and management. Saudi J Gastroenterol 2013;19(1):45–53.
22. Sawhney MS, Al-Bashir S, Cury MS, et al. International consensus guidelines for surgical resection of mucinous neoplasms cannot be applied to all cystic lesions of the pancreas. Clin Gastroenterol Hepatol 2009;7(12):1373–6.
23. Vege SS, Ziring B, Jain R, et al. Clinical Guidelines C, American Gastroenterology A. American gastroenterological association institute guideline on the diagnosis and management of asymptomatic neoplastic pancreatic cysts. Gastroenterology 2015;148(4):819–22 ; quize12-3.
24. ASoP Committee, Muthusamy VR, Chandrasekhara V, et al. The role of endoscopy in the diagnosis and treatment of cystic pancreatic neoplasms. Gastrointest Endosc 2016;84(1):1–9.
25. Elta GH, Enestvedt BK, Sauer BG, et al. ACG Clinical Guideline: Diagnosis and Management of Pancreatic Cysts. Am J Gastroenterol 2018;113(4):464–79.
26. Lim LG, Lakhtakia S, Ang TL, et al. Factors determining diagnostic yield of endoscopic ultrasound guided fine-needle aspiration for pancreatic cystic lesions: a multicentre Asian study. Dig Dis Sci 2013;58(6):1751–7.
27. Rogart JN, Loren DE, Singu BS, et al. Cyst wall puncture and aspiration during EUS-guided fine needle aspiration may increase the diagnostic yield of mucinous cysts of the pancreas. J Clin Gastroenterol 2011;45(2):164–9.
28. Lai R, Stanley MW, Bardales R, et al. Endoscopic ultrasound-guided pancreatic duct aspiration: diagnostic yield and safety. Endoscopy 2002;34(9):715–20.
29. Brandwein SL, Farrell JJ, Centeno BA, et al. Detection and tumor staging of malignancy in cystic, intraductal, and solid tumors of the pancreas by EUS. Gastrointest Endosc 2001;53(7):722–7.
30. Bick BL, Enders FT, Levy MJ, et al. The string sign for diagnosis of mucinous pancreatic cysts. Endoscopy 2015;47(7):626–31.
31. Frossard JL, Amouyal P, Amouyal G, et al. Performance of endosonography-guided fine needle aspiration and biopsy in the diagnosis of pancreatic cystic lesions. Am J Gastroenterol 2003;98(7):1516–24.
32. Pais SA, Attasaranya S, Leblanc JK, et al. Role of endoscopic ultrasound in the diagnosis of intraductal papillary mucinous neoplasms: correlation with surgical histopathology. Clin Gastroenterol 2007;5(4):489–95.
33. Thornton GD, McPhail MJ, Nayagam S, et al. Endoscopic ultrasound guided fine needle aspiration for the diagnosis of pancreatic cystic neoplasms: a meta-analysis. Pancreatology 2013;13(1):48–57.
34. Thosani N, Thosani S, Qiao W, et al. Role of EUS-FNA-based cytology in the diagnosis of mucinous pancreatic cystic lesions: a systematic review and meta-analysis. Dig Dis Sci 2010;55(10):2756–66.
35. van der Waaij LA, van Dullemen HM, Porte RJ. Cyst fluid analysis in the differential diagnosis of pancreatic cystic lesions: a pooled analysis. Gastrointest Endosc 2005;62(3):383–9.
36. Hammel P, Levy P, Voitot H, et al. Preoperative cyst fluid analysis is useful for the differential diagnosis of cystic lesions of the pancreas. Gastroenterology 1995;108(4):1230–5.
37. McCarty TR, Garg R, Rustagi T. Pancreatic cyst fluid glucose in differentiating mucinous from nonmucinous pancreatic cysts: a systematic review and meta-analysis. Gastrointest Endosc 2021;94(4):698–712 e6.

38. Mohan BP, Madhu D, Khan SR, et al. Intracystic Glucose Levels in Differentiating Mucinous From Nonmucinous Pancreatic Cysts: A Systematic Review and Meta-analysis. J Clin Gastroenterol 2022;56(2):e131–6.

39. Al-Haddad M, DeWitt J, Sherman S, et al. Performance characteristics of molecular (DNA) analysis for the diagnosis of mucinous pancreatic cysts. Gastrointest Endosc 2014;79(1):79–87.

40. Sawhney MS, Devarajan S, O'Farrel P, et al. Comparison of carcinoembryonic antigen and molecular analysis in pancreatic cyst fluid. Gastrointest Endosc 2009; 69(6):1106–10.

41. Kim SG, Wu TT, Lee JH, et al. Comparison of epigenetic and genetic alterations in mucinous cystic neoplasm and serous microcystic adenoma of pancreas. Mod Pathol 2003;16(11):1086–94.

42. Wu J, Jiao Y, Dal Molin M, et al. Whole-exome sequencing of neoplastic cysts of the pancreas reveals recurrent mutations in components of ubiquitin-dependent pathways. Proc Natl Acad Sci U S A 2011;108(52):21188–93.

43. Moore PS, Zamboni G, Brighenti A, et al. Molecular characterization of pancreatic serous microcystic adenomas: evidence for a tumor suppressor gene on chromosome 10q. Am J Pathol 2001;158(1):317–21.

44. Selenica P, Raj N, Kumar R, et al. Solid pseudopapillary neoplasms of the pancreas are dependent on the Wnt pathway. Mol Oncol 2019;13(8):1684–92.

45. ASoP Committee, Forbes N, Coelho-Prabhu N, et al. Adverse events associated with EUS and EUS-guided procedures. Gastrointest Endosc 2022;95(1): 16–26 e2.

46. Facciorusso A, Mohan BP, Tacelli M, et al. Use of antibiotic prophylaxis is not needed for endoscopic ultrasound-guided fine-needle aspiration of pancreatic cysts: a meta-analysis. Expert Rev Gastroenterol Hepatol 2020;14(10):999–1005.

47. Balaban VD, Cazacu IM, Pinte L, et al. EUS-through-the-needle microbiopsy forceps in pancreatic cystic lesions: A systematic review. Endosc Ultrasound 2021; 10(1):19–24.

48. Tacelli M, Celsa C, Magro B, et al. Diagnostic performance of endoscopic ultrasound through-the-needle microforceps biopsy of pancreatic cystic lesions: Systematic review with meta-analysis. Dig Endosc 2020;32(7):1018–30.

49. Barresi L, Crino SF, Fabbri C, et al. Endoscopic ultrasound-through-the-needle biopsy in pancreatic cystic lesions: A multicenter study. Dig Endosc 2018;30(6): 760–70.

50. Yang D, Trindade AJ, Yachimski P, et al. Histologic Analysis of Endoscopic Ultrasound-Guided Through the Needle Microforceps Biopsies Accurately Identifies Mucinous Pancreas Cysts. Clin Gastroenterol Hepatol 2019;17(8):1587–96.

51. Mittal C, Obuch JC, Hammad H, et al. Technical feasibility, diagnostic yield, and safety of microforceps biopsies during EUS evaluation of pancreatic cystic lesions (with video). Gastrointest Endosc 2018;87(5):1263–9.

52. Crino SF, Bernardoni L, Brozzi L, et al. Association between macroscopically visible tissue samples and diagnostic accuracy of EUS-guided through-the-needle microforceps biopsy sampling of pancreatic cystic lesions. Gastrointest Endosc 2019;90(6):933–43.

53. Kovacevic B, Klausen P, Hasselby JP, et al. A novel endoscopic ultrasound-guided through-the-needle microbiopsy procedure improves diagnosis of pancreatic cystic lesions. Endoscopy. Nov 2018;50(11):1105–11.

54. Yang D, Samarasena JB, Jamil LH, et al. Endoscopic ultrasound-guided through-the-needle microforceps biopsy in the evaluation of pancreatic cystic lesions: a multicenter study. Endosc Int Open 2018;6(12):E1423–30.

55. de Jong DM, Stassen PMC, Groot Koerkamp B, et al. The role of pancreatoscopy in the diagnostic work-up of intraductal papillary mucinous neoplasms: a systematic review and meta-analysis. Endoscopy 2023;55(1):25–35.

56. Arnelo U, Siiki A, Swahn F, et al. Single-operator pancreatoscopy is helpful in the evaluation of suspected intraductal papillary mucinous neoplasms (IPMN). Pancreatology 2014;14(6):510–4.

57. van der Wiel SE, Stassen PMC, Poley JW, et al. Pancreatoscopy-guided electrohydraulic lithotripsy for the treatment of obstructive pancreatic duct stones: a prospective consecutive case series. Gastrointest Endosc 2022;95(5):905–914 e2.

58. Saghir SM, Mashiana HS, Mohan BP, et al. Efficacy of pancreatoscopy for pancreatic duct stones: A systematic review and meta-analysis. World J Gastroenterol 2020;26(34):5207–19.

59. Saftoiu A, Napoleon B, Arcidiacono PG, et al. Do we need contrast agents for EUS? Endosc Ultrasound 2020;9(6):361–8.

60. Fusaroli P, Serrani M, De Giorgio R, et al. Contrast Harmonic-Endoscopic Ultrasound Is Useful to Identify Neoplastic Features of Pancreatic Cysts (With Videos). Pancreas 2016;45(2):265–8.

61. Hocke M, Cui XW, Domagk D, et al. Pancreatic cystic lesions: The value of contrast-enhanced endoscopic ultrasound to influence the clinical pathway. Endosc Ultrasound 2014;3(2):123–30.

62. Yamashita Y, Ueda K, Itonaga M, et al. Usefulness of contrast-enhanced endoscopic sonography for discriminating mural nodules from mucous clots in intraductal papillary mucinous neoplasms: a single-center prospective study. J Ultrasound Med 2013;32(1):61–8.

63. Krishna SG, Brugge WR, Dewitt JM, et al. Needle-based confocal laser endomicroscopy for the diagnosis of pancreatic cystic lesions: an international external interobserver and intraobserver study (with videos). Gastrointest Endosc 2017; 86(4):644–654 e2.

64. Konda VJ, Meining A, Jamil LH, et al. A pilot study of in vivo identification of pancreatic cystic neoplasms with needle-based confocal laser endomicroscopy under endosonographic guidance. Endoscopy 2013;45(12):1006–13.

65. Napoleon B, Lemaistre Al, Pujol B, et al. A novel approach to the diagnosis of pancreatic serous cystadenoma: needle-based confocal laser endomicroscopy. Endoscopy 2015;47(1):26–32.

Pancreatic Cyst Fluid Analysis

Pradeep K. Siddappa, MBBS, Walter G. Park, MD, MS*

KEYWORDS

- Pancreatic cyst • Biomarkers • Intraductal papillary mucinous neoplasms
- Cyst fluid

KEY POINTS

- Cyst fluid cytology is highly specific for the diagnosis of malignancy associated with pancreatic cyst.
- Newer cyst fluid markers such as glucose, KRAS, and GNAS are more sensitive and specific in differentiating mucinous and non-mucinous cysts compared with carcinoembryonic antigen.
- Deoxyribonucleic acid (DNA) mutation markers such as TP53 and methylation markers can be used to accurately predict patients with high-risk lesions (high-grade dysplasia/malignancy).

BACKGROUND

Introduction

Pancreatic cysts (PCs) are increasingly discovered due to a routine use of sensitive cross-sectional imaging techniques such as computed tomography (CT) and MRI.[1] Most cysts harbor neoplastic potential with the most common type being intraductal papillary mucinous neoplasms (IPMN).[2] Other cysts with malignant potential include mucinous cystic neoplasm (MCN), cystic neuroendocrine tumor (cNET) and solid pseudopapillary neoplasm (SPN). It is estimated that 15% of patients with pancreatic ductal adenocarcinoma (PDAC) evolve from a precursor mucinous cystic lesion.[3] PDAC has an overall 5-year survival rate of 10% and is projected to become the second leading cause of cancer-related mortality by 2030.[4] Because of its dismal prognosis, an early detection and management of these precursor lesions is crucial to prevent their progression to malignancy.

CURRENT MANAGEMENT OF PANCREATIC CYSTS

Multiple societies have issued guidelines for the management of PCs.[5–9] Unfortunately most of the recommendations from published guidelines are based on low

Division of Gastroenterology & Hepatology, Stanford University, Stanford, CA, USA
* Corresponding author. 300 Pasteur Drive, H0206B, Stanford, CA 94305.
E-mail address: wgpark@stanford.edu

Gastrointest Endoscopy Clin N Am 33 (2023) 599–612
https://doi.org/10.1016/j.giec.2023.03.006
1052-5157/23/© 2023 Elsevier Inc. All rights reserved.

giendo.theclinics.com

quality of evidence. Almost half of patients with high-grade dysplasia/malignancy are missed by using the guidelines alone for management of PCs.[10,11] Moreover, approximately 20% of patients who undergo guideline-directed management undergo unnecessary surgery and suffer significant complications.[12,13] In a retrospective multicenter study by Xu and colleagues, the 2015 American Gastroenterological Association (AGA), the 2012 International consensus criteria, and the 2010 American College of Radiology guidelines were compared in their ability to predict high-grade dysplasia/malignancy in resected PCs. Using these guidelines, resection of the cysts would have missed underlying high-grade dysplasia/malignancy in 92.7%, 26.8%, and 46.3% of patients, respectively.[14] Current imaging tools such as CT, MRI, and endoscopic ultrasound (EUS), are inadequate to accurately distinguish the different cyst types and malignant/high-grade dysplastic cyst from benign cysts. Although EUS offers an excellent resolution of PCs, their ability to distinguish mucinous from non-mucinous cysts and to detect the presence of underlying malignancy is poor, ranging between 40% and 90%.[15] This is further affected by the subjective nature of the procedure.[16]

The advent of "big-data" analysis from high-throughput multi-omic platforms has opened the door for the discovery of multiple biomarkers in different disease states.[17] PC fluid has been mined for potential diagnostic and prognostic biomarkers to differentiate cyst types as well as to triage them to interventions by identifying high-grade dysplasia/malignant lesions. In this review, the authors summarize the diagnostic performance and utility of published cyst fluid biomarkers to differentiate mucinous from non-mucinous cysts as well as the more significant question of identifying lesions with underlying high-grade dysplasia or malignancy.

Advances in Cyst Fluid Analysis in Mucinous Cysts

Cytology
Cytology is the most traditional approach to cyst fluid analysis that historically has been of limited yield due to low cellularity of the aspirated fluid.[18] The detection of mucinous cysts from non-mucinous cysts by cytopathology can be difficult due to gastrointestinal tract contamination during sampling.[19] In a large multicenter retrospective study, cytology was diagnostically useful in only 29% of patients.[20] In a large prospective study by Brugge and colleagues, cyst fluid cytology had a sensitivity to detect mucinous lesions of 35% and specificity of 83% when compared with the surgical pathology report.[21] In a recent systematic review by Tanaka and colleagues, cytology (13 studies, $n = 743$ patients) had an odds ratio (OR) of 11 to detect malignant lesions with a sensitivity and specificity of 57% and 84%, respectively.[22] EUS-guided brushing of the cyst wall to detect intracellular mucin (ICM) has been evaluated to increase the sensitivity of cytology in the diagnosis of PCs greater than 20 mm. ICM was detected in 62% of brushings sample compared with 23% of plain fine needle aspiration (FNA) samples.[23] In a recent randomized controlled trial (RCT) comparing EUS-guided brushings to EUS FNA cytology in patients with pancreatic cysts greater than 15 mm, the diagnostic accuracy of the brushings was only 44.8% compared with 41.1% in the FNA group ($P = .5$).[24]

Protein biomarkers
Any change in the genome associated with the neoplastic process leads to a parallel change in protein expression. This differential expression of proteins makes them ideal as biomarkers of disease states. Protein biomarkers include some of the oldest and newest cyst fluid biomarkers.

Carcinoembryonic antigen

The two types of mucinous neoplasms (IPMN and MCN) are lined by endodermal-derived columnar epithelium which produces carcinoembryonic antigen (CEA). Non-mucinous cystic neoplasms such as SPN and cNET are lined by non-endoderm-derived cuboidal epithelium.[25] Lewandrowski and colleagues and Hammel and colleagues identified that CEA and cancer (CA) 72 to 4 were elevated in cyst fluid from MCN.[26,27] Brugge and colleagues performed a prospective multicenter study where CEA, CA 72 to 4, CA 125, CA 19 to 9, and CA 15 to 3 were measured in the PC fluid collected at the time of EUS. Compared with a histological diagnosis, the overall accuracy of CEA (79%) to differentiate mucinous from non-mucinous cysts was significantly better than EUS morphology (51%) and cytology (59%).[21] At a cutoff of greater than 800 ng/mL, the specificity of the marker increases to 98% but with lower sensitivity (48%).[28] However, the higher accuracies reported in earlier studies have not been replicated.[29] Further, there is no correlation between cyst fluid CEA level and dysplasia status in patients with mucinous PCs.[21,30,31] Although elevated CEA levels can predict mucinous cysts, extremely low levels of CEA in the cyst fluid can rule out mucinous cysts. Cyst fluid CEA level less than 5 ng/mL has been shown to predict pseudocysts and serous cystadenoma (SCA) with a sensitivity and specificity of 50% and 95%, respectively[28] (**Table 1**).

Amylase

Amylase is an enzyme produced by the exocrine pancreatic gland. Its proposed diagnostic utility was to differentiate pseudocysts; however, subsequent studies have shown this to be less reliable. Park and colleagues showed that cyst fluid amylase was elevated in IPMN, pseudocysts, MCN, and PDAC. At a cutoff of 5680 IU/L, the sensitivity, specificity, and diagnostic accuracy of cyst fluid amylase to differentiate pseudocysts from non-pseudocysts were 89%, 45%, and 54%, respectively (area under the curve [AUC] = 0.69).[32] Although cyst fluid amylase can be elevated in IPMNs, as they communicate with the pancreatic duct, amylase has not been shown to differentiate IPMNs from MCNs[21,30,31,33] (see **Table.1**).

Monoclonal antibody Das-1

A 40-kDa protein (Das-1) was identified in human colon extracts to react specifically to an immunoglobulin from the colon tissue from a patient with ulcerative colitis.[34] The murine antibody against this antigen, now called monoclonal antibody Das-1 (mAb Das-1), was used to detect Barrett's epithelium and esophageal adenocarcinoma.[35] In a pilot study, Das and colleagues performed a sandwich enzyme linked immunoabsorbent assay (ELISA) to detect mAb Das-1 in PC fluid of patients with IPMN. The sensitivity and specificity of mAb Das-1 to differentiate high-grade/malignant lesions form the intermediate/low-grade lesions was 85% and 95%, respectively.[36] Their findings were validated in a multicenter study where the sensitivity and specificity of mAb Das-1 to identify high-risk cyst lesions (PC with invasive carcinoma, high-grade IPMN/ MCN, intermediate-grade Intestinal IPMN) was 88%, and 99%, respectively[37] (**Table 2**). mAb Das-1 may improve the management of high-risk PCs pending widespread use in clinical practice.

Inflammatory Markers

All cancers, including PDAC, stimulate immune response. Cytokine changes suggestive of Th1 and Th2 immune activity has been shown to differentiate between PDAC and chronic pancreatitis in pancreatic juice and serum.[38,39] Maker and colleagues showed Interleukin-1b cytokine levels to be significantly elevated in the high-risk group compared with those with low-/moderate-grade IPMN[40] (see **Table 2**). Prostaglandin E2 (PGE2) is an inflammatory cytokine which is highly

Table 1
Validated diagnostic markers in the pancreatic cyst fluid to differentiate between different types of cysts

Biomarker	Cutoff	Sensitivity	Specificity	Comments	Reference
CEA	≥192 ng/ml	60.4%	88.6%	Mucinous cysts	Khan et al,[29] 2022
	>800 ng/mL	48%	98%	Mucinous cysts	van der Waaij et al,[28] 2005
	<5 ng/mL	50%	95%	SCA and pseudocyst	van der Waaij et al,[28] 2005
CA 19-9	<37 U/mL	19%	98%	SCA and pseudocyst	van der Waaij et al,[28] 2005
Amylase	<250U/L	44%	98%	SCA, mucinous cysts	van der Waaij et al,[28] 2005
MUC5AC:WGA, MUC5AC:BGH and Endorepellin:WGA	Elevation in any of the 2 proteins	87%	100%	Mucinous cysts	Cao et al,[44] 2013
Glucose	≤66 mg/dL	94%	64%	Mucinous cysts	Park et al,[72] 2013
Kynurenine	< 34,000 (abundance level)	90%	100%	Mucinous cysts	Park et al,[72] 2013
KRAS mutation	Presence of mutation	71%	89%	Mucinous cysts	McCarty et al,[60] 2021
GNAS mutation	Presence of mutation	46%	98%	Mucinous cysts	McCarty et al,[60] 2021
KRAS and/or GNAS mutation	Presence of mutation	94%	91%	Mucinous cysts	McCarty et al,[60] 202
VEGF-A	>5000 pg/mL	100%	83.7%	SCN	Car et al,[44] 2017

Table 2
Prognostic markers in the pancreatic cyst fluid to identify patients with high-risk lesions (high-grade dysplasia/cancer)

Biomarker	Cutoff	Sensitivity	Specificity	Comments	Reference
mAb Das-1	Optical density value of 0.1	88%	99%	High-risk pancreatic cystic lesions[a]	Das et al,[37] 2019
TP53/PIK3CA/PTEN in patients with KRAS/GNAS mutation	-	89%	100%	High grade (HG) IPMN/IPMN cancer/MCN cancer	Singhi et al,[61] 2018
IL-1b	>1.26 pg/mL	79%	95%	HG IPMN/IPMN cancer	Maker et al,[40] 2011
Cytology	-	57%	82%	HG IPMN/IPMN cancer	Tanaka et al,[22] 2019
KRAS		54%	46%	HG IPMN/IPMN cancer	Tanaka et al,[22] 2019
GNAS		29%	46%	HG IPMN/IPMN cancer	Tanaka et al,[22] 2019
CEA		68%	53%	HG IPMN/IPMN cancer	Tanaka et al,[22] 2019
DNA content in the cyst fluid					
• High DNA quantity		78%	53%	HG IPMN/IPMN cancer	Simpson et al,[59] 2018
• High DNA quality		48%	70%		
• High clonality loss of heterozygosity (HC LOH)[b]	≥75%	20%	98%		
• High-quantity DNA + KRAS + GNAS	-	67%	95%		
Methylated TBX15 and BMP3	-	90%	92%	HG IPMN/IPMN cancer	Majumder et al,[66] 2019

a Pancreatic cystic lesions with invasive carcinomas, high-grade dysplasia, or intestinal-type IPMNs with intermediate-grade dysplasia.
b High clonality loss of heterozygosity of tumor suppressor genes.

expressed in multiple cancers including PDAC.[41] In a validation study by Yip-Schneider and colleagues, PGE2 levels in the cyst fluid of patients with high-risk lesions were significantly higher compared with those with low-risk lesions. At a PGE2 cutoff level of 1.1 pg/μL, sensitivity and specificity to detect high-risk lesions was 63% and 79%, respectively.

Vascular Endothelial Growth Factor-A

Serous cystadenomas are the third most common PC neoplasms. As benign lesions, identification is clinically useful as these cysts warrant no further surveillance. The histopathology of serous cystic neoplasm (SCN) tissue is characterized by a prominent microvascular network.[42] Consequently, vascular endothelial growth factor-A (VEGF-A) was discovered as a specific cyst fluid biomarker for the diagnosis of SCN.[43] In a validation study by Carr and colleagues, cyst fluid VEGF-A, at a cutoff value of greater than 5000 pg/mL had a sensitivity of 100% and specificity of 83.7% to diagnose SCN. When VEGF-A was combined with a CEA level less than 10 ng/mL, the sensitivity and specificity to diagnose SCN changed to 95.5% and 100%, respectively[44] (see **Table 1**).

Other Protein Markers

High-mobility group (HMG) proteins are a family of nuclear proteins that bind to DNA and nucleosomes and affect structural and functional alterations to the chromatin. Overexpression of these proteins has been found in many malignant and benign neoplasms.[45] In a pilot study by DiMaio and colleagues, the median concentration of HMG-A2 protein was found to be significantly elevated in the cyst fluid of patients with high-grade IPMN (4.2 ng/mL) compared with low (0.6 ng/mL)/moderate-grade IPMN (1.55 ng/mL).[46]

Different glycoforms of proteins can act as markers of the underlying cyst pathology. In a study by Cao and colleagues, glycan alterations were seen in only two proteins: Endorepellin and MUC5AC. A three-marker panel was developed based on these proteins reactivity to wheat germ agglutinin and blood group H antibody and was able to distinguish mucinous from non-mucinous cysts with a sensitivity and specificity of 87% and 100%, respectively[47] (see **Table 1**).

Mass spectrometry is the most sensitive method for identification of protein biomarkers in a biological specimen. HOOK1, PTPN6, and CD55 are some of the novel protein biomarkers discovered using mass-spectrometry methods to detect high-grade malignant lesions.[48,49]

Molecular Markers

Although cellular components of the cyst fluid are minimal, they are a rich source of DNA exfoliated from the lining epithelium. The most common mutations seen in mucinous lesions such as IPMN and MCN are in oncogenes such as kirsten rat sarcoma virus (KRAS) and guanine nucleotide binding protein, alpha stimulating (GNAS), and in tumor suppressor genes such as RNF43, CDKN2A, PTEN, TP53, and SMAD4.[19] Mutation of TP53, PIK3CA (oncogene), deletions of PTEN, losses in CDKN2A, and SMAD4 are seen in high-grade dysplasia and PDAC.[50] Increased telomerase activity is also seen more often in IPMNs with high-grade dysplasia or IPMN cancer compared with low-grade lesions.[51] Allelic imbalance with predominance of mutant type allele leads to aggressive cancer phenotype.[52] GNAS is also an oncogene which encodes for the G-protein stimulating α subunit. Mutations in the gene lead to constitutive activation of the subunit protein leading to amplification of growth signaling. GNAS mutations are more specific to IPMNs and are rarely seen in MCNs. GNAS mutations are seen in 66% of patients with IPMN. Mutation in KRAS and GNAS is seen in more than 96% of patients with IPMN.[53] Patients with low-grade IPMN are likely to have multiple distinct driver mutations (KRAS and GNAS) suggesting a polyclonal origin, however, as they develop into high-grade dysplasia a single clone is selected and the heterogeneity disappears.[54]

Mutation Analysis

Next-generation sequencing (NGS) techniques require a much smaller quantity of cyst fluid and are capable of simultaneously evaluating multiple genes.[55,56] The amount of the shed DNA, its quality, mutations in oncogenes, and loss of heterozygosity of tumor suppressor genes have been investigated for their ability to distinguish different types of cysts and to predict the underlying grade of dysplasia[57,58] (see **Tables 1 and 2**). There is a correlation with the amount of DNA shed into the cyst fluid and the degree of dysplasia. In a retrospective study by Simpson and colleagues, cyst fluid cytology negative IPMN patients with an eventual diagnosis of high-grade dysplasia/malignancy (high-risk IPMN), either after resection or biopsy, who underwent cyst fluid molecular analysis were reviewed. High DNA quantity had a sensitivity and specificity of 78% and 53%, respectively, to identify high-risk IPMN. When taken together high-quantity DNA, KRAS, and GNAS mutations had a sensitivity and specificity of 67% and 95%, respectively.[59] In a recent meta-analysis by McCarty and colleagues, KRAS alone had a sensitivity and specificity of 62% and 97%, respectively; GNAS alone had a sensitivity and specificity of 31% and 100%, respectively, to differentiate mucinous from non-mucinous cysts. When combined KRAS and GNAS, sensitivity and specificity improved to 75% and 99%, respectively. In comparison, however, CEA alone had a sensitivity and specificity of 72% and 88%, respectively.[60]

Singhi and colleagues used targeted NGS (PancreaSeq) on 626 prospectively collected PC fluid samples. Mutations in KRAS, GNAS, NRAS, HRAS, BRAF, CTNNB1, TP53, PIK3CA, PTEN, and AKT1 genes were targeted by NGS. The pathology diagnosis was available for 102 patients (17%) who underwent surgery. NGS findings of KRAS/GNAS mutation in these patients had a sensitivity and specificity of 89% and 100% to detect a mucinous cyst. Genomic alterations in TP53, PIK3CA, and/or PTEN in patients with KRAS/GNAS mutations had a sensitivity and specificity of 79% and 95%, respectively, to detect advanced neoplasia.[61]

DNA Methylation Markers

Aberrant changes in DNA methylation are a feature of progression of neoplastic process to malignancy.[62] These changes have been shown to occur during the evolution of IPMN from low-grade dysplasia to cancer.[63,64] In a study by Hata and colleagues, PC fluid from patients who underwent surgery was analyzed to detect previously identified methylated DNA markers (MDMs) (SOX17, BNIP3, FOXE1, PTCHD2, SLIT2, EYA4, and SFRP1). As a single marker, methylated SOX17 had the best sensitivity and specificity (78.4% and 85.6%, respectively) to detect high-risk cystic lesions.[65] In a study by Majumder and colleagues, 19 novel differentially methylated regions were identified in the tissue of patients with PDAC, and high-grade dysplastic lesions compared with those with normal pancreatic tissue, benign cysts and cysts with low-grade dysplasia. Among 13 MDMs that were selected to be analyzed in cyst fluid, TBX15 and BMP3 had the highest AUC to differentiate patients with malignancy/high-grade dysplasia. In the validation cohort, the 2 MDM panel had a sensitivity and specificity of 90% and 92% to differentiate cases from controls (AUC = 0.93)[66] (see **Table 2**).

MicroRNAs

MicroRNAs (miRNAs) are a group of noncoding ribonucleic acid (RNAs) who primarily function as regulators of gene translation. They primarily act by mRNA degradation and translational repression.[67] The abnormal expression of miRNA is a feature of human malignancies and has also been described in PDACs.[68] In a pilot study by Ryu and colleagues, prospectively collected PC fluid from 40 patients who underwent surgical resection was evaluated for the presence of five miRNAs which were previously shown to be overexpressed in PDAC by quantitative reverse transcriptase PCR. Mucinous cysts showed a significant overexpression of miR-21, miR-221, and miR-17-3p, compared with non-mucinous cysts ($P < .01$). miR-21 had the highest median AUC (AUC = 0.89), with a sensitivity and specificity of 76% and 80%, respectively.[69] Matthaei and colleagues identified 37 candidate miRNAs in the PC fluid which differentiated low-grade IPMNs from high-grade IPMNs. Nine selected miRNAs using logistic regression model were able to differentiate cysts requiring resection (high-grade IPMN, pancreatic neuroendocrine tumors, and SPNs) from those requiring conservative management with a sensitivity and specificity of 89% and 100%, respectively.[70] Shirakami and colleagues evaluated for the presence of differentially expressed miRNAs in patients with IPMN cancer and IPMN adenoma and they found six miRNAs (miR-711, miR-3679-5p, miR-6126, miR-6780b-5p, miR-6798-5p, and miR-6879-5p) were significantly overexpressed in patients with IPMN cancer compared with IPMN adenoma.[71]

Other Molecular Markers

Telomerase enzyme expression may function as a marker of neoplastic progression which is conspicuous by its absence in normal tissue. In a study by Hata and colleagues, cyst fluid telomerase activity was elevated in patients with high-grade dysplasia/malignancy compared with those without. A telomerase cutoff value of $\geq$730 copies/L was able to accurately identify high-risk lesions with a sensitivity and specificity of 74.2% and 93.2%, respectively.[51]

Methylation markers, miRNA, and telomerase expression assays in PC fluid analysis are currently only reported in the research setting. These cyst fluid tests can soon become a part of the diagnostic armamentarium available for PCs.

Metabolic Markers

Glucose levels within the mucinous PCs have been found to be lower compared with non-mucinous cysts. Although the exact cause for this finding is not clear, this difference has been used as a marker to differentiate mucinous from non-mucinous cysts. At a cutoff of glucose level of 66 mg/dL, the sensitivity and specificity to differentiate mucinous from non-mucinous cysts was 94% and 64%, respectively (receiver operator curve [ROC] = 0.88).[72] In a study by Smith and colleagues, intracystic glucose was found to be a better differentiator of mucinous cysts from non-mucinous cysts compared with CEA levels. At a cutoff glucose of $\leq$25 mg/dL, the area under ROC for differentiation was significantly higher (0.96) compared with CEA at a cutoff of $\geq$192 ng/mL (0.81, $P = .003$). The sensitivity and specificity at the same cutoff for glucose and CEA were 88.1% and 91.2% and 62.7% and 88.2%, respectively.[73]

To further simplify, onsite glucometers have been used to measure glucose in the cyst fluid with success. In a study by Noia and colleagues, intracystic glucose measured onsite by glucometer was compared with laboratory-based colorimetry. They found an excellent correlation between the two measurements (ICC = 0.98). At a glucose cutoff level of 73 mg/dL onsite glucometry was able to distinguish mucinous from non-mucinous cysts with a sensitivity and specificity of 89% and 90%, respectively.[74] In a recent meta-analysis by McCarty and colleagues, cyst fluid glucose was compared with cyst fluid CEA to differentiate mucinous from non-mucinous cysts. The pooled sensitivity and specificity of the cyst fluid glucose alone to distinguish mucinous from non-mucinous cysts was 91% and 86%, respectively. Cyst fluid glucose had a better diagnostic accuracy compared with cyst fluid CEA level (94% vs 84%, respectively).[75]

SUMMARY

Cyst fluid analysis remains an important investigation to diagnose PCs. Currently used cyst fluid markers such as CEA, glucose, KRAS, and GNAS mutations analysis are more geared toward differentiation of mucinous from non-mucinous cysts. With the emergence of newer molecular markers, the prospect of differentiating high-risk from low-risk PCs appears promising. With improvement in sequencing technology, molecular tests are projected to become cheaper and more easily accessible to the masses. The adoption of multi-marker panels instead of individual markers will likely improve diagnostic accuracy and serve as a foundation for diagnosis and prognosis of PCs.

CLINICS CARE POINTS

- In sub-centimeter pancreatic cyst, performing EUS cyst fluid aspiration for analysis is unlikely to change management, and adequate yield may not be obtained.
- For patients with pancreatic cysts greater than 2 cm, it is reasonable to perform EUS-guided cyst fluid aspiration for analysis.
- If feasible "Next Generation Sequencing" DNA profiling of the cyst fluid should be prioritized as it will give you the most information.
- If DNA profiling is not available, measuring glucose or CEA can help differentiate mucinous from non-mucinous cysts.
- Because of the low cellularity in the cyst fluid sample, cytology is often of low diagnostic yield.

DISCLOSURE

W.G. Park and P.K. Siddappa have no relevant disclosures to this manuscript.

REFERENCES

1. Brugge WR, Lauwers GY, Sahani D, et al. Cystic neoplasms of the pancreas. N Engl J Med 2004;351(12):1218–26.
2. Munigala S, Javia SB, Agarwal B. Etiologic distribution of pancreatic cystic lesions identified on computed tomography/magnetic resonance imaging. Pancreas 2019;48(8):1092–7.
3. Singhi AD, Koay EJ, Chari ST, et al. Early Detection of Pancreatic Cancer: Opportunities and Challenges. Gastroenterology 2019;156(7):2024–40.
4. Siegel RL, Miller KD, Jemal A. Cancer statistics, 2020. CA A Cancer J Clin 2020; 70(1):7–30.

5. Tanaka M, Fernández-del Castillo C, Adsay V, et al. International consensus guidelines 2012 for the management of IPMN and MCN of the pancreas. Pancreatology 2012;12(3):183–97.

6. Tanaka M, Fernández-del Castillo C, Kamisawa T, et al. Revisions of international consensus Fukuoka guidelines for the management of IPMN of the pancreas. Pancreatology 2017;17(5):738–53.

7. Vege SS, Ziring B, Jain R, et al. American gastroenterological association institute guideline on the diagnosis and management of asymptomatic neoplastic pancreatic cysts. Gastroenterology 2015;148(4):819–22.

8. ESGoCTot Pancreas. European evidence-based guidelines on pancreatic cystic neoplasms. Gut 2018;67(5):789–804.

9. Elta GH, Enestvedt BK, Sauer BG, et al. ACG clinical guideline: diagnosis and management of pancreatic cysts. Journal of the American College of Gastroenterology 2018;113(4):464–79.

10. Ma GK, Goldberg DS, Thiruvengadam N, et al. Comparing American Gastroenterological Association pancreatic cyst management guidelines with Fukuoka consensus guidelines as predictors of advanced neoplasia in patients with suspected pancreatic cystic neoplasms. J Am Coll Surg 2016;223(5):729–37. e1.

11. Kaimakliotis P, Riff B, Pourmand K, et al. Sendai and Fukuoka consensus guidelines identify advanced neoplasia in patients with suspected mucinous cystic neoplasms of the pancreas. Clin Gastroenterol Hepatol 2015;13(10):1808–15.

12. Cho CS, Russ AJ, Loeffler AG, et al. Preoperative classification of pancreatic cystic neoplasms: the clinical significance of diagnostic inaccuracy. Ann Surg Oncol 2013;20(9):3112–9.

13. Lyman WB, Passeri M, Cochran A, et al. Discrepancy in postoperative outcomes between auditing databases: A NSQIP comparison. Am Surg 2018;84(8):1294–8.

14. Xu MM, Yin S, Siddiqui AA, et al. Comparison of the diagnostic accuracy of three current guidelines for the evaluation of asymptomatic pancreatic cystic neoplasms. Medicine 2017;96(35):e7900.

15. Scheiman JM, Hwang JH, Moayyedi P. American gastroenterological association technical review on the diagnosis and management of asymptomatic neoplastic pancreatic cysts. Gastroenterology 2015;148(4):824–48. e22.

16. Ahmad NA, Kochman ML, Brensinger C, et al. Interobserver agreement among endosonographers for the diagnosis of neoplastic versus non-neoplastic pancreatic cystic lesions. Gastrointest Endosc 2003;58(1):59–64.

17. Hasin Y, Seldin M, Lusis A. Multi-omics approaches to disease. Genome Biol 2017;18(1):83.

18. Centeno BA, Warshaw AL, Mayo-Smith W, et al. Cytologic Diagnosis of Pancreatic Cystic Lesions. Acta Cytol 1997;41(4):972–80.

19. Singhi AD, Wood LD. Early detection of pancreatic cancer using DNA-based molecular approaches. Nat Rev Gastroenterol Hepatol 2021;18(7):457–68.

20. Le Borgne J, de Calan L, Partensky C. Cystadenomas and cystadenocarcinomas of the pancreas: a multiinstitutional retrospective study of 398 cases. French Surgical Association. Ann Surg 1999;230(2):152–61.

21. Brugge WR, Lewandrowski K, Lee-Lewandrowski E, et al. Diagnosis of pancreatic cystic neoplasms: a report of the cooperative pancreatic cyst study. Gastroenterology 2004;126(5):1330–6.

22. Tanaka M, Heckler M, Liu B, et al. Cytologic Analysis of Pancreatic Juice Increases Specificity of Detection of Malignant IPMN-A Systematic Review. Clin Gastroenterol Hepatol 2019;17(11):2199–211, e21.

23. Al-Haddad M, Gill K, Raimondo M, et al. Safety and efficacy of cytology brushings versus standard fine-needle aspiration in evaluating cystic pancreatic lesions: a controlled study. Endoscopy 2010;42(2):127–32.

24. Lariño-Noia J, de-la-Iglesia D, Iglesias-García J, et al. Endoscopic ultrasound cytologic brushing vs endoscopic ultrasound-fine needle aspiration for cytological diagnosis of cystic pancreatic lesions. A multicenter, randomized open-label trial. Rev Esp Enferm Dig 2018;110(8):478–84.

25. van Huijgevoort N, Del Chiaro M, Wolfgang CL, et al. Diagnosis and management of pancreatic cystic neoplasms: current evidence and guidelines. Nat Rev Gastroenterol Hepatol 2019;16(11):676–89.

26. Lewandrowski KB, Southern JF, Pins MR, et al. Cyst fluid analysis in the differential diagnosis of pancreatic cysts. A comparison of pseudocysts, serous cystadenomas, mucinous cystic neoplasms, and mucinous cystadenocarcinoma. Ann Surg 1993;217(1):41–7.

27. Hammel P, Levy P, Voitot H, et al. Preoperative cyst fluid analysis is useful for the differential diagnosis of cystic lesions of the pancreas. Gastroenterology 1995;108(4):1230–5.

28. van der Waaij LA, van Dullemen HM, Porte RJ. Cyst fluid analysis in the differential diagnosis of pancreatic cystic lesions: a pooled analysis. Gastrointest Endosc 2005;62(3):383–9.

29. Khan I, Baig M, Bandepalle T, et al. Utility of Cyst Fluid Carcinoembryonic Antigen in Differentiating Mucinous and Non-mucinous Pancreatic Cysts: An Updated Meta-Analysis. Dig Dis Sci 2022;67(9):4541–8.

30. Cizginer S, Turner BG, Bilge AR, et al. Cyst fluid carcinoembryonic antigen is an accurate diagnostic marker of pancreatic mucinous cysts. Pancreas 2011;40(7):1024–8.

31. Ngamruengphong S, Bartel MJ, Raimondo M. Cyst carcinoembryonic antigen in differentiating pancreatic cysts: a meta-analysis. Dig Liver Dis 2013;45(11):920–6.

32. Park WG, Mascarenhas R, Palaez-Luna M, et al. Diagnostic performance of cyst fluid carcinoembryonic antigen and amylase in histologically confirmed pancreatic cysts. Pancreas 2011;40(1):42–5.

33. Thornton GD, McPhail MJ, Nayagam S, et al. Endoscopic ultrasound guided fine needle aspiration for the diagnosis of pancreatic cystic neoplasms: a meta-analysis. Pancreatology 2013;13(1):48–57.

34. Das KM, Sakamaki S, Vecchi M, et al. The production and characterization of monoclonal antibodies to a human colonic antigen associated with ulcerative colitis: cellular localization of the antigen by using the monoclonal antibody. J Immunol 1987;139(1):77–84.

35. Das KM, Prasad I, Garla S, et al. Detection of a shared colon epithelial epitope on Barrett epithelium by a novel monoclonal antibody. Ann Intern Med 1994;120(9):753–6.

36. Das KK, Xiao H, Geng X, et al. mAb Das-1 is specific for high-risk and malignant intraductal papillary mucinous neoplasm (IPMN). Gut 2014;63(10):1626–34.

37. Das KK, Geng X, Brown JW, et al. Cross validation of the monoclonal antibody Das-1 in identification of high-risk mucinous pancreatic cystic lesions. Gastroenterology 2019;157(3):720–30. e2.

38. Noh KW, Pungpapong S, Wallace MB, et al. Do cytokine concentrations in pancreatic juice predict the presence of pancreatic diseases? Clin Gastroenterol Hepatol 2006;4(6):782–9.

39. Seicean A, Popa D, Mocan T, et al. Th1 and Th2 profiles in patients with pancreatic cancer compared with chronic pancreatitis. Pancreas 2009;38(5):594–5.

40. Maker AV, Katabi N, Qin LX, et al. Cyst fluid interleukin-1beta (IL1beta) levels predict the risk of carcinoma in intraductal papillary mucinous neoplasms of the pancreas. Clin Cancer Res 2011;17(6):1502–8.

41. Yip-Schneider MT, Barnard DS, Billings SD, et al. Cyclooxygenase-2 expression in human pancreatic adenocarcinomas. Carcinogenesis 2000;21(2):139–46.

42. Reid MD, Choi HJ, Memis B, et al. Serous Neoplasms of the Pancreas: A Clinicopathologic Analysis of 193 Cases and Literature Review With New Insights on Macrocystic and Solid Variants and Critical Reappraisal of So-called "Serous Cystadenocarcinoma. Am J Surg Pathol 2015;39(12):1597–610.

43. Yip-Schneider MT, Wu H, Dumas RP, et al. Vascular Endothelial Growth Factor, a Novel and Highly Accurate Pancreatic Fluid Biomarker for Serous Pancreatic Cysts. J Am Coll Surg 2014;218(4):608–17.

44. Carr RA, Yip-Schneider MT, Dolejs S, et al. Pancreatic cyst fluid vascular endothelial growth factor A and carcinoembryonic antigen: a highly accurate test for the diagnosis of serous cystic neoplasm. J Am Coll Surg 2017;225(1):93–100.

45. Hock R, Furusawa T, Ueda T, et al. HMG chromosomal proteins in development and disease. Trends Cell Biol 2007;17(2):72–9.

46. DiMaio CJ, Weis-Garcia F, Bagiella E, et al. Pancreatic cyst fluid concentration of high-mobility group A2 protein acts as a differential biomarker of dysplasia in intraductal papillary mucinous neoplasm. Gastrointest Endosc 2016;83(6):1205–9.

47. Cao Z, Maupin K, Curnutte B, et al. Specific glycoforms of MUC5AC and endorepellin accurately distinguish mucinous from nonmucinous pancreatic cysts. Mol Cell Proteomics 2013;12(10):2724–34.

48. Do M, Han D, Wang JI, et al. Quantitative proteomic analysis of pancreatic cyst fluid proteins associated with malignancy in intraductal papillary mucinous neoplasms. Clinical proteomics 2018;15:17.

49. Do M, Kim H, Shin D, et al. Marker identification of the grade of dysplasia of intraductal papillary mucinous neoplasm in pancreatic cyst fluid by quantitative proteomic profiling. Cancers 2020;12(9):2383.

50. Singhi AD, Nikiforova MN, McGrath K. DNA testing of pancreatic cyst fluid: is it ready for prime time? Lancet Gastroenterology & Hepatology 2017;2(1):63–72.

51. Hata T, Dal Molin M, Suenaga M, et al. Cyst Fluid Telomerase Activity Predicts the Histologic Grade of Cystic Neoplasms of the PancreasTelomerase Activity in Pancreatic Cyst Fluid. Clin Cancer Res 2016;22(20):5141–51.

52. Krasinskas AM, Moser AJ, Saka B, et al. KRAS mutant allele-specific imbalance is associated with worse prognosis in pancreatic cancer and progression to undifferentiated carcinoma of the pancreas. Mod Pathol 2013;26(10):1346–54.

53. Wu J, Matthaei H, Maitra A, et al. Recurrent GNAS mutations define an unexpected pathway for pancreatic cyst development. Sci Transl Med 2011;3(92):92ra66.

54. Fischer CG, Guthrie VB, Braxton AM, et al. Intraductal papillary mucinous neoplasms arise from multiple independent clones, each with distinct mutations. Gastroenterology 2019;157(4):1123–37. e22.

55. Tsiatis AC, Norris-Kirby A, Rich RG, et al. Comparison of Sanger sequencing, pyrosequencing, and melting curve analysis for the detection of KRAS mutations: diagnostic and clinical implications. J Mol Diagn 2010;12(4):425–32.

56. Jones M, Zheng Z, Wang J, et al. Impact of next-generation sequencing on the clinical diagnosis of pancreatic cysts. Gastrointest Endosc 2016;83(1):140–8.

57. Winner M, Sethi A, Poneros JM, et al. The role of molecular analysis in the diagnosis and surveillance of pancreatic cystic neoplasms. J Pancreas 2015;16(2): 143–9.

58. Shen J, Brugge WR, Dimaio CJ, et al. Molecular analysis of pancreatic cyst fluid: a comparative analysis with current practice of diagnosis. Cancer 2009;117(3): 217–27.

59. Simpson RE, Cockerill NJ, Yip-Schneider MT, et al. DNA profile components predict malignant outcomes in select cases of intraductal papillary mucinous neoplasm with negative cytology. Surgery 2018;164(4):712–8.

60. McCarty TR, Paleti S, Rustagi T. Molecular analysis of EUS-acquired pancreatic cyst fluid for KRAS and GNAS mutations for diagnosis of intraductal papillary mucinous neoplasia and mucinous cystic lesions: a systematic review and meta-analysis. Gastrointest Endosc 2021;93(5):1019–33. e5.

61. Singhi AD, McGrath K, Brand RE, et al. Preoperative next-generation sequencing of pancreatic cyst fluid is highly accurate in cyst classification and detection of advanced neoplasia. Gut 2018;67(12):2131–41.

62. Jones PA, Baylin SB. The fundamental role of epigenetic events in cancer. Nat Rev Genet 2002;3(6):415–28.

63. Hong S-M, Omura N, Vincent A, et al. Genome-Wide CpG Island Profiling of Intraductal Papillary Mucinous Neoplasms of the PancreasGenome-Wide CpG Island Methylation of Pancreatic IPMNs. Clin Cancer Res 2012;18(3):700–12.

64. Nones K, Waddell N, Song S, et al. Genome-wide DNA methylation patterns in pancreatic ductal adenocarcinoma reveal epigenetic deregulation of SLIT-ROBO, ITGA2 and MET signaling. Int J Cancer 2014;135(5):1110–8.

65. Hata T, Dal Molin M, Hong SM, et al. Predicting the Grade of Dysplasia of Pancreatic Cystic Neoplasms Using Cyst Fluid DNA Methylation Markers. Clin Cancer Res 2017;23(14):3935–44.

66. Majumder S, Taylor WR, Yab TC, et al. Novel methylated DNA markers discriminate advanced neoplasia in pancreatic cysts: marker discovery, tissue validation, and cyst fluid testing. Am J Gastroenterol 2019;114(9):1539.

67. O'Brien J, Hayder H, Zayed Y, et al. Overview of MicroRNA Biogenesis, Mechanisms of Actions, and Circulation. Front Endocrinol 2018;9. https://doi.org/10.3389/fendo.2018.00402.

68. Szafranska A, Davison T, John J, et al. MicroRNA expression alterations are linked to tumorigenesis and non-neoplastic processes in pancreatic ductal adenocarcinoma. Oncogene 2007;26(30):4442–52.

69. Ryu JK, Matthaei H, Dal Molin M, et al. Elevated microRNA miR-21 levels in pancreatic cyst fluid are predictive of mucinous precursor lesions of ductal adenocarcinoma. Pancreatology 2011;11(3):343–50.

70. Matthaei H, Wylie D, Lloyd MB, et al. miRNA Biomarkers in Cyst Fluid Augment the Diagnosis and Management of Pancreatic CystsmiRNA Signatures in Pancreatic Cyst Fluid. Clin Cancer Res 2012;18(17):4713–24.

71. Shirakami Y, Iwashita T, Uemura S, et al. Micro-RNA analysis of pancreatic cyst fluid for diagnosing malignant transformation of Intraductal papillary mucinous neoplasm by comparing Intraductal papillary mucinous adenoma and carcinoma. J Clin Med 2021;10(11):2249.

72. Park WG, Wu M, Bowen R, et al. Metabolomic-derived novel cyst fluid biomarkers for pancreatic cysts: glucose and kynurenine. Gastrointest Endosc 2013;78(2): 295–302. e2.

73. Smith ZL, Satyavada S, Simons-Linares R, et al. Intracystic glucose and carcinoembryonic antigen in differentiating histologically confirmed pancreatic mucinous neoplastic cysts. Am J Gastroenterol 2022;117(3):478–85.

74. Noia JL, Mejuto R, Oria I, et al. Rapid diagnosis of mucinous cystic pancreatic lesions by on-site cyst fluid glucometry. Surg Endosc 2022;36(4):2473–9.

75. McCarty TR, Garg R, Rustagi T. Pancreatic cyst fluid glucose in differentiating mucinous from nonmucinous pancreatic cysts: a systematic review and meta-analysis. Gastrointest Endosc 2021;94(4):698–712. e6.

Surveillance of Pancreatic Cystic Neoplasms

Ankit Chhoda, MD[a], Julie Schmidt, APRN[b], James J. Farrell, MD[b,*]

KEYWORDS

- Pancreatic cyst • Surveillance • Pancreatic cancer • IPMN

KEY POINTS

- Expanded utilization and improved sensitivity of cross-sectional imaging and an overall aging population have substantially contributed to the clinical burden of pancreatic cysts.
- Mucinous pancreatic cysts (MCNs and IPMNs) inherent risk of malignant progression. Among the at-risk lesions which lack features suggestive of advanced neoplasia at baseline, radiologic or endoscopic surveillance is recommended.
- Surveillance of pancreatic cysts relies on consensus guidelines which generally focus on morphology, surgical indications and have varying surveillance intervals and modalities.

INTRODUCTION

Pancreatic cystic neoplasms (PCNs), especially incidental asymptomatic ones seen on noninvasive CT or MRI imaging, remain a common clinical challenge but rarely lead to pancreatic cancer. Their frequency and clinical uncertainty related to cancer risk are a source of angst among patients and their health care providers. PCNs can be broadly classified into those with little or no risk of malignancy such as pseudocysts and serous cystadenoma (SCA),[1] those with definite malignancy, such as cystic degeneration in pancreatic ductal adenocarcinoma (PDAC), and those with a variable risk of developing malignancy including mucinous cysts such as intraductal papillary mucinous cystic neoplasms (IPMNs) or mucinous cystic neoplasms (MCNs).[2] Mucinous cysts represent the predominant premalignant lesions. There are many other uncommon types of pancreatic cysts, and the clinically important ones sometimes requiring surveillance include cystic neuroendocrine neoplasms.

Although patients with pseudocysts and serous cystadenoma are typically managed conservatively, and those patients with overt evidence of advanced neoplasia (defined as high-grade dysplasia [HGD] or invasive cancer) including in

[a] Division of Gastroenterology, Beth Israel Deaconess Medical Center, Boston, MA, USA; [b] Yale Multidisciplinary Pancreatic Cyst Clinic (Yale MPaCC), Yale Center for Pancreatic Disease, Section of Digestive Disease, Yale University School of Medicine, New Haven, CT, USA
* Corresponding author. Yale Center for Pancreatic Disease, Section of Digestive Diseases, Yale University School of Medicine, LMP 1080, 15 York Street, New Haven, CT 06510.
E-mail address: james.j.farrell@yale.edu

Gastrointest Endoscopy Clin N Am 33 (2023) 613–640
https://doi.org/10.1016/j.giec.2023.03.010
1052-5157/23/© 2023 Elsevier Inc. All rights reserved.

the setting of IPMN and MCNs are typically managed by surgical resection, most incidental cysts typically are mucinous especially IPMNs, which have a low variable risk of malignancy and so may be managed by surveillance depending on their risk stratification. This is considered a safer and better option than the alternative of surgical resection, the only currently accepted treatment option.

The definite diagnosis and malignant risk stratification of these presumed mucinous cysts are challenging. However, for many cysts, often a presumed or suspected diagnosis is all that is possible, especially when managing potential branch-duct IPMNs (BD-IPMNs). Hence, important clinical questions pertaining to surgery, surveillance, or stopping surveillance are often made with imperfect diagnoses of both cyst type and risk of malignancy. As the only widely accepted treatment for PCNs with advanced neoplasia is surgical resection, the clinical challenge in 2023 is to accurately preoperatively diagnose them and their malignant potential before deciding about surgery, surveillance, or doing nothing. The absence of reliable imaging or biomarkers to predict advanced neoplasia in pancreatic cysts has necessitated the need for clinical guidelines to guide their management. This review will focus on current concepts in the surveillance of newly diagnosed pancreatic cysts focusing on low-risk BD-IPMNs those without worrisome features (WFs) (acute pancreatitis, mural nodules <5 mm, main duct size 5-9 mm, abrupt change in caliber of main pancreatic duct, increased serum level of CA19–9, rapid cyst growth, cyst size >3 cm, or lymphadenopathy) and high-risk stigmata (HRS) (solid pancreas mass, dilated main pancreatic duct, or jaundice), including a review of current clinical guidelines on surveillance.

PANCREAS CYSTIC NEOPLASM SURVEILLANCE: GOALS AND CHALLENGES

The challenges of PCN surveillance are compounded by the likely large numbers of pancreatic cysts eligible for surveillance. Although the overall prevalence of pancreatic cyst (PC) ranges from 3% to 15% in the United States, the frequency of incidentally discovered cysts among patients undergoing cross-sectional CT or MRI imaging for unrelated indications may be as high as 49-71%.[3–8] The vast majority of identified incidental cysts, although likely to be premalignant mucinous types of cysts, never will truly benefit from surgery and never develop into cancer. However, owing to their variable and often unpredictable risk of malignancy, surveillance is required.

Surveillance is defined as the ongoing follow-up of patients at increased risks of disease. It should be differentiated from screening, which is typically used in average risk population to stratify into higher and lower risk of disease. For patients with PCNs, surveillance aims to differentiate patients who would benefit from surgical intervention (eg, those with mucinous-type cysts and advanced neoplasia) from those who may benefit from ongoing surveillance (eg, those mucinous type of cysts with low-grade dysplasia [LGD]) or even the cessation of surveillance. The goals are dependent on the patient and the pancreatic cyst features being surveyed.

There are many potential benefits to PCN surveillance including finding the cancer at an early stage when it is easier to treat and has a better prognosis and outcome, preventing the development of cancer by findings changes (eg, HGD) which if left untreated would become cancer, and reassuring a surveyed patient if the results of surveillance are "normal" or stable. However, in PCN surveillance, due to the lack of perfect imaging and diagnostic tools to both accurately diagnose and risk-stratify pancreatic cysts, there are also several limitations including tests suggesting advanced neoplasia (a false positive) and resulting surgery when there might not be one, tests not detecting advanced neoplasia at all even though it is present (a false negative), and additional surveillance tests leading to more tests and procedures that may be harmful and expensive, even possibly for patients who do not need surveillance. Finally, in contrast to management of other gastrointestinal malignancies (eg, polypectomy for colonic polyps), the decision for pursuing or deferring pancreatic surgical resection (currently the only accepted treatment option for at-risk pancreatic cyst patients) has more implications. Although the mortality rate from pancreatic resection for pancreatic cysts is up to 2.1%, even in expert centers, surgical morbidity which includes exocrine and/or endocrine pancreatic insufficiency has been reported in 30% of the population. Alternatively, deferred or delayed surgical treatment may risk interval progression of advanced neoplasia and deprive the patient of survival benefits of surveillance. Their large numbers combined with the limitation of current diagnostic strategies and treatment options represent the challenge of surveillance in this population.

ELIGIBILITY FOR PANCREATIC CYST SURVEILLANCE: WHO?

Decision-making in PCN surveillance, preferably performed in a multidisciplinary environment, takes into account both PCN and patient-based factors to weigh the relative risks and benefits of initiating or stopping a PCN surveillance strategy.

Pancreatic Cystic Neoplasm Factors

Many decisions about surveillance are made without having a definite tissue diagnosis or malignancy stratification, relying on a combination of morphologic features and clinical guidelines to determine the type of PC, and when necessary, the grade of malignancy.

Main and mixed duct intraductal papillary mucinous neoplasm
The risk of malignant transformation in main duct and mixed IPMNs is similar, and they are managed in a similar manner.[9–12] Treatment of main-duct or mixed-duct IPMN is surgical resection, typically a partial resection, but on occasion, a total pancreatectomy.[13] The short-term and long-term consequences of a pancreatic resection in these often elderly or frail individuals need to be weighed carefully against the potential benefit. Occasionally in the absence of a definite diagnosis of invasive malignancy, patients with main- or mixed-duct IPMN are closely and safely surveyed with both noninvasive (contrast enhanced CT or MRI) and invasive imaging (endoscopic ultrasound [EUS] and endoscopic retrograde cholangiopancreatography [ERCP] with pancreatoscopy).[14–18]

Branch duct-intraductal papillary mucinous neoplasm
BD-IPMNs that account for most asymptomatic incidental PCs are all considered premalignant, but the risk varies based on the size, associated features (eg, nodules), multiplicity, and the underlying epithelial subtype. The overall risk of carcinomatous transformation in BD-IPMN is currently estimated to be between 1% and 2% per year in surveillance studies.[5,19–22] Multiple recent large surveillance studies of presumed BD-IPMN, with follow-up longer than 5 years, support a very high disease-specific 5-year survival for patients with low-risk BD-IPMNs (without WFs) in the realm of 96%-98%, the persistent and often late (after 5 years) risk of developing WFs and even HRS in otherwise low-risk IPMNs (about 5%), the late persistence of the risk of cancer (0–4%) after 5 and 10 years of surveillance, and the potential value of using baseline cyst size or cyst rate of growth to predict progression of morphology and cancer in the setting of IPMN (**Table 1**).[18,23–34] Presumed BD-IPMNs with epithelial nodule are often referred for surgery. However, patients with small intracystic nodules less than 5 mm may be surveyed safely with EUS, often using EUS-guided microforceps biopsy or contrast-enhanced EUS to more closely image them.

Table 1
Clinical outcomes of large-sized cohorts (>300 pts) of presumed IPMNs undergoing surveillance

Age, Year	Study Design	Follow-up (month)	Surveillance Modality	Age	Sample Size	WF	HRS	Guideline	High-Grade Dysplasia	IPMN-Derived PC	Concomitant PC	Mortality
Broughton et al,[142] 2016, Canada	Retrospective cohort	17.3	CT, MRI, EUS	65.2	450	N.R.	N.R.	ICG 2012	0	5 UC	-	DSM: 0 / EPM: 0
Chung et al,[143] 2013, Korea	Retrospective cohort	27.1	CT, MRI, EUS	62	793	N.R.	N.R.	ICG 2006	0	4	2	DSM: 0 / EPM: 0
Del Chiaro et al,[144] 2017, Sweden	Prospective cohort	31	CT, MRI, EUS	75.1	395	-	41	EG 2011	10	2	2	DSM: 4 / EPM: 29
Han et al,[145] 2021, Korea	Retrospective cohort	50	EUS, CT, & MRI	63.6	1450	43	270	ICG 2017	0	11 UC	-	N.R. / N.R.
Keane et al,[146] 2020, UK	Retrospective cohort	85	CT, MRCP, ERCP, EUS	67	570		245	N.R.	10	0	0	DSM: 7 / EPM: 2
Kim, 2017, Korea	Retrospective cohort	46.1	CT, MRCP, & EUS.	61.7	553	0	12	ICG 2012	0	2	0	N.R. / N.R.
Kwong et al,[138] 2016, USA	Retrospective cohort	87	CT, MRI, MRCP, and EUS	66	310	-	4	AGA	2	3	0	DSM: 3 / EPM: 26
Lawrence et al,[28] 2017, USA	Prospective cohort	85.2	CT, MRI, EUS,	66	2472	N.R.	N.R.	ICG 2012	15	58	0	DSM: 30 / EPM: 260
Lawson et al,[25] 2015, USA	Retrospective cohort	49.5	CT, MRI, EUS	67	404	1	0	ICG 2012	0	1	0	DSM: 1 / EPM: 10
Lee et al,[147] 2021, USA	Retrospective cohort	96	CT, MRCP, & EUS.	68	982		100	ICG 2017	0	5	0	DSM: 4# / EPM: 147#
Marchiengi et al,[148] 2019, Italy	Retrospective cohort	62	MRI/MRCP	64.5	1036	4	40	ICG 2012	1	11	0	DSM: 4 / EPM: 20
Moris et al,[149] 2017, USA	Retrospective cohort	36	EUS and MRI	67.5	431	-	6	ICG 2012	3	5 UC	0	N.R. / N.R.
Mukewar et al,[150] 2017, USA	Retrospective cohort	58.8	CT, MRI, MRCP, EUS	65.8	802	-	87	ICG 2012	0	15	0	N.R. / N.R.

Ohno et al,[151] 2018, Japan	Prospective cohort	32.5	CT, EUS, MRI, & MRCP	66	664	N.R.	N.R.	ICG 2012	0	3	6	DSM: 4 EPM: 14
Oyama et al,[32] 2020, Japan	Retrospective cohort	72	EUS, ERCP	67.5	1404	N.R.	N.R.	ICG 2012	0	38	30	N.R. N.R.
Pandey et al,[152] 2019, USA	Retrospective cohort	50	MRI and CT	68	390	-	12	ACR	2	1	0	N.R. N.R.
Park, 2019, Korea	Retrospective cohort	63.6	CT, EUS, MRI, & MRCP	56.4	427	2	9	ICG 2017	0	1 UC	0	N.R. N.R.
Pergolini et al,[23] 2017, USA	Retrospective Cohort	82	EUS, MRI, & MRCP	66	577	53	142	ICG 2012	15	21	7	DSM: 5 N.R.
Yoshioka et al,[153] 2020, Japan	Retrospective cohort	60.36	CT, MRCP	67.2	1030	-	39	ICG 2012	0	16, 9 UC	15	N.R. N.R.

Abbreviations: ACR, American College of Radiology; AGA, American Gastroenterology Association; CT, contrast tomography; DSM, disease-specific mortality; EG, European Guidelines; EPM, extrapancreatic mortality; ERCP, endoscopic retrograde cholangiopancreatography; EUS, endoscopic ultrasound; HGD, high-grade dysplasia; HRS, high-risk stigmata; ICG, International Consensus Guidelines; IPMC, IPMN-derived pancreatic cancer; MRCP, magnetic resonance cholangiopancreatography; MRI, magnetic resonance imaging; N.R., not recorded; PC, pancreatic cancer; UC, unclassified; WF, worrisome features.

BD-IPMNs maybe multifocal in 21% to 41% of patients.[35] This "field defect" has implications not only for diagnosis but also for both long-term surveillance and postoperative surveillance. Concomitant PDAC remote from the IPMN of interest influences the need for imaging the entire pancreas during surveillance.[35,36] However, more recent data suggest that the rate of concomitant PDAC in the setting of IPMN could be as high as 18% (from molecular pathology series) and up to 28% (from surgical series).[37–39] Although IPMN-derived carcinomas correlate with IPMN size and main pancreatic duct diameter, there are no radiologic IPMN cyst-related risk factors (eg, size, mural nodules, presence of cancer) for the development of these concomitant PDACs. These findings support the importance of carefully reviewing the entire pancreatic parenchyma in addition to the cyst during PCN surveillance.[36,37,40,41]

Mucinous cystic neoplasm

In general, all suspected MCNs exceeding 4 cm in size and any suspected MCN which has a mural nodule or is symptomatic should undergo resection.[19,42–44] Surveillance can be pursued for presumed MCNs less than 3 cm in size in the absence of WFs or HRS that characterize indications for resection in IPMN disease.[45–47] In 3- to 4-cm lesions suspected to be MCN, the risks of empiric resection with a low likelihood of finding invasive disease should be balanced with the need for long-term surveillance. As the natural history of MCN growth is not well understood, adherence to a surveillance regimen is important; this can be quite prolonged as a diagnosis typically occurs in the fourth or fifth decade of life. An important exception to surveillance exists in female patients still pursuing childbirth. The threshold growth during pregnancy has been reported, with resultant tumor rupture, and elective resection of presumed MCNs should be pursued in such patients.[48–50]

Nonmucinous pancreatic cystic neoplasms

Data have shown that malignancy associated with SCAs are an exceedingly rare entity and have minimal importance in determining candidacy for surgery in SCN.[51] Instead, the main criteria for intervention in SCN are lesion size, diagnostic uncertainty, and the presence of symptoms, with the remainder being candidates for surveillance or not. Surveillance studies of the natural history of SCN show slow growth over time, which can range from 2 to 6 mm per year on average (range: 1.2 to 19.8 mm per year), with larger lesions growing faster than smaller ones.[52–54] In asymptomatic patients with both imaging and endoscopic sampling findings confirming a diagnosis of SCN, cessation of surveillance is an attractive option, especially for lesions less than 4 cm in size that are unlikely to grow substantially. For larger or questionable SCNs where the diagnosis is uncertain even after EUS imaging and cyst fluid analysis, we favor at least 1 follow-up study 1-2 years following the diagnosis to assess the rate of growth and confirm the diagnosis before ending surveillance.[42,55] In such cases, patients should be thoroughly counseled on the signs or symptoms that should prompt a return for subsequent workup in the future. A theoretical reason to consider ongoing intermitted surveillance for large proven pancreatic-head SCN is to obtain a diagnosis of main pancreatic duct obstruction early and intervene before the development of body and tail gland atrophy and possible exocrine and endocrine dysfunction.[1,42,56]

Several series have, however, demonstrated cystic pancreatic endocrine neoplasms (CPENs) with malignant potential.[57–60] Similar to all endocrine pancreatic tumors, malignancy is difficult to predict based on biopsy alone (either cytology or core biopsy), and so surgical resection is recommended for most patients.[61–63] Evolving data and current international guidelines support the concept of safe observation of small (<2 cm) nonfunctioning pancreatic neuroendocrine tumors (PNETs)[64,65] although this is countered by surgical series with low rates of lymph node positivity even in small PNETs.[66-69] Whether this extends to CPEN as well is unclear; however, it may certainly be considered for patients who are poor surgical candidates or in advanced age. In one series of 12 patients with asymptomatic cystic PNETs who were conservatively managed with clinical and imaging follow-up because of a small tumor size or because of their advanced age or comorbidities, 10 (83.3%) had stable clinical/tumor burden on CT/EUS during a median follow-up of 12.5 months (range 1.2–61.9 months).[70]

As patients with solid pseudopapillary neoplasm (SPN) are typically young and this pancreatic cyst carries a low risk of malignant behavior, nonoperative surveillance is not typically recommended. Conservative nonoperative management for lymphoepithelial cysts and cystic lymphangiomas are appropriate when the correct diagnosis is made, and premalignant or malignant cystic neoplasms have been excluded.[71-73] However, it may be difficult to differentiate from other PCNs, and so the diagnostic uncertainty often necessitates surgical resection for more common precancerous cysts.[74,75]

Indeterminate pancreatic cysts

There are clinical situations where despite an extensive workup (including molecular analysis of pancreatic cyst fluid), no definite or highly suspicious diagnosis can be made. Typically, the challenge is differentiating a pseudocyst (which may also arise in response to an IPMN) from a BD-IPMN or other mucinous cyst, where there is no obvious history of pancreatitis or risk factors for pancreatic disease. Other examples differentiating a macrocystic SCA from a MCN with the typical cytology or very low carcinoembryonic antigen (CEA) are not seen despite nonviscous cyst fluid. For these cases, both long-term and short-term surveillance can proceed indefinitely or until a more definite diagnosis is made or the cyst resolves on imaging. Often its during the surveillance period that more definitive information may be obtained.[76]

Postoperative Surveillance for Pancreatic Cysts

Postoperative pancreatic cyst surveillance represents a very specific population in PCN surveillance where the recommendations for surveillance can be refined based on detailed knowledge of the resected pathology.

Mucinous cysts with cancer

For patients with either an IPMN or MCN cancer, the postoperative surveillance is influenced by the prognosis associated with the cancer and the treatment plan. Postoperative imaging in this scenario is primarily focused on looking for postoperative complications and cancer recurrence. Surveillance of the residual glands may document existing cysts, the development of new cyst, pancreatic duct dilatation, or concomitant PDAC.[77]

Intraductal papillary mucinous neoplasm without cancer

For patients who have undergone surgical resection of either an IPMN with either LGD or HGD, postoperative surveillance is essential for monitoring the residual gland for the presence of existing cyst, new cyst development (15–25% risk), or concomitant cancer although the overall risks for subsequent cancer development in the residual gland are rare. This is based on the concept that IPMN is a field defect and affects the entire gland with recurrence rates of up to 31% reported in individuals with HGD. There is evidence to suggest that the presence of HGD in the resection specimen (including at the resection margin) carries a much high risk of significant disease in the residual gland compared with patients with LGD, warranting perhaps closer surveillance.

Patients with noninvasive IPMN should be monitored based on the findings of the residual pancreas. The largest remaining cyst should dictate surveillance strategies per recent guidelines, ranging from 6 to 24 months of intervals.[77-79]

Mucinous cystic neoplasm without cancer
Following resection and in the absence of mucinous cystadenocarcinoma, no direct surveillance is required as the risk of MCN recurrence is extremely low.

Nonmucinous cysts
Except in cases of Von Hippel-Lindau syndrome, resected SCNs do not recur. Thus, no surveillance is required following successful surgery for SCN. Although certain surgical series for CPENs show no recurrence reported up to 5 years, other studies have reported rates of recurrence of 12% observed anywhere from 7 to 41 months after complete resection even when pathology showed a benign disease.[70] This suggests the need for long-term surveillance in patients with CPENs after surgical resection. In addition, patients with CPENs in the setting of multiple endocrine neoplasia will require close ongoing surveillance even after surgical resection of their most worrisome pancreatic cyst. The main difference between pancreatic SPN and pancreatic adenocarcinoma is the very low recurrence rate of approximately 4% to 5% after surgical resection for pancreatic SPN, supporting the role of postoperative surveillance in this group of patients. Several factors have been proposed to predict tumor recurrence in SPN including age (older age), gender (older age), EUS biopsy, and Ki-67 status.[80,81]

Patient Factors

There are several patient factors that may influence decisions to pursue or stop surveillance in patients who would normally be recommended for surgery and also for those who would normally be surveyed. For example, it is generally believed that surveillance should not be pursued in a cancer risk population if the planned intervention, in this case pancreas surgical resection, would not ultimately be considered, or if the patients has a limited life expectancy.

Age
Age is commonly used by other cancer surveillance guidelines to determine starting or stopping surveillance. However, defining a specific age cutoff for pancreatic cyst surveillance is a "double-edged sword." With increasing age comes the increased morbidity and mortality associated with the surgical intervention, but also the increased risk of malignancy.[22,82,83] Evidence-based Markov models comparing competing management strategies for asymptomatic pancreatic cysts, including surgery, surveillance, and stopping surveillance, have demonstrated that as patients aged and pancreatic cysts got smaller, stopping the surveillance maximizes quality-adjusted life years across all age groups for any cyst less than 3 cm in size. This is likely due to the poor quality of life experienced postoperatively, often outweighing the minimal benefit derived from surgical resection In the aging population.[84]

Comorbidities
It is unlikely that age alone is sufficient to guide treatment decisions for management of pancreatic cysts, and other factors influencing risk of surgical intervention and overall life expectancy, such as a patient's comorbidity, will become more important. Several validated comorbidity tools such as the Charlson Age Adjusted Comorbidity index (CACI) or an adult comorbidity evaluation 27 (ACE-27) score are accurate at assessing life expectancy in a given patient population.[85,86] Patients with multiple

comorbidities have an 11-fold higher risk of non-IPMN-related death within 3 years. Its known that the risk of pancreaticoduodenectomy mortality increases from 1% to 2.9% when the CACI is greater than 7 in expert pancreatic surgical centers.[87] The risk of non-IPMN mortality exceeding the IPMN cancer-specific mortality for patients with moderate or severe comorbidities has been reported by several studies, including in PCN surveillance studies.[88–90] In a large unselected group of patients with low-risk presumed pancreatic BD-IPMNs undergoing surveillance, comorbidity was influenced by the presence of associated malignancy and chronic liver disease. When these were removed, significant comorbidities persisted and were responsible for the majority of overall mortality, with very few contributions from disease-specific mortality.[91]

Surgical and surveillance risks

Related to the issue of comorbidity are patient risks related of surgical resection either now or in the surveillance future. In addition to risks of mortality related to surgery, there are significant postsurgical morbidities including postoperative diabetes that need to be considered before undertaking surgical resection. Even for main-duct IPMN or BD-IPMN with HRS or WF in poor surgical candidates, the risks of surgical resection may far outweigh the actual risks of malignant progression, justifying a surveillance approach in this population.[14–18] If the patients are considered to be at too high risk of surgery, then it is often argued that they should not even be surveyed. However, under certain circumstances, surveillance may be helpful. For example, if the definite diagnoses of an invasive malignancy influence decision for surgery or open the options for chemotherapy, then it can be helpful to continue surveillance in this population. Surgical intervention then needs to be balanced by harm related to surveillance. Although surveillance imaging with MRI or CT scanning is considered safe, in a study of 909 patients with pancreatic cysts who underwent endoscopci ultrasound - fine needle aspiration (EUS-FNA), a systematic review quantified EUS-FNA-related complications to be 2.75%, including pancreatitis followed by abdominal pain and intracystic hemorrhage.[92]

Patient anxiety and preferences

Patient concern and preference is also an important consideration in determining whether or not to start or stop PCN surveillance. The detection of a pancreatic cysts and awareness of associated PDAC risk may cause substantial anxiety and fear. This perceived cancer risk as well as procedural distress constitute the psychological harm of cyst surveillance.[93] While there are conflicting data about levels of cancer worry and anxiety in patients undergoing pancreatic cyst surveillance, there are currently little data on patient preference in pancreas cyst surveillance strategies.[94–97] The psychological burden of pancreatic cyst surveillance was first quantified among 47 patients undergoing EUS evaluation using State-Trait Anxiety Inventory, and "some" and "a lot" of stress was observed in 60% and 23% of patients, respectively.[94] Psychological burden among pancreatic cyst patients was also investigated in an International Classification of Diseases 10th Revision-based pancreatic cyst registry. This cross-sectional study reported low prevalence of anxiety (median 4 [1–6]) and depression (median 2 [1–4]) among PC patients.[95] In addition, a substantial gap in patients' knowledge of their type of cyst and its potential consequences and implications was reported.[95] One recent prospective study on this topic confirms how little patients know about the relative risks of their PCNs and how much they rely on health care workers for guidance on the subject when deciding between invasive surveillance with EUS and surgical management.[95] What patients are willing to accept in terms of lifelong surveillance, compared with other demands on their time and health care finances, remains unknown. Other factors influencing patients' willingness to stop cessation, such as acceptance of major surgery and fear of underlying malignancy, have not been well studied for pancreatic cysts.

Diabetes

It is increasingly appreciated that new-onset diabetes, especially type 2 diabetes mellitus (DM), is a risk factor for the development of PDAC. Data including a recent large meta-analysis demonstrate the association between the development of DM and both the morphologic progression of pancreatic cysts as well as the development of cancer.[98–100] Some clinical guidelines have incorporated new-onset DM as a WF necessitating closer imaging and surveillance.

Family history of pancreatic cancer

A combination of significant family history of pancreatic cancer (defined as greater than 2 affected family members with PDAC) and certain inherited germline mutations is known to be associated an increased risk of PDAC. The exact interplay between family history, germline genetics, and PCNs still remains to be clarified.[101] Some studies suggest that a family history of pancreatic cancer and germline mutations are associated with a higher risk of morphologic progression and cancer risk in pancreatic cysts, hence justifying closer and prolonged surveillance.[102] However, other studies have not been able to demonstrate a strong correlation to justify a change in cyst surveillance based on a limited family history of PDAC. The study by Nehra and colleagues[103] based on 324 resected IPMN cases showed that among patients with familial history, concomitant PDAC occurred more frequently but had similar IPMN characteristics. A similar observation of significantly higher concomitant PCs (17.6% vs 2.1%, $P = .01$) among IPMN patients with one first degree relative were observed by Mandai and colleagues.[104] Thus, for early detection of concomitant PCs, individuals with 1 or more affected first-degree relatives have a higher risk and deserve more aggressive surveillance. Surveillance for shorter intervals should also be performed for IPMN patients with a family history of familial PDAC (ie, >1 first-degree relatives with PDAC) although whether these patients are susceptible to more aggressive IPMNs remains unclear.[103]

Immunosuppression

Although considered risk factors for hematologic malignancies, there is very little evidence to support the role of immunosuppression in increasing or decreasing the risk of progression or cancer development in patients with pancreatic cysts undergoing surveillance.[105,106]

Resource utilization

Owing to associated health resource expenditure, cost-effectiveness of pancreatic cyst surveillance has been an important area for clinical investigation and will likely impact health system planning for PC surveillance. The cost-effectiveness of pancreatic cyst surveillance, especially in the long term, is not yet fully established. Adherence to higher-intensity surveillance guidelines, that is, revised International Consensus Guidelines (ICG), would impose higher economic burden than American Gastroenterology Association (AGA) guidelines. A study based on the Monte Carlo simulation model compared outcomes of surveillance by IAP versus AGA guidelines and revealed a significantly higher costs ($168.3 million vs $89.4 million) but lower missed cancers (71% vs 49%) among patients.[107]

Analysis of actual health care utilization data at a single-center cross-sectional study of presumed BD-IPMN patients observed a significant association of high image resource utilization (HRU) with initial cyst size and rapid cyst growth over first 2 years.[108] Interestingly, cost-effectiveness of surveillance as compared to nonsurveillance or operative treatment ("do nothing") improves substantially ($100,000/quality adjusted life year) if overtreatment of low-risk cysts is avoided.[109] Thus, increasing the specificity of surveillance is a promising step toward higher cost-effectiveness and lower HRU.

PANCREAS CYSTIC NEOPLASM SURVEILLANCE: MODALITIES

Once a decision has been made to survey a patient with a PCN, a decision has to be made how to balance the use of noninvasive testing and imaging such as abdominal ultrasound, MRI, or CT with invasive studies including EUS, ERCP, and pancreatoscopy. The role and value of blood-based surveillance tools such as HgBA1C and CA19-9 also need to be considered.

Cross-Sectional Imaging: Transabdominal Ultrasound, MRI, and Computerized Tomography

In PCN surveillance, MRI is preferred because of the lack of ionizing radiation, its noninvasive nature, the better resolution for smaller cysts, and the greatest accuracy in evaluating communication between a cyst and the main pancreatic duct.[110,111] However, several controversies still exist with MRI imaging for pancreatic cysts. First, adding intravenous (IV) contrast to the MRI protocol improves parenchymal imaging and can be useful for detecting both concomitant mass as well as nodules associated with cysts or duct, and hence differentiating from mucinous globules. The American College of Radiology (ACR) guidelines and most centers favor MRI with contrast as preferred for surveillance imaging. However, the addition of IV contrast adds cost, imaging time, and potentially risk. There are several short MRI imaging protocols that do not use IV contrast and have been shown to be useful in imaging pancreatic cysts for surveillance.[111]

Another major issue relates to quality improvement and standardization processes for imaging and reporting with MRI or CT. One of the goals of surveillance is to detect changes in cyst and pancreatic duct morphology, in addition to looking for the development of masses. Several studies have demonstrated the interobserver and intraobserver variability associated with PCN surveillance imaging. One study noted a difference of 4 mm each between cyst measurements by EUS and CT scan and between EUS and MRI scan. Moreover, between two cross-sectional modalities, CT and MRI scans, a 3-mm difference between cyst measurements was observed.[112] Interobserver variability is another important factor, and a 2.8-fold difference in follow-up recommendation was observed in an investigation of focal PCN lesions. This variation occurred despite controlling for patient-related, radiologist-related, and lesion characteristics.[113]

Hence, imaging performance and reporting should be formalized in any prospective cyst imaging surveillance program, through the use of an accepted reporting protocol. The ACR guideline recommendations define reporting criteria for pancreatic cysts that radiologists should adhere to when reading cross-sectional imaging and outline surveillance schedules based on the cyst and patient characteristics. An important aspect of the ACR recommendations is consensus guidelines on protocol optimization for CT/MRI and standardization of radiologic reporting. For example, there are 6 reporting criteria that radiologists should adhere to when reading cross-sectional imaging for PCLs: cyst morphology and location, cyst size, possible communication with the main pancreatic duct, presence of WFs, or HRS, growth on follow-up examination, and multiplicity.[20] Standardization of imaging thus can serve as an important measure to reduce heterogeneity and impact on imaging HRU. After the introduction of measurement standards in one study, a significant reduction in median variability (4.0 mm to 3.3 mm [$P < .01$]) and improvement in interobserver agreement (0.59 to 0.65 [$P = .04$]) was observed after 6 weeks of training.[114]

There will be times when a patient cannot undergo an MRI scan because of availability or patient preference. Under those circumstances, a good-quality pancreas protocol CT scan with IV contrast is an alternative and has been shown to be suitable for certain key pancreatic imaging features. The ACR guidelines note similar sensitivities and specificities of MRI with contrast-enhanced sequences or multiphase multiple-detector high-resolution CT, which can be used for diagnostic or surveillance purposes.[24] CT may be prioritized if there is high suspicion for cancer, and assessment of vascular involvement or metastatic disease is needed.

Currently, there is no indication for the use of PET/CT scans in pancreatic cyst surveillance although they have been used in initial cystic neoplasms workup.[115] In some countries, transabdominal ultrasound is used as part of a surveillance imaging program especially when body habitus allows for detailed imaging of the pancreas using regular abdominal ultrasound.[116]

Endoscopic Surveillance

Although more invasive than MRI or CT, EUS is the most sensitive test to identify a solid component, intracystic nodule, and allows one to perform cyst fluid analysis for cytology and tumor and molecular markers, as well as cyst wall biopsy. The diagnostic potential of EUS may be improved during surveillance using novel modalities such as contrast-enhanced EUS needle-based confocal laser end microscopy and EUS-guided microforceps biopsy.[1,117–122] Although EUS and other endoscopic tools are frequently used in the initial diagnosis and workup of patients with pancreatic cysts, including all cysts greater than 2 cm per most guidelines, there is a relatively smaller role for EUS in routine surveillance of low-risk presumed BD-IPMNs, with an increased role for noninvasive imaging. More frequently, EUS may also be used in surveillance alternating with MRI or CT imaging in patients who are considered to be at a higher risk of developing cancer but who have elected to forego surgery in the absence of a definitive diagnosis of cancer or HGD such as in main-duct IPMN or presumed BD-IPMN greater than 3 cm with or without small intracystic epithelial nodules. During PCN surveillance, EUS is used for further clarification and to rule out associated masses or nodules in patients who develop WFs. The role of subsequent EUS-FNA and cyst fluid analysis purely in surveillance has been studied. It may encourage changes in management if there is evidence of a cancer or HGD or if the tumor marker profile or molecular analysis changes the initial diagnosis.[76] There does not appear to be a definite role for serial surveillance pancreatic cyst fluid analysis to justify its routine use in surveillance other than for when a pancreatic cyst EUS is indicated.[123]

There is a limited role for ERCP and pancreatoscopy in the routine surveillance of patients with pancreatic cysts, with it being used primarily for main-duct and mixed-duct IPMN surveillance to assist in detecting and biopsy intraductal nodularity.

CA19-9

An elevated serum CA19-9 is considered a WF although the real value utility of this biomarker in pancreatic cyst surveillance is unclear because of its low sensitivity and specificity for detecting pancreatic malignancy.[124,125] Nonetheless it is typically included in pancreatic cyst surveillance and acted upon with more frequent imaging including EUS imaging when it is elevated or rises during surveillance.

HgBA1c

Similarly, there has been increased recognition of the risk associated between new-onset type 2 diabetes and pancreatic cancer. Although the risk is low and is typically within the 3 years after the onset of the DM, there are now credible links between new-onset diabetes and the progression of pancreatic cyst neoplasms. To this extent, most PCN surveillance protocols now include serial HgBA1c to screen for either diabetes or glucose intolerance. However, it must be stated that because of the very high prevalence of type 2 DM in the general population, any increase in glucose is more than likely related to DM and not necessarily an underlying pancreas malignancy or progression of a pancreatic cyst under surveillance.

PANCREAS CYST NEOPLASM SURVEILLANCE CONTROVERSY: STOPPING FOR CYST STABILITY?

With the existing challenges of accurately characterizing BD-IPMNs, the determination of optimal duration of surveillance especially among stable, small, low-risk BD-IPMNs is an area of controversy. The assumption of persistent malignant risk, carcinogenesis being a stochastic event, lack of an understanding of the biology of malignant progression, and finally, the fear of concomitant PCs support lifelong surveillance. However, surveillance cessation is favored by low rates of malignant change especially among small cysts less than 1.5 cm in size, socioeconomic offsets, procedural risks associated with, and EUS as well as therapeutic resection.[126] The specific decision to stop surveillance of presumed low-risk BD-IPMNs (those without either WFs or HRS) is controversial and needs to balance the real risk of malignancy or developing malignancy (0.007 per person-years of follow-up) and IPMN-related mortality (0.9%), with the patient's life expectancy, quality of life expectations, and mortality from non-pancreatic-related causes.[19,22] The concept of stopping surveillance for small cysts which show stability after 2 years, in any age group, has been also suggested by the ACR and after 5 years of cyst stability by the AGA guidelines.[35,39,127,128]

In a recent multicenter prospective Japanese study of 1404 patients with IPMN, there was a cumulative incidence of pancreatic cancer of 3.3% at 5 years, 6.6% at 10 years, and 15% at 15 years. The risk of developing pancreatic cancer was 10-fold higher in this group than in age-match control subjects.[32] The risk of malignancy based on this and other presumed BD-IPMN surveillance studies has been quantified in a recent meta-analysis, which revealed that among 100 individuals with BD-IPMNs with initial 5 years of size stability, extended surveillance over the next 5 years would yield 2 PCs but progress to WF/HRS in 19 patients.[129]

For now, there are not enough data to support stopping surveillance universally after 5 or even 10 years of "stability" although there is a pressing need to reign in costly surveillance strategies without supporting outcomes data. A hope in the era of precision medicine is that a combination of patient factors (age, comorbidity state, preference), cyst factors (histology subtype, presence or absence of WF/HRS, duration of surveillance), and more predictive pancreatic cyst fluid biomarkers will provide a more nuanced and informed decision-making process for stopping pancreatic cyst surveillance, especially for patients with very small presumed BD-IPMNs.[130–132]

PANCREATIC CYSTIC NEOPLASM SURVEILLANCE: COMPARING THE CLINICAL GUIDELINES

The absence of reliable imaging and biomarkers to predict advanced neoplasia in pancreatic cysts has necessitated the development of several clinical guidelines (revised ICG(2017), American College of Gastroenterology (ACG) AGA, ACR, and European Pancreatic Cyst Guidelines) to assist the clinician and patient in decision-making for surveillance.[19,133–135] In the case of surveillance, guidance on type, interval, and cessation of surveillance are often provided.[19,127,133,136] One of the major criticism of the current set of guidelines is the very-low-quality evidence available upon which to develop and generate these guidelines. This results in several recommendations being based primarily on expert opinion in the absence of data. Several efforts are being made to improve this, but for now, we are beholden to the current set of guidelines.

Endoscopic Ultrasound in Pancreatic Cystic Neoplasm Surveillance

The revised ICG support EUS during surveillance for further evaluation of all patients with WFs, as well as routine use in surveillance for cysts greater than 3 cm, whereas the AGA guidelines only recommend EUS for patient with pancreatic cysts greater than 3 cm and who have either a solid mass or a dilated main pancreatic duct. The European guidelines are nonspecific on EUS use including in surveillance.

The Worrisome Feature "Rate of Growth" During Pancreatic Cystic Neoplasm Surveillance

Rapid cyst growth has been emphasized as a WF among the revised ICG 2017, European, ACR, and ACG guidelines. ACR guidelines stratified rapid growth based on the initial lesion size, that is, among cysts, <0.5 cm was represented by a 100% increase; among cysts, $\geq$0.5 cm and <1.5 cm, a 50% increase; and for cysts $\geq$1.5 cm, a 20% increase in long-axis diameter was considered as rapid growth. Other consensus guidelines use absolute size cutoffs (including 5 mm/2 years [revised ICG], 5 mm/year [EG], 3 mm/year [ACG]) as thresholds to define rapid IPMN growth. Interestingly, these recommendations were based on select cohort studies demonstrating significant association of rapid cyst growth with HGD/invasive carcinoma.[137,138] Thus, rapid cyst growth as a WF necessitates EUS evaluation and surveillance intensification.[38,46] In contrast to all the other guidelines, AGA recommended that an increase in the size of the cyst was not a statistically significant risk factor for malignancy.

Surgical Referral During Pancreatic Cystic Neoplasm Surveillance

The AGA guidelines are more stringent than the revised ICG guidelines when it comes to recommending surgical evaluation during surveillance, requiring the presence of 2 of 3 features (cyst size greater than 3 cm, a solid component, or a dilated main pancreatic duct), or if EUS finds suspicious or positive cytology, or confirms a dilated main pancreatic duct or solid lesion. The other guidelines including revised ICG, ACG, and European guidelines recommend surgery if any high-risk features are present. During the PCN surveillance, guidelines support patients with features proving or concerning for either HGD or cancer being referred for multidisciplinary management involving gastroenterology and surgical care at centers with high volume of pancreatic surgical expertise.

Surveillance Regimens

The revised ICG use a combination of CT, MRI, and EUS imaging during surveillance with the modality and the interval being based on the size of the cyst (**Table 2**). Following the ICG guidelines, patients with BD-IPMNs and worrisome features are recommended to undergo EUS. More frequent surveillance imaging is recommended in patients with less than 2-cm BD-IPMNs and mural nodules larger than 5 mm, main duct involvement, or positive cytology on EUS. In patients with BD-IPMNs of 2 cm or greater and mural

Table 2
Clinical guidelines approach to surveillance of pancreatic cystic neoplasms without high-risk or worrisome features at diagnosis

Cyst Size	2015 AGA Guidelines	2017 ICG Guidelines	2018 European Guidelines	2018 ACG Guidelines	2017 ACR Guidelines
<1 cm	MRI at 1 year, then every 2 years	CT/MRI in 6 months, then every 2 years if stable	EUS/MRI & CA19–9 for 1 year; then annually	MRI every 2 years, lengthen if stable	Cysts <1.5 cm: MRI/CT 1 year
1–2 cm	MRI at 1 year, then every 2 years	CT/MRI Q6 months for 1 year; annually for 2 years; lengthen if stable	EUS/MRI & CA19–9 Q6months for 1 year; then annually	MRI annually for 2 yrs., then every 2 years	Cysts 1.5–2.5 cm: MRI/CT Q6months x4, then lengthen if stable
2–3 cm	MRI at 1 year, then every 2 years	EUS in Q3-6 months; lengthen to every year with alternating MRI/EUS as appropriate	EUS/MRI & CA19–9 Q6months for 1 year; then annually	EUS/MRI Q6months for 3 years then annually	Cysts ≥ 2.5 cm: MRI/CT annually for 10 years
≥3 cm	MRI at 1 year, then every 2 years	Close surveillance; alternate MRI/EUS 3–6 months	EUS/MRI & CA19–9 Q6 months for 1 year; then annually	EUS/MRI Q6 months for 3 yrs. then annually	As above

Abbreviations: MRI, magnetic resonance imaging.

nodules of 5 mm or larger, main-duct involvement, or positive cytology on EUS, surgical consideration is more strongly recommended, especially for young and surgically fit patients. According to revised ICG, BD-IPMNs that do not require immediate resection should undergo active surveillance with short-interval follow-up initially (3–6 months from diagnosis) and then extended according to specific size-based intervals if stable. However, individual surveillance recommendations may depend on the presence of worrisome features.

The AGA guidelines favor using MRI annually for all cyst recommending the use of EUS for patients who develop morphologic change during surveillance. The European guidelines suggest either MRI or EUS in routine surveillance. The ACG guidelines provide size-based recommendations on active surveillance strategies for patients with IPMNs/MCNs that do not require immediate resection.[19] The ACR recommendations stratify surveillance recommendations by patient age, tumor size, and involvement of the main PD with further refinement according to internal growth or development of concerning features. There are variable proposed surveillance schedules for patients with stable cysts smaller than 2.5 cm. For patients with cysts small than 2.5 cm with interval growth, worrisome features or HRS EUS-FNA is recommended.[5,21,22] For patients with cysts larger than 2.5 cm, interval growth, worrisome features, or HRS, EUS-FNA and surgical consultation are recommended. With ACR guidelines, patients older than 80 years are recommended to undergo less-frequent screening over a shorter overall surveillance period, whereas patients younger than 65 years are recommended to undergo more frequent surveillance imaging. In general, surveillance should continue for 10 years even if cysts are stable and have low risk or until the patient is no longer a surgical candidate.

Stopping Surveillance

Stopping surveillance after stable cyst imaging for 5 years is a recommendation of the AGA guidelines, and after 10 years of stability in low-risk cysts, or sooner if the patients reaches 80 years of age after stability, or until the patients is no longer a surgical candidate is the recommendations of the ACR (**Table 3**). This issue of ceasing surveillance is not addressed in the other PCN clinical guidelines.[88] The ACG guidelines recommend that patients fit for surgery should continue surveillance until they are no longer surgical candidates, and that patients older than 75 years should undergo surveillance imaging only after discussion with the multidisciplinary team.

Postoperative Surveillance

For patients who underwent pancreatic resections, heterogeneity in the surveillance recommendations among various consensus guidelines is noted (**Table 4**). Both the revised ICG and European guidelines recommend ongoing postoperative surveillance of the residual tissue whether dysplasia is present or not in the resection specimen. According to the revised ICG guidelines, all patients who undergo surgical resection of IPMNs should continue surveillance until they are no longer surgical candidates. The European guidelines after resection surveillance recommendations vary by PCN subtype and the extent of surgery performed. However, the AGA guidelines do recommend MRI surveillance every 2 years after resection of a PCN with advanced neoplasia (malignancy or HGD). The AGA guidelines do not recommend ongoing surveillance for patients after resection if there is no evidence of invasive cancer or dysplasia on resection. Per the ACG guidelines: patients who undergo surgical resection for benign nonmucinous lesions (SCAs, pseudocyst) do not require postoperative surveillance; patients with resected solid pseudo papillary neoplasms should undergo yearly surveillance for 5 years; patients with resected MCNs without associated

Table 3
Guidelines approach for stopping surveillance based on cyst stability

Guidelines	Recommendation	Strength of Recommendation
2015 AGA Guidelines	Stop surveillance after 5 years if no significant change.	Conditional
2017 ICG Guidelines	Lifelong surveillance	Not reported
2018 European Guidelines	No rational term for termination of surveillance	Very weak recommendation Strong agreement
2018 ACG guidelines	Insufficient evidence to support discontinuing surveillance after 5≥ years in patients who are still surgically fit.	Conditional recommendation; very low quality of evidence
2017 ACR Guidelines	For most patients, 10-year follow-up recommended. patients > 80 years at Q2year imaging for 2 years and stop if stable or patient no longer surgical candidate	Not reported

Table 4
Guidelines approach to postoperative surveillance of pancreatic cysts

Histology of Resected Specimen	2015 AGA Guidelines	2017 ICG Guidelines	2018 European Guidelines	2018 ACG Guidelines	2017 ACR Guidelines
IPMN with Cancer	MRI Q2 years	Identical to the follow-up for resected PDAC	Identical to the follow-up for resected PDAC	Continue surveillance	No recommendations
IPMN with HGD	MRI Q2 years	MRI/CT at 6 months	IPMN with high-grade dysplasia or MD-IPMN:MRI/EUS Q6months for 2 years.	Continue surveillance	No recommendations
IPMN with LGD	No surveillance	MRI/CT at 6 months	Identical to the follow-up for nonresected IPMN	Continue surveillance	No recommendations
MCN with cancer	MRI Q2 years	Identical to PDAC follow-up	Identical to the follow-up for resected PDAC	MRI annually × 5 years	No recommendations
MCN without cancer	No surveillance	No recommendations	No recommendations	No surveillance	No recommendations
Serous cystadenoma	No surveillance	No recommendations	No recommendations	No surveillance	No recommendations
Cystic pancreatic neuroendocrine tumor	No recommendations	No recommendations	No recommendations	No recommendations	No recommendations
Solid-pseudopapillary neoplasm	No recommendations	No recommendations	No recommendations	MRI annually x 5 years	No recommendations

Abbreviations: EUS, endoscopic ultrasound; ICG, International Consensus Guidelines; IPMN, intraductal papillary mucinous neoplasm; MCN, Mucinous cystic neoplasm; MRCP, magnetic resonance cholangiopancreatography; MRI, magnetic resonance imaging.

adenocarcinoma do not require continued surveillance, but MCNs with advanced neoplasia should undergo surveillance for 5 years; patients with resected IPMNs should continue surveillance of the remaining pancreas regardless of whether advanced neoplasia was present on pathology. The ACR guidelines do not comment on postresection surveillance strategies. The surveillance intervals in the postoperative setting variy with the different guidelines with most recommending surveillance every 6 months, for 2 years and then yearly for patient with HGD in the resected pancreas.

PANCREATIC CYST SURVEILLANCE: FUTURE DIRECTIONS

A greater understanding of the biology and natural history of progression of pancreatic cysts is needed to improve our PCN surveillance strategies.[139] This in turn may permit the development and validation of a blood-based approach for pancreatic cyst diagnosis and stratification, as well as refining pancreatic cyst fluid biomarkers for prediction of natural history purposes.[140] Further studies on the role of chemoprevention and even PCN ablation to alter the natural history of PCNs may impact on how we survey these patients Additional prospective studies such as the ACRIN-ECOG 2185 which is a prospective randomized controlled trial comparing a high-intensity surveillance program with a low-intensity testing program will provide very valuable, needed, and detailed clinical outcome information on pancreatic cysts surveillance, which will allow for a more reasoned discussions about the intensity of surveillance, use of valuable resources, and when to consider stopping surveillance.[141]

DISCLOSURE

The authors have nothing to disclose.

REFERENCES

1. Jais B, Rebours V, Malleo G, et al. Serous cystic neoplasm of the pancreas: a multinational study of 2622 patients under the auspices of the International Association of Pancreatology and European Pancreatic Club (European Study Group on Cystic Tumors of the Pancreas). Gut 2016;65(2):305–12.
2. Berman JJ, Albores-Saavedra J, Bostwick D, et al. Precancer: a conceptual working definition – results of a Consensus Conference. Cancer Detect Prev 2006;30(5):387–94.
3. Gardner TB, Glass LM, Smith KD, et al. Pancreatic cyst prevalence and the risk of mucin-producing adenocarcinoma in US adults. Am J Gastroenterol 2013; 108(10):1546–50.
4. de Jong K, Nio CY, Hermans JJ, et al. High prevalence of pancreatic cysts detected by screening magnetic resonance imaging examinations. Clin Gastroenterol Hepatol 2010;8(9):806–11.
5. Laffan TA, Horton KM, Klein AP, et al. Prevalence of unsuspected pancreatic cysts on MDCT. AJR Am J Roentgenol 2008;191(3):802–7.
6. Kimura W, Nagai H, Kuroda A, et al. Analysis of small cystic lesions of the pancreas. Int J Pancreatol 1995;18(3):197–206.
7. Lee KS, Sekhar A, Rofsky NM, et al. Prevalence of incidental pancreatic cysts in the adult population on MR imaging. Am J Gastroenterol 2010;105(9):2079–84.
8. Mella JM, Gomez EJ, Omodeo M, et al. Prevalence of incidental clinically relevant pancreatic cysts at diagnosis based on current guidelines. Gastroenterol Hepatol 2018;41(5):293–301.

9. Adsay NV, Conlon KC, Zee SY, et al. Intraductal papillary-mucinous neoplasms of the pancreas: an analysis of in situ and invasive carcinomas in 28 patients. Cancer 2002;94(1):62–77.

10. Fukushima N, Mukai K, Sakamoto M, et al. Invasive carcinoma derived from intraductal papillary-mucinous carcinoma of the pancreas: clinicopathologic and immunohistochemical study of eight cases. Virchows Arch 2001;439(1):6–13.

11. Kloppel G. Clinicopathologic view of intraductal papillary-mucinous tumor of the pancreas. Hepato-Gastroenterology 1998;45(24):1981–5.

12. Cuillerier E, Cellier C, Palazzo L, et al. Outcome after surgical resection of intraductal papillary and mucinous tumors of the pancreas. Am J Gastroenterol 2000;95(2):441–5.

13. Fernández-del Castillo C, NV A. Intraductal papillary mucinous neooplasms of the pancreas. Gastroenterology 2010;139:708–13.

14. Kim TH, Song TJ, Lee SO, et al. Main duct and mixed type intraductal papillary mucinous neoplasms without enhancing mural nodules: Duct diameter of less than 10 mm and segmental dilatation of main pancreatic duct are findings support surveillance rather than immediate surgery. Pancreatology 2019;19(8): 1054–60.

15. Vanella G, Crippa S, Archibugi L, et al. Meta-analysis of mortality in patients with high-risk intraductal papillary mucinous neoplasms under observation. Br J Surg 2018;105(4):328–38.

16. Sakai A, Masuda A, Eguchi T, et al. Clinical outcome of conservatively managed pancreatic intraductal papillary mucinous neoplasms with mural nodules and main duct dilation. J Gastroenterol 2021;56(3):285–92.

17. Roch AM, DeWitt JM, Al-Haddad MA, et al. Nonoperative management of main pancreatic duct-involved intraductal papillary mucinous neoplasm might be indicated in select patients. J Am Coll Surg 2014;219(1):122–9.

18. Crippa S, Bassi C, Salvia R, et al. Low progression of intraductal papillary mucinous neoplasms with worrisome features and high-risk stigmata undergoing non-operative management: a mid-term follow-up analysis. Gut 2017; 66(3):495–506.

19. Tanaka M, Fernández-del Castillo C, Adsay V, et al. International consensus guidelines 2012 for the management of IPMN and MCN of the pancreas. Pancreatology 2012;12(3):183–97.

20. Farrell JJ, Fernandez-del Castillo C. Pancreatic cystic neoplasms: management and unanswered questions. Gastroenterology 2013;144(6):1303–15.

21. Ooka K, Rustagi T, Evans A, et al. Surveillance and outcomes of nonresected presumed branch-duct intraductal papillary mucinous neoplasms: a meta-analysis. Pancreas 2017;46(7):927–35.

22. Crippa S, Capurso G, Camma C, et al. Risk of pancreatic malignancy and mortality in branch-duct IPMNs undergoing surveillance: A systematic review and meta-analysis. Dig Liver Dis 2016;48(5):473–9.

23. Pergolini I, Sahora K, Ferrone CR, et al. Long-term risk of pancreatic malignancy in patients with branch duct intraductal papillary mucinous neoplasm in a referral center. Gastroenterology 2017;153(5):1284–1294 e1281.

24. Mukewar S, de Pretis N, Aryal-Khanal A, et al. Fukuoka criteria accurately predict risk for adverse outcomes during follow-up of pancreatic cysts presumed to be intraductal papillary mucinous neoplasms. Gut 2017;66(10):1811–7.

25. Lawson RD, Hunt GC, Giap AQ, et al. Pancreatic cysts suspected to be branch duct intraductal papillary mucinous neoplasm without concerning features have

low risk for development of pancreatic cancer. Ann Gastroenterol 2015;28(4): 487–94.

26. Gausman V, Kandel P, Van Riet PA, et al. Predictors of progression among low-risk intraductal papillary mucinous neoplasms in a multicenter surveillance cohort. Pancreas 2018;47(4):471–6.

27. Crippa S, Pezzilli R, Bissolati M, et al. Active surveillance beyond 5 years is required for presumed branch-duct intraductal papillary mucinous neoplasms undergoing non-operative management. Am J Gastroenterol 2017;112(7): 1153–61.

28. Lawrence SA, Attiyeh MA, Seier K, et al. Should patients with cystic lesions of the pancreas undergo long-term radiographic surveillance?: results of 3024 patients evaluated at a single institution. Ann Surg 2017;266(3):536–44.

29. Han Y, Lee H, Kang JS, et al. Progression of pancreatic branch duct intraductal papillary mucinous neoplasm associates with cyst size. Gastroenterology 2018; 154(3):576–84.

30. Kayal M, Luk L, Hecht EM, et al. Long-term surveillance and timeline of progression of presumed low-risk intraductal papillary mucinous neoplasms. AJR Am J Roentgenol 2017;209(2):320–6.

31. Marchegiani G, Andrianello S, Pollini T, et al. Trivial" cysts redefine the risk of cancer in presumed branch-duct intraductal papillary mucinous neoplasms of the pancreas: a potential target for follow-up discontinuation? Am J Gastroenterol 2019;114(10):1678–84.

32. Oyama H, Tada M, Takagi K, et al. Long-term risk of malignancy in branch-duct intraductal papillary mucinous neoplasms. Gastroenterology 2020;158(1): 226–237 e225.

33. Lee BS, Nguyen AK, Tekeste TF, et al. Long-term follow-up of branch-duct intraductal papillary mucinous neoplasms with No change in first 5 Years of diagnosis. Pancreatology 2021;21(1):144–54.

34. Balduzzi A, Marchegiani G, Pollini T, et al. Systematic review and meta-analysis of observational studies on BD-IPMNS progression to malignancy. Pancreatology 2021. S1424-3903(21)00148-4.

35. Farrell JJ. Prevalence, Diagnosis and Management of Pancreatic Cystic Neoplasms: Current Status and Future Directions. Gut Liver 2015;9(5):571–89.

36. Tanaka M. Intraductal papillary mucinous neoplasm of the pancreas as the main focus for early detection of pancreatic adenocarcinoma. Pancreas 2018;(47): 544–50.

37. Felsenstein MN, Masica M, Masica DL. IPMNs with co-occurring invasive cancers: neighbours but not always relatives. Gut 2018;67(9):1652–62.

38. Lafemina J, Katabi N, Klimstra D. Malignant progression in IPMN: a cohort analysis of patients initially selected for resection or observation. Ann Surg Oncol 2013;20(2):440–7.

39. Oyama H, Tada M, Takagi K, et al. Long-term risk of malignancy in branch duct intraductal papillary mucinous neoplasms. Gastroenterology 2020;158(1): 226–37.

40. Yamaguchi KKS, Hatori T, Maguchi H, et al. Pancreatic ductal adenocarcinoma derived from IPMN and pancreatic ductal adenocarcinoma concomitant with IPMN. Pancreas 2011;40(4):571–80.

41. Torisu YT, Kinoshita K, Tomita Y, et al. Pancreatic cancer screening in patients with presumed branch-duct intraductal papillary mucinous neoplasms. World J Clin Oncol 2019;10(2):67–74.

42. European Study Group on Cystic Tumours of the P. European evidence-based guidelines on pancreatic cystic neoplasms. Gut 2018;67(5):789–804.
43. Nilsson LN, Keane MG, Shamali A, et al. Nature and management of pancreatic mucinous cystic neoplasm (MCN): a systematic review of the literature. Pancreatology 2016;16(6):1028–36.
44. Ethun CG, Postlewait LM, McInnis MR, et al. The diagnosis of pancreatic mucinous cystic neoplasm and associated adenocarcinoma in males: an eight-institution study of 349 patients over 15 years. J Surg Oncol 2017; 115(7):784–7.
45. Crippa S, Salvia R, Warshaw AL, et al. Mucinous cystic neoplasm of the pancreas is not an aggressive entity: lessons from 163 resected patients. Ann Surg 2008;247(4):571–9.
46. Park JW, Jang JY, Kang MJ, et al. Mucinous cystic neoplasm of the pancreas: is surgical resection recommended for all surgically fit patients? Pancreatology 2014;14(2):131–6.
47. Allen PJ, D'Angelica M, Gonen M, et al. A selective approach to the resection of cystic lesions of the pancreas: results from 539 consecutive patients. Ann Surg 2006;244(4):572–82.
48. Kosumi K, Takamori H, Hashimoto D, et al. Mucinous cystic neoplasm of the pancreas activated during pregnancy. Surg Case Rep 2015;1(1):13.
49. Takashima S, Wato M, Inaba T, et al. A case of pancreatic mucinous cystic neoplasm that enlarged during pregnancy and was resected after childbirth. Nihon Shokakibyo Gakkai Zasshi 2014;111(9):1789–97.
50. Naganuma S, Honda K, Noriki S, et al. Ruptured mucinous cystic neoplasm with an associated invasive carcinoma of pancreatic head in a pregnant woman: report of a case and review of literature. Pathol Int 2011;61(1):28–33.
51. Friebe V, Keck T, Mattern D, et al. Serous cystadenocarcinoma of the pancreas: management of a rare entity. Pancreas 2005;31(2):182–7.
52. Tseng JF, Warshaw AL, Sahani DV, et al. Serous cystadenoma of the pancreas: tumor growth rates and recommendations for treatment. Ann Surg 2005;242(3): 413–9 [discussion: 419-421].
53. Chalian H, Tore HG, Rezai P, et al. MDCT evaluation of the growth kinetics of serous and benign mucinous cystic neoplasms of the pancreas. Cancer Imag 2011;11:116–22.
54. El-Hayek KM, Brown N, O'Rourke C, et al. Rate of growth of pancreatic serous cystadenoma as an indication for resection. Surgery 2013;154(4):794–800 [discussion: 800-792].
55. Das A, Wells CD, Nguyen CC. Incidental cystic neoplasms of pancreas: what is the optimal interval of imaging surveillance? Am J Gastroenterol 2008;103(7): 1657–62.
56. Le Borgne J, de Calan L, Partensky C. Cystadenomas and cystadenocarcinomas of the pancreas: a multiinstitutional retrospective study of 398 cases. French Surgical Association. Ann Surg 1999;230(2):152–61.
57. Davtyan H, Nieberg R, Reber HA. Pancreatic cystic endocrine neoplasms. Pancreas 1990;5(2):230–3.
58. Kamisawa T, Fukayama M, Koike M, et al. A case of malignant cystic endocrine tumor of the pancreas. Am J Gastroenterol 1987;82(1):86–9.
59. Fernandez-del Castillo C, Warshaw AL. Cystic tumors of the pancreas. Surg Clin North Am 1995;75(5):1001–16.
60. Singhi AD, Chu LC, Tatsas AD, et al. Cystic pancreatic neuroendocrine tumors: a clinicopathologic study. Am J Surg Pathol 2012;36(11):1666–73.

61. Gaujoux S, Tang L, Klimstra D, et al. The outcome of resected cystic pancreatic endocrine neoplasms: a case-matched analysis. Surgery 2012;151:518–25.
62. Boninsegna L, Partelli S, D'Innocenzio MM, et al. Pancreatic cystic endocrine tumors: a different morphological entity associated with a less aggressive behavior. Neuroendocrinology 2010;92:246–51.
63. Bordeianou L, Vagefi PA, Sahani DV, et al. Cystic pancreatic endocrine neoplams: a distinct tumor type? J Am Coll Surg 2008;206:1154–8.
64. Lee LC, Grant CS, Salomao DR, et al. Small, nonfunctioning, asymptomatic pancreatic neuroendocrine tumors (PNETs): Role for nonoperative management. Surgery 2012;152(6):965–74.
65. Gaujoux S, Partelli S, Maire F, et al. Observational study of natural history of small sporadic nonfunctioning pancreatic neuroendocrine tumors. J Clin Endocrinol Metab 2013;98(12):4784–9.
66. Haynes AB, Deshpande V, Ingkakul T, et al. Implications of incidentally discovered, nonfunctioning pancreatic endocrine tumors: short-term and long-term patient outcomes. Arch Surg 2011;146(5):534–8.
67. Kuo EJ, Salem RR. Population-level analysis of pancreatic neuroendocrine tumors 2 cm or less in size. Ann Surg Oncol 2013;20(9):2815–21.
68. Kunz PL, Reidy-Lagunes D, Anthony LB, et al. Consensus guidelines for the management and treatment of neuroendocrine tumors. Pancreas 2013;42(4):557–77.
69. Falconi M, Eriksson B, Kaltsas G, et al. ENETS consensus guidelines update for the management of patients with functional pancreatic neuroendocrine tumors and non-functional pancreatic neuroendocrine tumors. Neuroendocrinology 2016;103(2):153–71.
70. Ridtitid W, Halawi H, DeWitt JM, et al. Cystic pancreatic neuroendocrine tumors: outcomes of preoperative endosonography-guided fine needle aspiration, and recurrence during long-term follow-up. Endoscopy 2015;47(7):617–25.
71. Khristenko E, Garcia EE, Gaida MM, et al. Lymphoepithelial cyst of the pancreas: can common imaging features help to avoid resection? Langenbeck's Arch Surg 2023;408(1):82.
72. Bihari C, Rastogi A, Rajesh S, et al. Cystic lymphangioma of pancreas. Indian J Surg Oncol 2016;7(1):106–9.
73. Coe A, Conway J, Evans J, et al. The yield of EUS-FNA in undiagnosed upper abdominal adenopathy is very high. J Clin Ultrasound 2013;41(4):210–3.
74. Jathal A, Arsenescu R, Crowe G, et al. Diagnosis of pancreatic cystic lymphangioma with EUS-guided FNA: report of a case. Gastrointest Endosc 2005;61(7):920–2.
75. Bhatia V, Rastogi A, Saluja SS, et al. Cystic pancreatic lymphangioma. The first report of a preoperative pathological diagnosis by endoscopic ultrasound-guided cyst aspiration. JOP 2011;12(5):473–6.
76. Madhani K, Yousaf M, Aamar A, et al. Impact of endoscopic ultrasound on diagnosis and management of presumed mucinous neoplasms when done for pancreatic cyst morphology change on non-invasive surveillance imaging. Endosc Int Open 2019;7(4):E389–95.
77. Correa-Gallego C, Miyasaka Y, Hozaka Y, et al. Surveillance after resection of non-invasive intraductal papillary mucinous neoplasms (IPMN). A systematic review. Pancreatology 2023;23(3):258–65.
78. Miller JR, Meyer JE, Waters JA, et al. Outcome of the pancreatic remnant following segmental pancreatectomy for non-invasive intraductal papillary mucinous neoplasm. HPB 2011;13(11):759–66.

79. Abraham SC, Klimstra D, Wilentz RE, et al. *Solid-pseudopapillary tumors of teh pancreas* are genetically distinct from pancreatic ductal adenocarcinomas and almost always harbor beta-catenin mutations. Am J Pathol 2002;160:1361–9.

80. Karsenti D, Caillol F, Chaput U, et al. Safety of endoscopic ultrasound-guided fine-needle aspiration for pancreatic solid pseudopapillary neoplasm before surgical resection: a european multicenter registry-based study on 149 patients. Pancreas 2020;49(1):34–8.

81. Serra S, Chetty R. Revision 2: an immunohistochemical approach and evaluation of solid pseudopapillary tumour of the pancreas. J Clin Pathol 2008; 61(11):1153–9.

82. Rodriguez JR, Salvia R, Crippa S, et al. Branch-duct intraductal papillary mucinous neoplasms: observations in 145 patients who underwent resection. Gastroenterology 2007;133(1):72–9 [quiz: 309-310].

83. Pelaez-Luna M, Chari ST, Smyrk TC, et al. Do consensus indications for resection in branch duct intraductal papillary mucinous neoplasm predict malignancy? A study of 147 patients. Am J Gastroenterol 2007;102(8):1759–64.

84. Weinberg BM, Spiegel BM, Tomlinson JS, et al. Asymptomatic pancreatic cystic neoplasms: maximizing survival and quality of life using Markov-based clinical nomograms. Gastroenterology 2010;138(2):531–40.

85. Charlson M, Szatrowski TP, Peterson J, et al. Validation of a combined comorbidity index. J Clin Epidemiol 1994;47(11):1245–51.

86. Piccirillo JF, Tierney RM, Costas I, et al. Prognostic importance of comorbidity in a hospital-based cancer registry. JAMA 2004;291(20):2441–7.

87. Fernandez-del Castillo C, Morales-Oyarvide V, McGrath D, et al. Evolution of the whipple procedure at the massachusetts general hospital. Surgery 2012;152(3 Suppl 1):S56–63.

88. Sahora K, Ferrone CR, Brugge WR, et al. Effects of comorbidities on outcomes of patients with intraductal papillary mucinous neoplasms. Clin Gastroenterol Hepatol 2015;13(10):1816–23.

89. Kawakubo K, Tada M, Isayama H, et al. Risk for mortality from causes other than pancreatic cancer in patients with intraductal papillary mucinous neoplasm of the pancreas. Pancreas 2013;42(4):687–91.

90. Kwok K.N., Eunis W. and Wu B., Comorbidities should be considered in the management of pancreatic cystic neoplasms, *Gastroenterology,* 146 (5), 2014, S-25.

91. Chhoda A, Yousaf MN, Madhani K, et al. Comorbidities drive the majority of overall mortality in low-risk mucinous pancreatic cysts under surveillance. Clin Gastroenterol Hepatol 2022;20(3):631–640 e631.

92. Wang KX, Ben QW, Jin ZD, et al. Assessment of morbidity and mortality associated with EUS-guided FNA: a systematic review. Gastrointest Endosc 2011; 73(2):283–90.

93. Overbeek KA, Kamps A, van Riet PA, et al. Pancreatic cyst surveillance imposes low psychological burden. Pancreatology 2019;19(8):1061–6.

94. Shieh FK, Siddiqui UD, Padda M, et al. Anxiety and perception of cancer risk in patients undergoing endoscopic ultrasonography for pancreas cystic lesions. Pancreas 2013;42(3):548–9.

95. Verma D, Kwok KK, Wu BU. Patient preferences for management of cystic neoplasms of the pancreas: a cross-sectional survey study. Pancreas 2017;46(3): 352–7.

96. Marinelli V, Secchettin E, Andrianello S, et al. Psychological distress in patients under surveillance for intraductal papillary mucinous neoplasms of the

pancreas: the "Sword of Damocles" effect calls for an integrated medical and psychological approach a prospective analysis. Pancreatology 2020;20(3): 505–10.

97. Nieminen H, Roine R, Ristimaki A, et al. Health-related quality of life and anxiety levels among patients under surveillance for intraductal papillary mucinous neoplasm. BMC Gastroenterol 2023;23(1):14.

98. Schweber AB, Brooks C, Agarunov E, et al. New onset diabetes predicts progression of low risk pancreatic mucinous cysts. Pancreatology 2020;20(8): 1755–63.

99. Sofi AA, Ahmad S, Peerzada M, et al. Diabetes mellitus and the risk of progression or malignancy of pancreatic cystic neoplasms in patients undergoing surveillance: a systematic review and meta-analysis. Pancreatology 2022;22(8): 1195–201.

100. Yamaguchi A, Tazuma S, Tamaru Y, et al. Long-standing diabetes mellitus increases concomitant pancreatic cancer risk in patients with intraductal papillary mucinous neoplasms. BMC Gastroenterol 2022;22(1):529.

101. Dbouk M, Brewer Gutierrez OI, Lennon AM, et al. Guidelines on management of pancreatic cysts detected in high-risk individuals: an evaluation of the 2017 Fukuoka guidelines and the 2020 International Cancer of the Pancreas Screening (CAPS) consortium statements. Pancreatology 2021;21(3):613–21.

102. Abe K, Kitago M, Kosaki K, et al. Genomic analysis of familial pancreatic cancers and intraductal papillary mucinous neoplasms: a cross-sectional study. Cancer Sci 2022;113(5):1821–9.

103. Nehra D, Oyarvide VM, Mino-Kenudson M, et al. Intraductal papillary mucinous neoplasms: does a family history of pancreatic cancer matter? Pancreatology 2012;12(4):358–63.

104. Mandai K, Uno K, Yasuda K. Does a family history of pancreatic ductal adenocarcinoma and cyst size influence the follow-up strategy for intraductal papillary mucinous neoplasms of the pancreas? Pancreas 2014;43(6):917–21.

105. Liu K, Joshi V, van Camp L, et al. Prevalence and outcomes of pancreatic cystic neoplasms in liver transplant recipients. World J Gastroenterol 2017;23(48): 8526–32.

106. Sugawara T, Franco SR, Ishida J, et al. Prevalence and progression of intraductal papillary mucinous neoplasms of the pancreas in solid organ transplant recipients: a systematic review. Am J Transplant 2023;23(3):429–36.

107. Lobo JM, Scheiman JM, Zaydfudim VM, et al. Clinical and economic outcomes of patients undergoing guideline-directed management of pancreatic cysts. Am J Gastroenterol 2020;115(10):1689–97.

108. Yousaf MN, Zhang Z, Chhoda A, et al. Su1459 – imaging resource utilization in active pancreatic cyst surveillance. Gastroenterology 2019;156(6):S-559.

109. Sharib J, Esserman L, Koay EJ, et al. Cost-effectiveness of consensus guideline based management of pancreatic cysts: the sensitivity and specificity required for guidelines to be cost-effective. Surgery 2020;168(4):601–9.

110. Luk L, Hecht EM, Kang S, et al. Society of abdominal radiology disease focused panel survey on clinical utilization of incidental pancreatic cyst management recommendations and template reporting. J Am Coll Radiol 2021;18(9): 1324–31.

111. Hecht EM, Khatri G, Morgan D, et al. Intraductal papillary mucinous neoplasm (IPMN) of the pancreas: recommendations for standardized imaging and reporting from the society of abdominal radiology IPMN disease focused panel. Abdom Radiol (NY) 2021;46(4):1586–606.

112. Maimone S, Agrawal D, Pollack MJ, et al. Variability in measurements of pancre-atic cyst size among EUS, CT, and magnetic resonance imaging modalities. Gastrointest Endosc 2010;71(6):945–50.

113. Ip IK, Mortele KJ, Prevedello LM, et al. Focal cystic pancreatic lesions: assess-ing variation in radiologists' management recommendations. Radiology 2011; 259(1):136–41.

114. Dunn DP, Brook OR, Brook A, et al. Measurement of pancreatic cystic lesions on magnetic resonance imaging: efficacy of standards in reducing inter-observer variability. Abdom Radiol (NY) 2016;41(3):500–7.

115. Serafini S, Sperti C, Brazzale AR, et al. The role of positron emission tomography in clinical management of intraductal papillary mucinous neoplasms of the pancreas. Cancers 2020;12(4).

116. Yu MH, Kim JH, Kang HJ, et al. Transabdominal Ultrasound for follow-up of inci-dentally detected low-risk pancreatic cysts: a prospective multicenter study. AJR Am J Roentgenol 2021;216(6):1521–9.

117. Lisotti A, Napoleon B, Facciorusso A, et al. Contrast-enhanced EUS for the char-acterization of mural nodules within pancreatic cystic neoplasms: systematic re-view and meta-analysis. Gastrointest Endosc 2021;94(5):881–889 e885.

118. Yamashita Y, Ueda K, Itonaga M, et al. Usefulness of contrast-enhanced endo-scopic sonography for discriminating mural nodules from mucous clots in intra-ductal papillary mucinous neoplasms: a single-center prospective study. J Ultrasound Med 2013;32(1):61–8.

119. Krishna SG, Modi RM, Kamboj AK, et al. In vivo and ex vivo confocal endomi-croscopy of pancreatic cystic lesions: a prospective study. World J Gastroen-terol 2017;23(18):3338–48.

120. Kadayifci A, Atar M, Basar O, et al. Needle-based confocal laser endomicro-scopy for evaluation of cystic neoplasms of the pancreas. Dig Dis Sci 2017; 62(5):1346–53.

121. Napoleon B, Lemaistre AI, Pujol B, et al. In vivo characterization of pancreatic cystic lesions by needle-based confocal laser endomicroscopy (nCLE): propo-sition of a comprehensive nCLE classification confirmed by an external retro-spective evaluation. Surg Endosc 2016;30(6):2603–12.

122. Nakai Y, Iwashita T, Park DH, et al. Diagnosis of pancreatic cysts: EUS-guided, through-the-needle confocal laser-induced endomicroscopy and cystoscopy trial: DETECT study. Gastrointest Endosc 2015;81(5):1204–14.

123. Rahal MA, DeWitt JM, Patel H, et al. Serial EUS-Guided FNA for the surveillance of pancreatic cysts: a study of long-term performance of tumor markers. Dig Dis Sci 2022;67(11):5248–55.

124. Morales-Oyarvide V, Fong ZV, Fernandez-Del Castillo C, et al. Intraductal papil-lary mucinous neoplasms of the pancreas: strategic considerations. Visc Med 2017;33(6):466–76.

125. Wang W, Zhang L, Chen L, et al. Serum carcinoembryonic antigen and carbo-hydrate antigen 19-9 for prediction of malignancy and invasiveness in intraduc-tal papillary mucinous neoplasms of the pancreas: a meta-analysis. Biomed Rep 2015;3(1):43–50.

126. Ciprani D, Weniger M, Qadan M, et al. Risk of malignancy in small pancreatic cysts decreases over time. Pancreatology 2020;20(6):1213–7.

127. Berland LL, Silverman SG, Gore RM, et al. Managing incidental findings on abdominal CT: white paper of the ACR incidental findings committee. J Am Col Radiol 2010;7:754–73.

128. Khannoussi W, Vullierme MP, Rebours V, et al. The long term risk of malignancy in patients with branch duct intraductal papillary mucinous neoplasms of the pancreas. Pancreatology 2012;12(3):198–202.
129. Chhoda A, Singh S, Sheth AH, et al. Benefit of extended surveillance of low-risk pancreatic cysts after 5-year stability: a systematic review and meta-analysis. Clin Gastroenterol Hepatol 2022. S1542-3565(22)00450-5.
130. Farrell JJ. Editorial: stopping pancreatic cyst surveillance? Am J Gastroenterol 2017;112(7):1162–4.
131. Farrell JJ. Does pancreatic cyst stability justify stopping intraductal papillary mucinous neoplasm surveillance? Gastroenterology 2020;158(1):44–6.
132. Paik KY, Choi SH, Heo JS, et al. Solid tumors of the pancreas can put on a mask through cystic change. World J Surg Oncol 2011;9:79.
133. Tanaka M, Chari S, Adsay V, et al. International consensus guidelines for management of intraductal papillary mucinous neoplasms and mucinous cystic neoplasms of the pancreas. Pancreatology 2006;6(1–2):17–32.
134. Del Chiaro M, Verbeke C, Salvia R, et al. European experts consensus statement on cystic tumours of the pancreas. Dig Liver Dis 2013;45(9):703–11.
135. Vege SS, Ziring B, Jain R, et al. Clinical Guidelines C, American Gastroenterology A. American gastroenterological association institute guideline on the diagnosis and management of asymptomatic neoplastic pancreatic cysts. Gastroenterology 2015;148(4):819–22 [quize:812-813].
136. Italian Association of Hospital G, Endoscopists, Italian Association for the Study of the P, et al. Italian consensus guidelines for the diagnostic work-up and follow-up of cystic pancreatic neoplasms. Dig Liver Dis 2014;46(6):479–93.
137. Kang MJ, Jang JY, Lee KB, et al. Long-term prospective cohort study of patients undergoing pancreatectomy for intraductal papillary mucinous neoplasm of the pancreas: implications for postoperative surveillance. Ann Surg 2014;260(2):356–63.
138. Kwong WT, Hunt GC, Fehmi SM, et al. Low rates of malignancy and mortality in asymptomatic patients with suspected neoplastic pancreatic cysts beyond 5 years of surveillance. Clin Gastroenterol Hepatol 2016;14(6):865–71.
139. Hernandez S, Parra ER, Uraoka N, et al. Diminished immune surveillance during histologic progression of intraductal papillary mucinous neoplasms offers a therapeutic opportunity for cancer interception. Clin Cancer Res 2022;28(9):1938–47.
140. Zhang C, Al-Shaheri FN, Alhamdani MSS, et al. Blood-based diagnosis and risk stratification of patients with pancreatic intraductal papillary mucinous neoplasm (IPMN). Clin Cancer Res 2022.
141. Weinberg DS, Gatsonis C, Zeh HJ, et al. Comparing the clinical impact of pancreatic cyst surveillance programs: A trial of the ECOG-ACRIN cancer research group (EA2185). Contemp Clin Trials 2020;97:106144.
142. Broughton J, Lipschitz J, Cantor M, et al. Determining the natural history of pancreatic cystic neoplasms: a Manitoban cohort study. HPB (Oxford) 2016;18(4):383–8.
143. Chung JW, Chung MJ, Park JY, et al. Clinicopathologic features and outcomes of pancreatic cysts during a 12-year period. Pancreas 2013;42(2):230–8.
144. Del Chiaro M, Ateeb Z, Hansson MR, et al. Survival Analysis and Risk for Progression of Intraductal Papillary Mucinous Neoplasia of the Pancreas (IPMN) Under Surveillance: A Single-Institution Experience. Ann Surg Oncol 2017;24(4):1120–6.

145. Han Y, Jang JY, Oh MY, et al. Natural history and optimal treatment strategy of intraductal papillary mucinous neoplasm of the pancreas: Analysis using a nomogram and Markov decision model. J Hepatobiliary Pancreat Sci 2021; 28(2):131–42.

146. Keane MG, Dadds HR, El Sayed G, et al. Clinical and radiological features that predict malignant transformation in cystic lesions of the pancreas: a retrospective case note review. AMRC Open Res 2020;1:4. https://doi.org/10.12688/amrcopenres.12860.2.

147. Lee BS, Nguyen AK, Tekeste TF, et al. Long-term follow-up of branch-duct intraductal papillary mucinous neoplasms with No change in first 5 Years of diagnosis. Pancreatology 2021;21(1):144–54.

148. Marchegiani G, Andrianello S, Pollini T, et al. "Trivial" Cysts Redefine the Risk of Cancer in Presumed Branch-Duct Intraductal Papillary Mucinous Neoplasms of the Pancreas: A Potential Target for Follow-Up Discontinuation? Am J Gastroenterol 2019;114(10):1678–84.

149. Moris M, Raimondo M, Woodward TA, et al. International Intraductal Papillary Mucinous Neoplasms Registry: Long-Term Results Based on the New Guidelines. Pancreas 2017;46(3):306–10.

150. Mukewar S, de Pretis N, Aryal-Khanal A, et al. Fukuoka criteria accurately predict risk for adverse outcomes during follow-up of pancreatic cysts presumed to be intraductal papillary mucinous neoplasms. Gut 2017;66(10):1811–7.

151. Ohno E, Hirooka Y, Kawashima H, et al. Natural history of pancreatic cystic lesions: A multicenter prospective observational study for evaluating the risk of pancreatic cancer. J Gastroenterol Hepatol 2018;33(1):320–8.

152. Pandey P, Pandey A, Luo Y, et al. Follow-up of Incidentally Detected Pancreatic Cystic Neoplasms: Do Baseline MRI and CT Features Predict Cyst Growth? Radiology 2019;292(3):647–54.

153. Yoshioka T, Shigekawa M, Ikezawa K, et al. Risk Factors for Pancreatic Cancer and the Necessity of Long-Term Surveillance in Patients With Pancreatic Cystic Lesions. Pancreas 2020;49(4):552–60.

Risk Models for Pancreatic Cyst Diagnosis

Alice Cattelani, MD[a], Giampaolo Perri, MD[a], Giovanni Marchegiani, MD, PhD[a], Roberto Salvia, MD, PhD[a], Stefano Francesco Crinò, MD[b,*]

KEYWORDS

- Pancreatic cystic neoplasm • IPMN • Pancreatic cancer

KEY POINTS

- Clinical decision-making for pancreatic cysts is based mostly on morphological features.
- Correct identification of malignancy-associated characteristics allows to reduce significant diagnostic errors.
- New reliable biomarkers are necessary to optimize risk models for malignant progression of pancreatic cysts.

INTRODUCTION

The overall prevalence of undefined pancreatic cysts (PCs) in the general population ranges from 2.6% to 15%, increasing with age to 37% in patients older than 80 years.[1,2] In clinical practice PCs are often incidentally discovered due to the extensive use of high-quality cross-sectional imaging in clinical practice.[3]

According to the latest World Health Organization classification PCs are divided into benign, premalignant, and malignant lesions.[4]

This classification is based on histopathological features, which are often difficult to determine precisely without surgical resection. Therefore, discriminating against these entities could be challenging, and in clinical practice the conundrum remains to discriminate each patient's malignancy risk and to decide whether to proceed with surveillance or undergo surgery. There has been increasing evidence on how most of the PCs do not eventually harbor associated invasive cancer or high-grade dysplasia (HGD), despite being advised for resection.[5–7] On the other hand, in many patients the risk of progression to malignancy during surveillance remains challenging to exclude with absolute certainty. The timing of resection could be categorized according to final pathology as "too early" (low-grade dysplasia), "too late" (invasive cancer), and "timely" (intermediate-grade dysplasia and HGD).[8] The challenge for

[a] Department of General and Pancreatic Surgery, The Pancreas Institute, University of Verona Hospital Trust, Verona, Italy; [b] Gastroenterology and Digestive Endoscopy Unit, The Pancreas Institute, G.B. Rossi University Hospital, Verona, Italy
* Corresponding author. Gastroenterology and Digestive Endoscopy Unit, Verona University Hospital (Borgo Roma), Piazzale Scuro 10, Verona 37134, Italy.
E-mail address: stefanofrancesco.crino@aovr.veneto.it

Gastrointest Endoscopy Clin N Am 33 (2023) 641–654
https://doi.org/10.1016/j.giec.2023.03.011
1052-5157/23/© 2023 Elsevier Inc. All rights reserved.
giendo.theclinics.com

clinicians is to identify the "timely" target of the surgical resection. Unfortunately, in real life PCs, and in particular intraductal papillary mucinous neoplasms (IPMNs), resemble the Schrödinger's cat[9]: unless the observer (surgeon) opens the box (patient's belly), the cat (IPMNs) is both alive (low-grade) and dead (high-grade) at the same time.[10] Only observational studies may identify further dynamic predictors of malignant transformation, with the aim of identifying with better accuracy HGD before the occurrence of cancer.

In the attempt to guide the clinicians in their everyday practice, expert consensus policies regarding the PCs' management have been condensed into guidelines, as summarized in **Fig. 1**.[11–14] Guidelines summarize predictors of malignant progressions that should be interpreted as dynamics predictors. The correct identification of malignancy-associated characteristics allows to reduce significant diagnostic error. Indeed, several studies showed that even at high-volume centers, preoperative diagnosis seems to be not correct in approximatively one-third of incidentally discovered PCs that underwent resection.[3,15] For this reason, several different invasive and noninvasive imaging modalities are applied routinely during the diagnostic workup to assess PCs' morphology, such as contrast-enhanced computed tomography (CT), MRI with magnetic resonance cholangiopancreatography (MRCP), contrast-enhanced ultrasonography, and endoscopic ultrasonography (EUS) with cyst fluid aspirate.

In this narrative review, the current knowledge regarding PC's morphologic features will be presented, correlating their presence to the estimated risk of malignancy and discussing available diagnostic tools to minimize clinically relevant diagnostic errors.

DIAGNOSTIC TOOLS
Radiology

CT and MRI are used to characterize PCs. Unfortunately, the accuracy of radiological images to identify PCs subtypes remains low, the accuracy of MRI to predict a specific

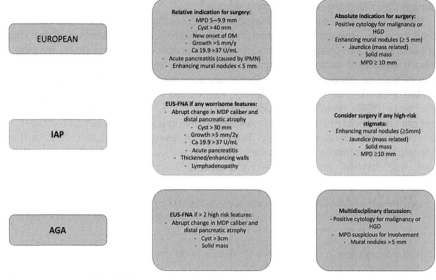

Fig. 1. International Guidelines on PCs. Ca 19.9, carbohydrate antigen 19-9; DM, mellitus diabetes; EUS-FNA, endoscopic ultrasound fine-needle aspiration; HGD, high-grade dysplasia; MPD, main pancreatic duct.

diagnosis varies between 50% and 86%, and the accuracy of CT in establishing a specific diagnosis ranges between 39% and 61.4%.[16] The sensitivities of MRI/MRCP for assessing main pancreatic duct (MPD) communication and internal septations have been reported to be 91% and 100%, respectively.[17] MRI is also more sensitive than CT to identify the presence of solid component or a mural node (MN) and to identify multifocal PCs.[18,19]

Endoscopy

EUS with or without fine-needle aspiration (FNA) is considered an ideal diagnostic modality for pancreatic cystic lesions, as it provides high-resolution images of PCs. In fact, EUS permits to accurately measure cyst size; clearly visualize the presence of septations, calcifications, or mural nodules; and assess the MPD diameter. In addition, it evaluates the PC's communications with MPD or its side branches.

EUS is recommended, as a second-line examination in addition to CT/MRI, when a radiological diagnosis of malignancy is not conclusive and/or whenever a PCs has clinical or radiological features of concern.[11,13,20] Guidelines offer guidance of whom to select for EUS-FNA based on the presence of specific risk features. The Fukuoka guideline recommends EUS for patients with any one of these clinical or radiologic worrisome features (pancreatitis, size $\geq$ 3 cm, enhancing nodule < 5 mm, main pancreatic duct 5–9 mm, thick cyst wall, abrupt change in main pancreatic duct diameter with upstream parenchymal atrophy, lymphadenopathy, elevated serum carbohydrate antigen (CA) 19-9, cyst growth $\geq$ 5 mm/2 years).[13] In a similar way, the European evidence-based guidelines (EEG) suggest EUS for patients with radiologic or clinical features of concern for malignancy (MPD $\geq$ 5 mm, size increase $\geq$ 5 mm/year, presence of mural nodule or solid component, jaundice secondary to posterior cruciate ligament, new-onset diabetes, increased CA 19-9).[11] Instead, the American Gastroenterological Association (AGA) guideline suggests EUS only for cysts with 2 high-risk imaging features (size $\geq$ 3 cm, solid component, or dilated main pancreatic duct) or if significant changes develop in the cyst during surveillance.[12]

FNA is often performed to obtain definitive diagnosis when malignancy transformation is suspected, particularly when solid component or MN are presumed by radiological investigations. The addition of EUS-FNA to abdominal imaging significantly increases the overall accuracy for diagnosis of neoplastic PCs.[21]

Guidelines do not clearly underline when it is deemed necessary to perform FNA for PCs during an EUS evaluation; in fact indications for EUS or FNA are not strictly the same. However, it is reasonable to perform EUS-FNA in all situations with features associated to a high risk of malignancy or when a histopathological diagnosis may change the clinical decision.[22]

Contrast-enhanced harmonic EUS (CH-EUS) is considered by available literature not superior to EUS to characterize different types of PCs. However, the role of CH-EUS is fundamental to better characterize mural nodules.[23] In fact, CH-EUS differentiates mucin clots from MNs with sensitivity, specificity, positive predictive value, negative predictive value, and accuracy of 100%, 80%, 92%, 100%, and 94%, respectively.[24] Olar and colleagues showed how CH-EUS FNA through an enhancing mural nodule in PCs resulted positive for any dysplasia or malignancy in 100% of cases and HGD or malignancy in 76.9% of cases.[23]

Biomarkers

The analysis of the PC fluid (CF) could be useful to improve the diagnostic accuracy to differentiate mucinous versus nonmucinous PCs and to define the malignant potentiality; however, CF analysis alone has a low diagnostic surrender of approximately 50%.[22]

In fact, carcinoembryonic antigen (CEA) could be dosed in CF. Several studies demonstrate that CF CEA level is higher in malignant/potentially malignant cysts than in benign cysts.[25] Furthermore, a threshold of CEA greater than 192 ng/L is used to differentiate mucinous from nonmucinous cysts with sensitivity, specificity, and accuracy of 75%, 84%, and 79%, respectively.[26,27] In literature, there is not full agreement on the upper limit cut-off of CEA; it is generally agreed that CEA less than 5 ng/mL is highly specific for nonmucinous PCs, with specificity reaching 95%, and CEA greater than 800 ng/mL is highly specific for mucinous PCs, with a specificity of 98%.[28,29]

In malignant/potentially malignant cysts, a lower level of CF glucose has been found, markedly consumed, compared with benign cysts (21.5 vs 68.5). Cyst glucose concentration is more predictive of mucinous PCs than CEA, with a cyst fluid glucose level of less than <50 mg/dL indicating a mucinous cyst with a sensitivity of 91% and specificity of 75% versus 67% and 80%, respectively, for CEA in the same study population.[30] In a systematic review sensitivity, specificity, and accuracy associated with intracystic glucose testing was 91%, 86%, and 94%, respectively.[31] It is important to emphasize that glucose is a simple and cheap biomarker.[25]

CA 19-9 is a diagnostic and prognostic tumor biomarker for pancreatic adenocarcinoma.[32–34] The elevation of CA 19-9 has been associated with both HGD and invasive cancer.[13,35] Fukuoka guidelines consider the elevation of CA 19.9 as a worrisome feature, and the EEG considers it a relative criteria for resection.[11,13] The AGA guidelines describe the elevation of CA 19-9 as a concerning feature of malignancy during PC surveillance.[12] A single-center study shows that an elevated CA 19-9 level is associated with malignancy in IPMN. In fact, in patients with HGD or invasive cancer a CA 19-9 level greater than 37 U/m was found. Furthermore, this percentage increases to 79% using a cut-off value of 100 U/ml. In the same study the use of serum CEA was also evaluated, but a correlation between an elevation of this tumor biomarker and malignancy in IPMN was not found.[36] It is important to underline that this study is based on a surgical series and that serum CA 19.9 is more closely associated with invasive cancer rather than HGD.

In the recent years, the next-generation sequencing (NGS) analysis permits to evaluate mutated oncogenes in CF sample. In particular, guanine nucleotide-binding protein–alpha subunit (GNAS) and Kirsten rat sarcoma virus (KRAS) genes are the most common mutated oncogenes in pancreatic cancer, and these mutations tend to occur also in mucinous PC tumorigeneses. KRAS and GNAS analysis achieved a sensitivity, specificity, and diagnostic accuracy of 94%, 91%, and 97%, respectively.[37] Pancreatic ductal adenocarcinoma arising from mucinous PCs is associated with mutation of TP53, SMAD4, CTNNB1, and the mammalian target of rapamycin.[30]

Mutations in the multiple endocrine neoplasia 1 (MEN1) gene or loss of heterozygosity are related with pancreatic neuroendocrine tumors with sensitivity and specificity of 68% and 98%, respectively. Furthermore, mutations in the von Hippel–Lindau gene are related with serous cystadenomas (SCNs) with a sensitivity and specificity of 71% and 100%.[30]

NGS represent the future for PCs' risk stratification; however, these types of diagnostic tests are particularly expensive; larger studies are necessary to identify the most cost-effective, accurate, and easily performable option.

Cytology

The cytology of CF has a low diagnostic power, due to low cellularity of the CF. Researchers have developed new strategies to evaluate PCs at the cellular level.

Different studies reported a new technique based on an EUS needle cytology brush introduced through a 19-gauge needle[38,39]; this technique presents difficulty in advancing the brush through a 19-gauge needle; furthermore, a randomize controlled trial showed that it does not improve the diagnostic power compared with EUS FNA.[40] Owing to these evidences and to the difficult related with this technique, interest in the use of EUS needle cytology brush has decreased. Another technique is EUS-through-the-needle biopsy (EUS-TTNB); a microforceps device (a forceps < 1 mm in diameter) is advanced through a 19-gauge EUS needle. A recent analysis reported the diagnostic yield of EUS-TTNB to be 74% and a diagnostic performance of 80%, with an adverse event rate of 5%.[28]

CLINICAL AND MORPHOLOGICAL RISK FACTORS
Symptoms

In literature, several studies based on surgical series reported the rate of symptomatic PCs ranging from 44% to 80%.[37,41] In clinical practice, except for jaundice and acute pancreatitis, it is very difficult to correlate the symptoms, such as abdominal pain, with the presence of PCs. Marchegiani and colleagues demonstrated that 1 out 3 patients diagnosed with a PC experienced abdominal pain; however, this prevalence was similar in the control group (patients without PCs). Only the patients with PCs located in the body-tail reported an increased prevalence of symptoms.[42] In observational studies, the presence of symptoms range from 17% to 21%.[43,44] Guidelines classify jaundice as a "absolute indication" for surgery, as strictly correlated with the presence of an invasive malignant component. It is important to underline how, despite very rarely, benign cysts may also cause jaundice (ie, large SCN in the pancreatic head). Conversely, acute pancreatitis is a "relative indication" (RI) for surgery.

Size

The International Association of Pancreatology (IAP) and AGA guidelines set a dimensional cut-off greater than or equal to 30 mm as a "worrisome feature" (WF), an indication to perform EUS-FNA,[12,13] whereas EEG set a dimensional cut-off greater than or equal to 40 mm as an RI for surgery.[11] It is important to underline that both these cut-offs have been chosen arbitrarily, as in literature a strong correlation between dimension and malignancy of PCs does not exist. In fact, PCs dimensions are not always related to their potential malignancy, depending on their nature: SCNs are, for example, always benign regardless of their dimension, whereas solid pseudopapillary tumors are always malignant. The association between size and malignancy is particularly present in mucinous cysts, without a precise cut-off. In different surgical series, the presence of PC size greater than or equal to 30 mm had a positive predictive value for malignancy ranging between 27% and 33%.[45–48] A single-institution analysis of the results from a surveillance program for patients with IPMN demonstrated that branch duct IPMN less than 40 mm can be safely observed, in the absence of other risk factors.[49] The size alone is probably not an appropriate indication for surgery in the absence of other risks factor, as the probability of malignancy is very low in such cases.[48] Recently, the PC growth rate has been considered a more accurate parameter to predict malignant transformation, as probably a better expression of PC biology.[50] As a matter of fact, IAP guidelines, in the last version, included a rapid rate of cyst growth greater than 5 mm/2 year in the list of WFs.[13] The EEG also underline the importance of the cyst growth rate but with a different cut-off compared with IAP guidelines. In fact the EEG considered the PC size increase to greater than or equal to 5 mm/year as an RI for surgery.[11] A retrospective analysis of patients with branch duct IPMN followed-up for more than 5 years underlined the importance of individualized surveillance protocols based on initial PC size and rate of growth.[44] The use of a dynamic perspective and the role of growth rate are stressed also in a retrospective analysis by Marchegiani and colleagues. The investigators, in compliance with the IAP guidelines, dichotomized the growth rate at 2.5 mm/year and found that developing a high-risk stigmata (HRS) during surveillance resulted statistically associated with a growth rate greater than or equal to 2.5 mm/year.[50]

Mural Nodes or Solid Component

The presence of MNs is a predictor of malignancy in PCs, considered as a morphologic expression of tumor proliferation. The presence of MNs should be investigated with contrast-enhanced MRI or CT. In a retrospective study MRI, both with dynamic study and diffusion-weighted imaging, showed an accuracy of 89.01% in detection of solid mural nodules greater than or equal to 5 mm.[51] EUS should be considered whenever the presence of MNs in unclear and for differentiating MNs to mucin clots.[13] The misperception of mucin clots for MNs is a critical issue for the endoscopist; a way to solve this problem is evaluate the echogenicity. In fact, mucin clots are hypoechoic with a hyperechoic rim and smooth surface instead MNs are isohyperechoic with irregular margin.[52] CH-EUS permit to distinguish between these lesions. CH-EUS had a good sensitivity (88.2%) and relatively high specificity (79.1%) for the diagnosis of MNs harboring HGD or invasive carcinoma. The pooled sensitivity increased to 97.0% and the pooled specificity to 90.4% when a dedicated contrast-harmonic mode is used.[52] MNs are one of the strongest predictors of malignancy, but the evidence of MNs alone does not directly relate with the presence of pancreatic cancer. As a matter of fact, the size of the MNs seems to be proportionally related to the risk of malignancy.[53] A meta-analysis determinate that the presence and the size of MNs has a substantial role in predicting malignancy in IPMNs.[50] A dimensional cut-off is necessary and helpful to guide clinicals and balance the advantages and disadvantages of different management in patients with relevant surgical risk and high risk of postoperative morbidity. The 2017 IAP guidelines indicated surgical resection for an enhanced MNs greater than or equal to 5 mm, based on a systematic review and meta-analyses together with a surgical series, confirming that MNs are the strongest predictor of either HGD or invasive cancer for all types of IPMNs.[54]

Dilatation of Main Pancreatic Duct

The international guidelines recommend surgery for patients with MPD greater than or equal to 10 mm (EEG have a lover cut-off, recommending resection when MPD is larger than 6 mm), whereas for patients with MPD between 5 and 9 mm it is recommended to perform additional diagnostics, similar to EUS, to clarify the risk of malignancy.[11–13] In surgical series, the MPD dilatation represents an independent predictor of malignancy.[7] Del Chiaro and colleagues showed that MPD, even low levels from 5 mm to 9.9 mm, is the best predictor of high-grade IPMN or invasive IPMN. They performed additional analyses and found that MPD from 5 to 7 mm could be considered the more accurate cut-off to identify patients with the highest risk.[7] In tertiary referral centers EUS-FNA is a safe and feasible procedure and considering that MPD is a strong independent factor of malignancy, EUS-FNA should be performed to obtain adequate cytological analysis whenever feasible.[55]

It is important to underline that the presence of MPD could be associated with different conditions other than IPMNs, for example periampullary or intrapancreatic neoplasms occluding/invading the duct or benign conditions as chronic pancreatitis, pancreas divisum, and mucous secretion from IPMNs arising in branch ducts.

Marchegiani and colleagues showed that in patients kept under surveillance the presence of MPD dilatation alone does not increase the risk of malignancy. In fact, MPD dilatation seemed associated to elevate risk of malignancy only when associated to other features of malignancy.[56] Crippa and colleagues analyzed a cohort of 281 patients with WFs and high-risk stigmata (HRS) who did not underwent surgical resection for advanced age or significant comorbidities. This study showed that 83 patients with MPD between 5 and 9 mm had a 5-year disease-specific survival of 96%, despite harboring a WF.[57] A close follow-up with MRI and MRCP may be a reasonable choice for this patient with MPD dilatation alone.

A recent prospective study analyzed 774 healthy volunteers undergoing standardized whole-body MRI with MRCP; the investigators found that the MPD diameter is increasing with age and exceeds the conventional upper reference value of 3 mm in a significant percentage of healthy subjects, even in those younger than 65 years.[58]

GUIDELINES AS RISK MODELS

Three main guidelines exist on the management of PCs (see **Fig. 1**): (1) the IAP guidelines, published in 2006 and updated in 2012 and 2016; (2) the EEG published in 2013 and updated in 2017; and (3) the AGA guidelines published in 2015.[11–13]

All guidelines identify risk factors of malignancy that need immediate surgery (high-risk stigmata or absolute indication for surgery); these risk factors are jaundice, enhancing mural nodule greater than 5 mm, solid mass in the pancreas, MPD greater than or equal to 10 mm, HGD, or cancer on cytology. The international guidelines and the European guidelines also identify a second category of risk, named WFs or RIs for surgery. According to IAP guidelines WFs should be investigated with EUS-FNA, and consequently clinicians may consider both surgery and close surveillance. Close surveillance is indicated when patients have significant comorbidities or when EUS does not clearly show predictors of malignancy.[13] Instead, a more aggressive policy is recommended by EEG. Surgical resection is recommended when a single RI is present in surgically fit patients, or when 2 or more RIs are identified in patients with significant comorbidities, without performing EUS.[11] The indication for surgery is particularly controversial in case of presence of some WFs/RIs (as MPD between 5 and 9 mm). These guidelines are fundamental to guide and uniform the clinical practice; however, recommendations are based on expert opinions or scientific evidence based mostly on surgical series and on few observational studies. Surgical series overestimated the risk of developing malignancy; for this reason guidelines have high sensitivity and low specificity ergo high rate of surgical overtreatment.

Furthermore, conflicts exit between guidelines and clinical practices. In fact, a recent study using a simulation-based model built in a digital app underlined that a relevant number of clinicians do not follow the available guidelines. In particular, in 16% of cases the responders did not choose any of the available guidelines.[14]

In case of small and presumptive benign cysts, which represent most newly diagnosed PCs, there is no international nor interdisciplinary consensus regarding the follow-up duration or criteria for follow-up discontinuation. The standardization of age or surgical candidacy–based endpoints for surveillance up discontinuation is an important aspect for the correct allocation of limited health care resources.

An observational multicentric study focusing on a cohort of patients affected by IPMNs who crossed over from surveillance to surgery demonstrated how patients with a stable WF during follow-up carried the lowest risk of harboring HGD/invasive cancer. On the other hand, the development of an additional WF or HRS during surveillance was associated with a higher rate of HGD/invasive cancer at final pathological evaluation. The obstructive jaundice is the only feature associated with an increased rate of invasive cancer at final pathological examination when the risk factors are considered as a static entity. This study stresses the concept that the dynamic interpretation of risk factors over time seems to be the most effective way to predict the development of malignancy in patients with PCs.[59]

FUTURE RISK PREDICTORS

DNA-based testing has emerged as an adjunct to the assessment of PCs. A prospective study of DNA-based molecular testing of EUS-FNA–obtained preoperative CF supported the usage of NGS analysis in CF given the high sensitivity and specificity in classifying PCs, especially IPMNs, and in the diagnosis of IPMNs with advanced neoplasia. In **Table 1** sensitivities and specificities of molecular testing and other diagnostic modalities based on 102 surgically resected PCs are summarized.[60] Future studies are required to explore the integration of DNA-based molecular testing into current management guidelines.

Roth and colleagues identified a serum protein signature discriminating low- and high-risk IPMN analyzing serum proteome with an antibody microarray platform. This signature in conjunction with routine clinical parameters reliably risk stratifies IPMN with an accuracy of 93%. It is fundamental to highlight that this is a retrospective single-center study including patients with pathologically confirmed IPMN following surgical resection; future studies are required to assess the diagnostic accuracy of this serum protein classifier and multiparameter model.[61]

Pollini and colleagues studied the role of the immune system in the progression of IPMN. The investigators showed how the tumor immune microenvironment of IPMNs

Table 1
Sensitivities and specificities of molecular testing based on 102 surgically resected pancreatic cysts

Parameter	Sensitivity (95% CL)	Specificity (95% CL)
IPMNs		
KRAS and/or GNAS mutations	100% (0.92–1.00)	96% (0.84–0.99)
IPMNs with advances neoplasia		
TP53, PIK3CA, and/or PTEN alterations	88% (0.62–0.98)	95% (0.88–0.98)
KRAS and/or GNAS mutations with TP53, PIK3CA, and/or PTEN alterations	88% (0.62–0.98)	97% (0.89–0.99)
GNAS MAF >55% or TP53|PIK3CA|PTEN MAFs at least equal to KRAS|GNAS MAFs	100% (0.77–1.00)	100% (0.95–1.00)
IPMNs and MNCs		
KRAS and/or GNAS mutations	89% (0.62–0.98)	100% (0.88–1.00)
IPMNs and MCN with advances neoplasia		
TP53, PIK3CA, and/or PTEN alterations	79% (0.54–0.93)	95% (0.88–0.98)
KRAS and/or GNAS mutations with IP53, PIK3CA, and/or PTEN alterations	79% (0.54–0.93)	96% (0.89–0.99)
GNAS MAF >55% or TP53|PIK3CA|PTEN MAFs at least equal to KRAS|GNAS MAFs	89% (0.66–0.98)	100% (0.95–1.00)

Abbreviations: IPMN, intraductal papillary mucinous neoplasm; MAF, mutant allele; MCN, mucinous cystic neoplasm.

Adapted from Singhi AD, McGrath K, Brand RE, et al. Preoperative next-generation sequencing of pancreatic cyst fluid is highly accurate in cyst classification and detection of advanced neoplasia. *Gut.* 2018;67(12):2131-2141.

evolves during malignant progression; a cytotoxic immune response rich in CD8+ T cells and a paucity of suppressing immunocytes changes to an immunosuppressive environment when neoplasms progress from low-grade dysplasia to HGD and then to invasive carcinoma. This evidence suggests that therapies that support cytotoxic T cells could be ideal for IPMNs with low-risk disease, whereas treatments that target regulatory T cells, myeloid-derived suppressor cells, and inhibitory macrophages could play a role in reducing malignant progression and treating high-risk disease. However, further studies are needed.[62] Another important future skill is artificial intelligence combined with EUS; in fact, EUS provides an image consisting of pixel that it is processed and organized by deep learning with algorithm to differentiate and stratify PCs. A recent study analyzed 5505 images from 28 PCs and correctly identified mucinous versus nonmucinous PCs with 98.3% sensitivity, 98.9% specificity, and 98.5% accuracy.[63] Another study analyzed 3355 EUS images from 43 patients who underwent pancreatectomy, artificial intelligence differentiated between high- and low-grade IPMNs by analyzing EUS images with an accuracy of 99.6%.[64,65]

SURGICAL RISK MODELS FOR PANCREATIC CYSTS

The cautious, risk-based approach to PC described by this review is necessary in order to select for surgery of only candidates with appropriate oncological targets (HGD or invasive carcinoma), sparing the burden of unnecessary operations to patients who do not show clinical or radiographic signs of malignancy. Pancreatic surgery is indeed

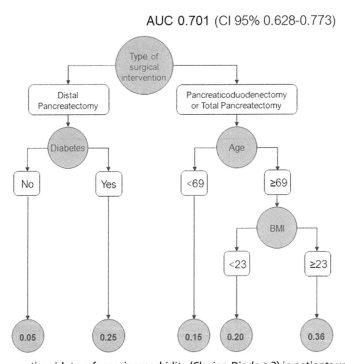

Fig. 2. Preoperative risk-tree for major morbidity (Clavien-Dindo ≥3) in patients undergoing pancreatic resection for IPMNs. BMI, body mass index. (*From* Marchegiani G, Crippa S, Perri G, et al. Surgery for Intraductal Papillary Mucinous Neoplasms of the Pancreas: Preoperative Factors Tipping the Scale of Decision-Making. Ann Surg Oncol. 2022;29(5):3206-3214.)

still burdened by high rates of major morbidity and mortality, and defining the surgical outcomes of pancreatectomy for PCs is important to identify independent predictors for major postoperative morbidity, and eventually have a preoperative disease-specific tool to predict the likelihood of major morbidity and postoperative pancreatic insufficiency. A recent bicentric study found that the overall major postoperative morbidity of pancreatic resection for IPMN is similar to that for other indications, in particular 23.9%. According to this study, the risk of major morbidity and postoperative pancreatic insufficiency in patients with IPMNs could be preoperatively stratified according to the type of intervention, based on the presence of preoperative diabetes, age, body mass index, and cyst size (**Fig. 2**). Being aware of such characteristics in the preoperative setting allows a proper surgical risk assessment that should drive counseling and personalize clinical decisions in surgical candidates, scaling the risk of malignancy with the surgical risk.

SUMMARY

In conclusion, despite the fact that an ideal test to discriminate malignancy in PCs does not yet exist, risk models to predict progression in PCs based on currently available predictors are able to minimize clinically relevant diagnostic errors. Regardless, future predictors are necessary to better understand the malignant progression of PCs.

CLINICS CARE POINTS

- Multifocality and communication between the cyst and the main pancreatic duct are highly suggestive of IPMN.
- Thruogh-the-needle biopsy is the only tool to retrieve histological specimens from the cyst wall, but the risk of adverse events is high in IPMN patients.[65]
- CH-EUS is the most sensitive investigation to differentiate mucus/debris from mural nodule or solid component.

DISCLOSURE

None.

REFERENCES

1. Lee KS, Sekhar A, Rofsky NM, et al. Prevalence of incidental pancreatic cysts in the adult population on MR imaging. Am J Gastroenterol 2010;105(9):2079–84.
2. Farrell JJ. Prevalence, Diagnosis and Management of Pancreatic Cystic Neoplasms: Current Status and Future Directions. Gut Liver 2015;9(5):571–89.
3. Correa-Gallego C, Ferrone CR, Thayer SP, et al. Incidental pancreatic cysts: do we really know what we are watching? Pancreatology 2010;10(2–3):144–50.
4. Nagtegaal ID, Odze RD, Klimstra D, et al. The 2019 WHO classification of tumours of the digestive system. Histopathology 2020;76(2):182–8.
5. Khoury RE, Kabir C, Maker VK, et al. What is the Incidence of Malignancy in Resected Intraductal Papillary Mucinous Neoplasms? An Analysis of Over 100 US Institutions in a Single Year. Ann Surg Oncol. Jun 2018;25(6):1746–51.
6. Attiyeh MA, Fernández-Del Castillo C, Al Efishat M, et al. Development and Validation of a Multi-institutional Preoperative Nomogram for Predicting Grade of

Dysplasia in Intraductal Papillary Mucinous Neoplasms (IPMNs) of the Pancreas: A Report from The Pancreatic Surgery Consortium. Ann Surg 2018;267(1): 157–63.

7. Del Chiaro M, Beckman R, Ateeb Z, et al. Main Duct Dilatation Is the Best Predictor of High-grade Dysplasia or Invasion in Intraductal Papillary Mucinous Neoplasms of the Pancreas. Ann Surg 2020;272(6):1118–24.

8. Tjaden C, Sandini M, Mihaljevic AL, et al. Risk of the Watch-and-Wait Concept in Surgical Treatment of Intraductal Papillary Mucinous Neoplasm. JAMA Surg 2021;156(9):818–25.

9. Schrödinger E. Die gegenwärtige Situation in der Quantenmechanik. Naturwissenschaften 1935;23:807–12.

10. Marchegiani G, Perri G, Salvia R. The quantum physics of intraductal papillary mucinous neoplasm of the pancreas. BJS Open 2022;6(3). https://doi.org/10.1093/bjsopen/zrac082.

11. ESGoCTot Pancreas. European evidence-based guidelines on pancreatic cystic neoplasms. Gut 2018;67(5):789–804.

12. Vege SS, Ziring B, Jain R, et al. American gastroenterological association institute guideline on the diagnosis and management of asymptomatic neoplastic pancreatic cysts. Gastroenterology 2015;148(4):819–22 [quiz: e12-3].

13. Tanaka M, Fernández-Del Castillo C, Kamisawa T, et al. Revisions of international consensus Fukuoka guidelines for the management of IPMN of the pancreas. Pancreatology 2017;17(5):738–53.

14. Marchegiani G, Balduzzi A, Pollini T, et al. The use of a mobile application to disseminate guidelines on cystic neoplasms of the pancreas - A snapshot study of 1000 case-simulations. Pancreatology 2021;21(8):1472–5.

15. Salvia R, Malleo G, Marchegiani G, et al. Pancreatic resections for cystic neoplasms: from the surgeon's presumption to the pathologist's reality. Surgery 2012;152(3 Suppl 1):S135–42.

16. Mohamed E, Jackson R, Halloran CM, et al. Role of Radiological Imaging in the Diagnosis and Characterization of Pancreatic Cystic Lesions: A Systematic Review. Pancreas 2018;47(9):1055–64.

17. Alwahbi O, Ghumman Z, van der Pol CB, et al. Pancreatic Cystic Lesions: Review of the Current State of Diagnosis and Surveillance. Can Assoc Radiol J 2022. https://doi.org/10.1177/08465371221130524. 8465371221130524.

18. Sahani DV, Kambadakone A, Macari M, et al. Diagnosis and management of cystic pancreatic lesions. AJR Am J Roentgenol 2013;200(2):343–54.

19. Waters JA, Schmidt CM, Pinchot JW, et al. CT vs MRCP: optimal classification of IPMN type and extent. J Gastrointest Surg 2008;12(1):101–9.

20. Ohno E, Hirooka Y, Itoh A, et al. Intraductal papillary mucinous neoplasms of the pancreas: differentiation of malignant and benign tumors by endoscopic ultrasound findings of mural nodules. Ann Surg 2009;249(4):628–34.

21. Khashab MA, Kim K, Lennon AM, et al. Should we do EUS/FNA on patients with pancreatic cysts? The incremental diagnostic yield of EUS over CT/MRI for prediction of cystic neoplasms. Pancreas 2013;42(4):717–21.

22. Lee LS. Updates in diagnosis and management of pancreatic cysts. World J Gastroenterol 2021;27(34):5700–14.

23. Olar MP, Bolboacă SD, Pojoga C, et al. Clinical Utility of the Contrast-Enhanced Endoscopic Ultrasound Guided Fine Needle Aspiration in the Diagnosis of Pancreatic Cyst. Diagnostics 2022;12(9). https://doi.org/10.3390/diagnostics12092209.

24. Yamashita Y, Ueda K, Itonaga M, et al. Usefulness of contrast-enhanced endoscopic sonography for discriminating mural nodules from mucous clots in intraductal papillary mucinous neoplasms: a single-center prospective study. J Ultrasound Med 2013;32(1):61–8.

25. Okasha HH, Abdellatef A, Elkholy S, et al. Role of endoscopic ultrasound and cyst fluid tumor markers in diagnosis of pancreatic cystic lesions. World J Gastrointest Endosc 2022;14(6):402–15.

26. Cizginer S, Turner BG, Bilge AR, et al. Cyst fluid carcinoembryonic antigen is an accurate diagnostic marker of pancreatic mucinous cysts. Pancreas 2011;40(7):1024–8.

27. Brugge WR, Lewandrowski K, Lee-Lewandrowski E, et al. Diagnosis of pancreatic cystic neoplasms: a report of the cooperative pancreatic cyst study. Gastroenterology 2004;126(5):1330–6.

28. van der Waaij LA, van Dullemen HM, Porte RJ. Cyst fluid analysis in the differential diagnosis of pancreatic cystic lesions: a pooled analysis. Gastrointest Endosc 2005;62(3):383–9.

29. Lopes CV. Cyst fluid glucose: An alternative to carcinoembryonic antigen for pancreatic mucinous cysts. World J Gastroenterol 2019;25(19):2271–8.

30. Paniccia A, Polanco PM, Boone BA, et al. Prospective, Multi-Institutional, Real-Time Next-Generation Sequencing of Pancreatic Cyst Fluid Reveals Diverse Genomic Alterations That Improve the Clinical Management of Pancreatic Cysts. Gastroenterology 2023;164(1):117–33.e7.

31. McCarty TR, Garg R, Rustagi T. Pancreatic cyst fluid glucose in differentiating mucinous from nonmucinous pancreatic cysts: a systematic review and meta-analysis. Gastrointest Endosc 2021;94(4):698–712.e6.

32. Lee KJ, Yi SW, Chung MJ, et al. Serum CA 19-9 and CEA levels as a prognostic factor in pancreatic adenocarcinoma. Yonsei Med J 2013;54(3):643–9.

33. Groot VP, Gemenetzis G, Blair AB, et al. Defining and Predicting Early Recurrence in 957 Patients With Resected Pancreatic Ductal Adenocarcinoma. Ann Surg 2019;269(6):1154–62.

34. Aoki S, Motoi F, Murakami Y, et al. Decreased serum carbohydrate antigen 19-9 levels after neoadjuvant therapy predict a better prognosis for patients with pancreatic adenocarcinoma: a multicenter case-control study of 240 patients. BMC Cancer 2019;19(1):252.

35. Del Chiaro M, Verbeke C, Salvia R, et al. European experts consensus statement on cystic tumours of the pancreas. Dig Liver Dis 2013;45(9):703–11.

36. Ciprani D, Morales-Oyarvide V, Qadan M, et al. An elevated CA 19-9 is associated with invasive cancer and worse survival in IPMN. Pancreatology 2020;20(4):729–35.

37. Masica DL, Dal Molin M, Wolfgang CL, et al. A novel approach for selecting combination clinical markers of pathology applied to a large retrospective cohort of surgically resected pancreatic cysts. J Am Med Inform Assoc 2017;24(1):145–52.

38. Lozano MD, Subtil JC, Miravalles TL, et al. EchoBrush may be superior to standard EUS-guided FNA in the evaluation of cystic lesions of the pancreas: preliminary experience. Cancer Cytopathol 2011;119(3):209–14.

39. Al-Haddad M, Raimondo M, Woodward T, et al. Safety and efficacy of cytology brushings versus standard FNA in evaluating cystic lesions of the pancreas: a pilot study. Gastrointest Endosc 2007;65(6):894–8.

40. Lariño-Noia J, de la Iglesia D, Iglesias-García J, et al. Endoscopic ultrasound cytologic brushing vs endoscopic ultrasound - fine needle aspiration for

cytological diagnosis of cystic pancreatic lesions. A multicenter, randomized open-label trial. Rev Esp Enferm Dig 2018;110(8):478–84.

41. Jang JY, Park T, Lee S, et al. Proposed Nomogram Predicting the Individual Risk of Malignancy in the Patients With Branch Duct Type Intraductal Papillary Mucinous Neoplasms of the Pancreas. Ann Surg 2017;266(6):1062–8.

42. Marchegiani G, Andrianello S, Miatello C, et al. The Actual Prevalence of Symptoms in Pancreatic Cystic Neoplasms: A Prospective Propensity Matched Cohort Analysis. Dig Surg 2019;36(6):522–9.

43. Mukewar S, de Pretis N, Aryal-Khanal A, et al. Fukuoka criteria accurately predict risk for adverse outcomes during follow-up of pancreatic cysts presumed to be intraductal papillary mucinous neoplasms. Gut 2017;66(10):1811–7.

44. Han Y, Lee H, Kang JS, et al. Progression of Pancreatic Branch Duct Intraductal Papillary Mucinous Neoplasm Associates With Cyst Size. Gastroenterology 2018; 154(3):576–84.

45. Sahora K, Mino-Kenudson M, Brugge W, et al. Branch duct intraductal papillary mucinous neoplasms: does cyst size change the tip of the scale? A critical analysis of the revised international consensus guidelines in a large single-institutional series. Ann Surg 2013;258(3):466–75.

46. Nguyen AH, Toste PA, Farrell JJ, et al. Current recommendations for surveillance and surgery of intraductal papillary mucinous neoplasms may overlook some patients with cancer. J Gastrointest Surg 2015;19(2):258–65.

47. Roch AM, Ceppa EP, DeWitt JM, et al. International Consensus Guidelines parameters for the prediction of malignancy in intraductal papillary mucinous neoplasm are not properly weighted and are not cumulative. HPB 2014;16(10): 929–35.

48. Robles EP, Maire F, Cros J, et al. Accuracy of 2012 International Consensus Guidelines for the prediction of malignancy of branch-duct intraductal papillary mucinous neoplasms of the pancreas. United European Gastroenterol J 2016; 4(4):580–6.

49. Del Chiaro M, Ateeb Z, Hansson MR, et al. Survival Analysis and Risk for Progression of Intraductal Papillary Mucinous Neoplasia of the Pancreas (IPMN) Under Surveillance: A Single-Institution Experience. Ann Surg Oncol 2017;24(4):1120–6.

50. Marchegiani G, Andrianello S, Pollini T, et al. Trivial" Cysts Redefine the Risk of Cancer in Presumed Branch-Duct Intraductal Papillary Mucinous Neoplasms of the Pancreas: A Potential Target for Follow-Up Discontinuation? Am J Gastroenterol 2019;114(10):1678–84.

51. D'Onofrio M, Tedesco G, Cardobi N, et al. Magnetic resonance (MR) for mural nodule detection studying Intraductal papillary mucinous neoplasms (IPMN) of pancreas: Imaging-pathologic correlation. Pancreatology 2021;21(1):180–7.

52. Lisotti A, Napoleon B, Facciorusso A, et al. Contrast-enhanced EUS for the characterization of mural nodules within pancreatic cystic neoplasms: systematic review and meta-analysis. Gastrointest Endosc 2021;94(5):881–9.e5.

53. Shimizu Y, Yamaue H, Maguchi H, et al. Predictors of malignancy in intraductal papillary mucinous neoplasm of the pancreas: analysis of 310 pancreatic resection patients at multiple high-volume centers. Pancreas 2013;42(5):883–8.

54. Marchegiani G, Andrianello S, Borin A, et al. Systematic review, meta-analysis, and a high-volume center experience supporting the new role of mural nodules proposed by the updated 2017 international guidelines on IPMN of the pancreas. Surgery 2018;163(6):1272–9.

55. Petrone MC, Magnoni P, Pergolini I, et al. Long-term follow-up of low-risk branch-duct IPMNs of the pancreas: is main pancreatic duct dilatation the most worrisome feature? Clin Transl Gastroenterol 2018;9(6):158.
56. Marchegiani G, Andrianello S, Morbin G, et al. Importance of main pancreatic duct dilatation in IPMN undergoing surveillance. Br J Surg 2018;105(13): 1825–34.
57. Crippa S, Bassi C, Salvia R, et al. Low progression of intraductal papillary mucinous neoplasms with worrisome features and high-risk stigmata undergoing non-operative management: a mid-term follow-up analysis. Gut 2017;66(3): 495–506.
58. Beyer G, Kasprowicz F, Hannemann A, et al. Definition of age-dependent reference values for the diameter of the common bile duct and pancreatic duct on MRCP: a population-based, cross-sectional cohort study. Gut 2023. https://doi.org/10.1136/gutjnl-2021-326106.
59. Marchegiani G, Pollini T, Andrianello S, et al. Progression vs Cyst Stability of Branch-Duct Intraductal Papillary Mucinous Neoplasms After Observation and Surgery. JAMA Surg 2021;156(7):654–61.
60. Singhi AD, McGrath K, Brand RE, et al. Preoperative next-generation sequencing of pancreatic cyst fluid is highly accurate in cyst classification and detection of advanced neoplasia. Gut 2018;67(12):2131–41.
61. Roth S, Bose P, Alhamdani MSS, et al. Noninvasive Discrimination of Low and High-risk Pancreatic Intraductal Papillary Mucinous Neoplasms. Ann Surg 2021;273(6):e273–5.
62. Pollini T, Adsay V, Capurso G, et al. The tumour immune microenvironment and microbiome of pancreatic intraductal papillary mucinous neoplasms. Lancet Gastroenterol Hepatol 2022;7(12):1141–50.
63. Vilas-Boas F, Ribeiro T, Afonso J, et al. Deep Learning for Automatic Differentiation of Mucinous versus Non-Mucinous Pancreatic Cystic Lesions: A Pilot Study. Diagnostics 2022;12(9). https://doi.org/10.3390/diagnostics12092041.
64. Schulz D, Heilmaier M, Phillip V, et al. Accurate prediction of histological grading of intraductal papillary mucinous neoplasia using deep learning. Endoscopy 2023. https://doi.org/10.1055/a-1971-1274.
65. Facciorusso A, Kovacevic B, Yang D, et al. Predictors of adverse events after endoscopic ultrasound-guided through-the-needle biopsy of pancreatic cysts: a recursive partitioning analysis. Endoscopy 2022;54(12):1158–68.

Innovation in the Surgical Management of Pancreatic Cystic Neoplasms

Same Operations, Narrower Indications, and an Individualized Approach to Decision-Making

Lauren E. Schleimer, MD[a], John A. Chabot, MD[b],
Michael D. Kluger, MD, MPH[c],*

KEYWORDS

- Pancreatic neoplasms • Intraductal papillary mucinous neoplasms
- Mucinous cystic neoplasms • Surgical procedures • Guidelines • Outcomes

KEY POINTS

- The major innovation in the surgical management of mucinous pancreatic cystic neoplasms has been narrowing the indications for operative intervention.
- Most mucinous pancreatic cystic neoplasms are managed with standard pancreatoduodenectomy or distal pancreatectomy, with controversy remaining around indications for total pancreatectomy and the role of parenchymal-sparing resection.
- Optimal decision-making incorporates clinical features, patient preferences and an individualized assessment of short-term and long-term risks and benefits.

Despite advances in the treatment of pancreatic ductal adenocarcinoma (PDAC), overall 5-year survival remains a dismal 11%.[1] This is due in part to the advanced nature of the disease on presentation and lack of viable screening modalities. Most PDAC are thought to originate from microscopic precursor lesions undetectable on imaging and clinically silent; others originate from certain pancreatic cystic neoplasms

[a] Department of Surgery, Columbia University Irving Medical Center, 177 Fort Washington Avenue, 8 Garden South, New York, NY 10032, USA; [b] Division of GI/Endocrine Surgery, Department of Surgery, Herbert Irving Pavilion, Columbia University Irving Medical Center, Columbia University, Vagelos College of Physicians & Surgeons, 161 Fort Washington Avenue, Suite 819, New York, NY 10032, USA; [c] Division of GI/Endocrine Surgery, Department of Surgery, Herbert Irving Pavilion, Columbia University Irving Medical Center, Columbia University, Vagelos College of Physicians & Surgeons, 161 Fort Washington Avenue, Suite 823, New York, NY 10032, USA
* Corresponding author.
E-mail address: mk2462@cumc.columbia.edu
Twitter: @lschleim (L.E.S.); @drkluger (M.D.K.)

Gastrointest Endoscopy Clin N Am 33 (2023) 655–677
https://doi.org/10.1016/j.giec.2023.03.003
1052-5157/23/© 2023 Elsevier Inc. All rights reserved.
giendo.theclinics.com

(PCNs). With increasing frequency and quality of abdominal imaging, a growing number of pancreatic cysts are incidentally diagnosed each year.[2] This has opened a window of opportunity for early intervention because the identification and resection of PCNs with malignant potential offers a means of preventing a deadly disease. Yet of the estimated 3 million patients with asymptomatic pancreatic cysts in the United States, a small minority of lesions poses a real threat of malignancy.[3]

Historically, the management of PCNs was operative. Most lesions were identified in symptomatic patients, and resection was the only reliable method of diagnosis and cancer prevention.[4,5] As diagnostic modalities improved, evidence for the safety of surveillance for select lesions accumulated. Guidelines were first developed in 2006 advocating for a more restrained approach,[6] and evolved to focus on targeting high-risk lesions for surgical management with judicious surveillance of lower risk lesions.[7–11]

Although minimally invasive approaches are now common, the actual operations have not fundamentally changed in decades. The operations performed for high-risk PCNs are standard oncologic resections—pancreatoduodenectomy, distal pancreatectomy, and total pancreatectomy.[12] Over the years, parenchymal-sparing resections (eg, enucleation, central pancreatectomy) have been proposed as alternatives to preserve pancreatic endocrine and exocrine function but their role in surgical management of PCNs has remained limited.[13] Controversy also remains around the indications for total pancreatectomy.[14]

Management of PCNs is dictated by balancing the risk of morbidity and mortality from pancreatic cancer against the morbidity and mortality of operative intervention. Thus, the primary targets for innovation in the surgical management of PCNs are individualized risk assessment and shared decision-making. In this article, we will review in broad strokes the developments in surgical management of PCNs, focusing on standards of care for operative intervention, including the extent of resection and operative approach. We will also review short-term and long-term outcomes of the surgical management of PCNs and discuss the importance of individualized risk–benefit assessment and shared decision-making.

EPIDEMIOLOGY OF PANCREATIC CYSTIC NEOPLASMS
Prevalence of Cysts

The increasing frequency and quality of diagnostic abdominal imaging has led to an explosion in diagnosis of PCNs. A 2019 meta-analysis estimated the pooled global prevalence of asymptomatic pancreatic cysts to be 8%[2]; however, retrospective series in the United States report up to 42% of individuals undergoing imaging for nonpancreatic indications have a pancreatic cyst, with estimates varying according to the setting, imaging modality and age of the population.[15,16] In one prospective study, full body MRI was performed on 1077 asymptomatic individuals identifying a weighted prevalence of pancreatic cysts of 48%. Among participants aged older than 80 years, the prevalence exceeded 75%.[17] Because imaging technology continues to improve, the prevalence of incidentally diagnosed cysts will continue to increase.[15]

Types of Cysts

Pancreatic cysts represent a variety of lesions including both neoplastic and nonneoplastic lesions. The WHO first published a classification of tumors of the pancreas in 1996,[18] with the most recent updates published in 2019.[19] Cystic lesions can be classified as nonneoplastic or neoplastic, and mucinous or nonmucinous. Nonneoplastic lesions include inflammatory pseudocysts; true nonneoplastic cysts are rare and include retention cysts and simple cysts. Among the neoplastic lesions, serous cystadenomas are nonmucinous and usually benign. Mucinous cystic neoplasms (MCNs) and intraductal papillary mucinous neoplasms (IPMNs) harbor malignant potential.[20] Less common nonmucinous neoplasms include cystic pancreatic neuroendocrine tumors and pseudopapillary neoplasms. Our focus in this article is the surgical management of PCNs with malignant potential, focusing on the mucinous lesions: MCNs and IPMNs.

IPMNs are dysplastic lesions of the ductal epithelium in communication with pancreatic ducts, characterized by dilated ducts and papillary projections. IPMNs are more common in men, with mean age of diagnosis in the sixth decade of life.[20] They are classified as main duct (MD-IPMNs) when greater than 5 mm segmental or diffuse dilation of the main pancreatic duct is present, branch duct (BD-IPMNs) when a mucinous cyst is in communication with a nondilated main pancreatic duct, or a mixed type (MT-IPMN) when both criteria are met.[7] Individuals may have multiple lesions throughout the pancreas and are at elevated risk of concomitant PDAC, suggesting the presence of IPMNs represents a "field defect" in which the entire ductal epithelium is at risk of dysplasia.[8]

MCNs are cystic adenomas occurring almost exclusively in women, typically diagnosed during the fourth and fifth decade of life.[20,21] MCNs are enveloped by a thick fibrous capsule containing ovarian-type stroma on pathology, and undergo malignant transformation through the adenoma to carcinoma sequence.[22] The vast majority occurs in the pancreatic body or tail and do not communicate with the ductal system.[21] Often MCNs are small, unifocal round cysts and may be difficult to differentiate from small BD-IPMNs on imaging.[21]

Although the true prevalence of each subtype of PCNs is not known, evidence from a 3-decade surgical series indicates IPMNs (51%) are the most frequently removed neoplastic cyst, followed by MCNs (16%), serous cystadenoma (13%), and pseudopapillary tumors (4%); up to 8% of resected lesions are nonneoplastic cysts including pseudocysts and true nonneoplastic cysts.[23] There has been a marked improvement in preoperative diagnostic accuracy over time. In the 1990s, concordance between the preoperative and final histopathologic diagnosis was only 45%; in the last decade, this has reached 80% and as high as 91% among patients who underwent EUS with cytology and molecular analysis.[23]

CURRENT GUIDELINES FOR OPERATIVE MANAGEMENT

Concerted efforts have been made to synthesize available evidence but no single uniform guideline for the management of PCNs yet exists. A recent review compared the 5 main guidelines[24]: the International Association of Pancreatology (IAP)[6-8] also known as Fukuoka guidelines, the European guidelines,[9] the American Gastroenterological Association (AGA) guidelines,[11] the American College of Gastroenterology (ACG) guidelines,[25] and the American College of Radiology (ACR) guidelines.[10,26] Each differs in its intended audience, patient population, type of cyst included, indications for operative intervention, and method and interval of surveillance.

Despite these extensive efforts, the predictive value of current guidelines remains suboptimal.[27,28]

Indications for Resection of Intraductal Papillary Mucinous Neoplasms

A comparison of the 2017 IAP and 2018 European guidelines' indications for surgery and recommended extent of resection for IPMNs is outlined in **Table 1**. Crippa and

Table 1
Current International Association of Pancreatology and European guidelines for the surgical management of intraductal papillary mucinous neoplasms

Guidelines	IAP, 2017[8]	European Consortium, 2018[9]
Risk stratification for surgery		
Elevated risk category	*Worrisome features*	*Relative indications*
Features	Cyst diameter ≥3 cm Enhancing mural nodule <5 mm Elevated Ca 19-9 MPD 5–9 mm Cyst growth rate ≥5 mm/2 y Abrupt change in caliber of MPD with distal atrophy Thickened/enhancing cyst walls Lymphadenopathy	Cyst diameter ≥4 cm Enhancing mural nodule <5 mm Elevated Ca 19-9 MPD 5–9.9 mm Cyst growth rate ≥5 mm/y New-onset diabetes mellitus Acute onset pancreatitis
Highest risk category	*High-risk stigmata*	*Absolute indications*
Features	Jaundice Enhancing mural nodule ≥5 mm MPD ≥10 mm	Jaundice Enhancing mural nodule ≥5 mm MPD ≥10 mm Solid mass Positive cytology for malignancy or high grade dysplasia
Extent of resection		
Whole gland involvement		
Diffuse MPD dilation	Pancreatoduodenectomy with frozen section to determine extent of resection if middle segment of MPD involved Consider total pancreatectomy if: • Young • Capable of managing pancreatic insufficiency • Definitive diagnosis • Larger degree of MPD dilation or presence of symptoms or mural nodules	Pancreatoduodenectomy with frozen section to determine extent of resection if MPD dilatation extends throughout pancreas Consider total pancreatectomy if: • Full length MPD dilatation with mural nodule in distal MPD • Familial pancreatic cancer

Multifocal BD-IPMN	Segmental resection to remove highest risk lesions with surveillance of remaining lesions Consider total pancreatectomy if strong family history of PDAC	Segmental resection to remove any high-risk lesions with frozen section to determine extent of resection and surveillance of remaining lesions Surveillance of cysts without concerning features
Parenchymal-sparing resection	Consider for BD-IPMN without clinical, radiologic, cytopathologic, or serologic suspicion of invasive carcinoma	Suitable only for low-risk lesions without risk factors
Margins	Additional resection only for high-grade dysplasia or malignancy Low grade dysplasia on margin acceptable	Additional resection only for high-grade dysplasia or malignancy Low grade dysplasia on margin acceptable

Abbreviations: BD-IPMN, branch-duct intraductal papillary mucinous neoplasm; IAP, International Association of Pancreatology; IPMN, intraductal papillary mucinous neoplasm; MPD, main pancreatic duct.

colleagues performed a retrospective review to assess the diagnostic accuracy of these two guidelines for pathologically confirmed IPMNs.[27] In their bi-institutional cohort, the malignancy rate for MD/MT-IPMNs and BD-IPMNs was 66% and 25%, respectively. Positive predictive values for diagnosing high-grade dysplasia or malignancy were 66% and 60% for the IAP and European guidelines, respectively.

The 2018 European guidelines offer absolute and relative indications for the surgical management of IPMNs (see **Table 1**). In healthy patients, the presence of even 1 relative indication justifies surgery, with a minimum of 2 for those with significant comorbidity.[9] Crippa and colleagues found the European guidelines were more sensitive, missing only 0.5% of IPMN-associated malignancy; however, overtreatment was common because 40% of patients had only low-grade dysplasia.

By contrast, the IAP guidelines had a lower rate of overtreatment for IPMNs (26%) but missed 10% of malignant IPMNs.[27] The 2017 IAP guidelines differentiate between "high-risk stigmata" and "worrisome features," incorporating endoscopic ultrasound (EUS) for further evaluation of lesions with worrisome features but no high-risk stigmata. EUS is used to differentiate mural nodules from accumulation of mucin, identify high-risk stigmata not seen on noninvasive imaging and perform cytology. Even if no worrisome features are present or EUS is equivocal, surgery is strongly considered for cysts 3 cm or greater in young, surgically fit patients and considered for cysts 2 cm or greater if patients would need prolonged surveillance.[8]

An earlier study evaluating the predictive value of the 2015 AGA, 2010 ACR, and 2012 IAP guidelines for malignancy in BD-IPMNs and asymptomatic MCNs highlighted the limitations of these guidelines for lesions with lower malignant potential than MD-IPMNs. The positive predictive values in this lower risk cohort ranged from 10% to 20%.[28] Notably, the 2015 AGA guidelines missed 93% of patients with high-grade dysplasia or malignancy, whereas the ACR and 2012 IAP guidelines missed 49% and 27%, respectively.

The 2015 AGA guidelines have also been criticized for calling to stop surveillance of stable cysts without high-risk features (ie, size <3 cm and without a solid component or dilated duct) after 5 years,[11] despite very-low quality of evidence.[29] The incidence of high-grade dysplasia or malignancy among patients with IPMNs continues to increase over time,[30–32] consistent with the underlying pathophysiology that makes age the greatest risk factor for both PCNs and PDAC. Stability at 5 years does not preclude malignant transformation, and the risk of PDAC among patients stable at 5 years remains elevated to 4 times the general population.[32] A large series of patients who underwent long-term surveillance of a BD-IPMNs per IAP guidelines found the cumulative incidence of PDAC was 3%, 7%, and 12% at 5, 10, and 15 years respectively, with a median time to surgery (5.7 years) that exceeded the period of surveillance for stable cysts recommended by the AGA.[31]

Indications for Resection of Mucinous Cystic Neoplasms

According to 2018 European guidelines, MCNs with size 4 cm or greater, high-risk features, or symptoms should undergo surgical resection. Resection may be considered depending on patients' age, comorbidity, surgical risk, and preference for lesions 3 to 4 cm.[9]

The IAP guidelines from 2012 reflected the historical precedent of resecting all MCNs in surgically fit patients regardless of size due to malignant potential and limited knowledge regarding their natural history. Since then, evidence has accumulated supporting lifelong surveillance for MCNs smaller than 4 cm.[9] A 2016 systematic review estimated the risk of adenocarcinoma at the time of resection of only 0.03% for lesions less than 4 cm.[21] The 2017 IAP update excluded the management of MCNs due to relatively few remaining controversies in their management, focusing exclusively on IPMNs.[8] The ACG guidelines recommended the same management strategy for MCNs and IPMNs, whereas the AGA and ACR guidelines do not direct surgical management according to type of cyst.[10,11,25]

Extent of Resection for Intraductal Papillary Mucinous Neoplasms

Of the available guidelines, only the IAP and European guidelines explicitly advise on the extent of resection for IPMNs.[8,9] Because the indications for surgery have narrowed to high risk lesions, the standard of care for most patients is oncologic resection—pancreatoduodenectomy, distal pancreatectomy, or total pancreatectomy—including lymph node dissection. There is a lack of consensus regarding the role of total pancreatectomy,[14] parenchymal-sparing resection, and the benefit of lymph node dissection.

Total pancreatectomy

Historically, total pancreatectomy has been avoided due to the life-altering morbidity of diabetes and exocrine insufficiency. Its applications have expanded in recent years with improvements in the management of these conditions.[33,34] In cases of MD-IPMNs or MT-IPMNs with diffuse main duct dilatation or multifocal BD-IPMNs involving the whole gland, total pancreatectomy offers a means of definitive diagnosis, treatment and cancer prevention. Unfortunately, overtreatment of lesions managed with total pancreatectomy is common—as many as 1 in 5 patients have either an unnecessary or too extensive resection based on ultimate pathologic findings.[35] Current IAP guidelines emphasize the importance of a definitive preoperative diagnosis and careful consideration of patients' ability to manage brittle diabetes and exocrine insufficiency postoperatively.[8]

A 2018 survey posed a series of case vignettes to international experts in pancreatic surgery regarding the management of MD-IPMNs and mixed-type IPMNs. Their findings demonstrated a lack of consensus about when total pancreatectomy is indicated.[14] Evidence suggests segmental resection for MD-IPMN/MT-IPMN is safe when no invasive component is present because only a minority of patients experience progression in the remnant requiring completion total pancreatectomy.[36] Both IAP and European guidelines prefer pancreatoduodenectomy over distal pancreatectomy for diffuse or middle segment pancreatic duct involvement in MD-IPMN or MT-IPMN when feasible. In this approach, frozen section analysis determines the extent of resection, up to total pancreatectomy if required to achieve margins negative for high-grade dysplasia.

Both IAP and European guidelines mention lowering the threshold for total pancreatectomy in patients with IPMNs and familial risk of pancreatic cancer, although the evidence to support this practice is weak. The IAP guidelines cite a single series of 49 surgical specimens for patients with familial risk who developed PDAC. When compared with patients with sporadic PDAC, there was a significantly higher prevalence of IPMNs and high-grade precursor lesions within the resected gland.[37] Patients with IPMNs and a family history of PDAC are at elevated risk of developing concurrent PDAC and extrapancreatic malignancies; however, biologic differences in the behavior of IPMNs in this population remain uncertain, and it is not conclusive whether altering management to favor total pancreatectomy is warranted.[38,39]

Extent of Resection for Mucinous Cystic Neoplasms

Because the vast majority of MCNs are located in the body/tail, most will be managed with distal pancreatectomy. The European guidelines recommend oncologic resection with lymphadenectomy and splenectomy if any concerning features are seen on imaging. Parenchymal-sparing resections may be considered in select patients undergoing resection of MCNs without suspicious features if long-term benefits outweigh higher short-term morbidity.[9]

Parenchymal-Sparing Resections

Various methods of parenchymal-sparing resection have been proposed as alternatives to formal anatomic resection. The most popular are central pancreatectomy and enucleation,[40] although other subsegmental resections including uncinatectomy, dorsal or ventral pancreatectomy, duodenum-preserving pancreatic head resection, and more have been reported.[41] Nevertheless, the vast majority of operations performed for PCNs are oncologic resections; according to the National Cancer Database (NCDB), 56% of operations for IPMNs or MCNs between 2010 and 2016 were pancreatoduodenectomy, 28% distal pancreatectomy, and 14% total pancreatectomy; only 2% of resections were classified as other.[12]

The 2018 European guidelines state parenchyma sparing resections are "suitable only for lesions with a very low probability of malignancy—for example in patients without risk factors who have a strong wish to be operated on."[9] The 2017 IAP guidelines make similar recommendation that limited or focal nonanatomic resections may only be considered for BD-IPMNs without evidence of invasive carcinoma, citing the increased risk of pancreatic fistula and recurrence due to residual neoplasm or intraoperative spillage of mucin.[8]

Central pancreatectomy

Central pancreatectomy is a parenchymal-sparing alternative to distal pancreatectomy for lesions in the body or neck of the pancreas.[41–43] A meta-analysis comparing the 2 procedures found lower rates of endocrine (4%) and exocrine (5%) insufficiency compared with distal pancreatectomy but higher postoperative morbidity (51%) including clinically significant (grade B/C) postoperative pancreatic fistula (POPF; 35%).[44] Postoperative mortality was estimated as less than 1%. As the procedure results in both a pancreatic ductal anastomosis and divided edge of the pancreas, it is unsurprising the risk of POPF is elevated. A propensity-matched series comparing central pancreatectomy to distal pancreatectomy found an objective measure of exocrine insufficiency (fecal elastase) was superior in central pancreatectomy when adequate parenchymal volume could be preserved; however, symptom severity and quality of life were not assessed.[45]

Enucleation

A 2019 systematic review examining enucleation of IPMNs found the vast majority of reported cases were low-risk BD-IPMNs for which surveillance would currently be recommended over surgery.[13] A 53% complication rate was reported, with 22% being major morbidity, and 27% of patients experiencing a clinically significant POPF. Endocrine (1%) and exocrine (8%) insufficiencies were rare. Investigations of quality of life after enucleation found similar results compared with age-matched controls.[46,47] A recent study reporting long-term follow-up after enucleation of 74 low-risk BD-IPMNs found nearly 20% of patients experienced recurrence, either at the enucleation site (5%) or in the remnant (13%) including an instance of IPMN-associated carcinoma at the enucleation site.[47] In their cohort, only BD-IPMN of less than 3 cm were considered for enucleation, with the final extent of resection determined by intraoperative frozen section; consequently, 96% of these low-risk lesions had low-grade dysplasia on final pathology. As there is no demonstrated survival advantage for resection of low-grade dysplasia, and resection does not spare patients from lifelong surveillance of the remnant, the actual benefit of surgical management to these patients is unclear.

Lymphadenectomy

A drawback of parenchymal-sparing resections is limited lymph node harvest. Lymph node metastasis is a key prognostic factor in PDAC, though more extensive lymph node dissections have not demonstrated a survival benefit.[48] In a series of more than 1000 resected IPMNs, Hirono and colleagues found of the 23% of patients with invasive IPMNs on pathology, approximately one-third had lymph node metastasis.[49] Notably, those with lymph node metastasis included patients with stage T1a disease. Although standard lymph node dissection is recommended based on current evidence, the value is prognostic stratification rather than any survival attributed to extirpation of nodes.

Other Considerations

Although consensus guidelines provide a helpful framework for decision-making, surgeons must consider many factors when determining the most appropriate course of management for an individual patient. Lesions with high-risk stigmata or absolute indications for surgery always warrant oncologic resection if managed operatively, but patient-specific factors should influence the surgical plan in lower-risk lesions. For example, a young patient with a central lesion may be a good candidate for central pancreatectomy to reduce the risk of postoperative diabetes and exocrine insufficiency if they can tolerate the short-term morbidity. In an older patient with preexisting diabetes, the benefit of parenchymal resection is less pronounced, and a standard resection may be preferred.

ESTIMATING THE BENEFITS AND HARMS OF SURGICAL INTERVENTION
Preventing Malignant Transformation

Genomic research has provided insight into the genetic alterations in PDAC and malignant transformation of IPMNs and MCNs. The transformation from an IPMN or MCN with high-grade dysplasia to invasive adenocarcinoma is estimated to take 3 to 7 years.[50] Estimates using administrative claims data suggest malignant transformation of pancreatic cysts is a rare event, with annual risk as low as 0.5%.[51] Although PDAC is biologically aggressive at the time of diagnosis, genomic timelines suggest a window for early intervention exists.[52,53] Elucidating the timing and markers of progression is of particular import for elderly patients in whom resection of premalignant lesions comes with greater risk and may confer less survival benefit. An estimated 15% of MCNs and 25% of IPMNs harbor malignancy at the time of surgical resection.[20] When high-grade dysplasia is included, the frequency increases. Because these estimates generally derived from series of surgically resected cysts, they are a better reflection of our ability to appropriately discriminate high-risk lesions than an estimate of the true prevalence of malignancy. If 42% of IPMNs selected for surgery harbor malignancy or high-grade dysplasia, then 58% of patients underwent surgery for a low-grade lesion for which surgery may have potentially been avoided at that point in their lives. A minority of patients undergoes an optimally timed resection—when high-grade dysplasia is present but no invasive carcinoma has developed.[54]

Because most high-risk lesions are resected, data on the natural history of unresected MD-IPMNs and MT-IPMNs are rare. The few studies that have reported on high-risk MD-IPMNs or MT-IPMNs where surgery was not offered due to medical comorbidity, borderline indication or patient refusal, found a rate of malignancy between 13% and 36% over median 30 to 54 months follow-up.[55–57] In a retrospective series of

424 patients with MCNs including 195 patients under surveillance, the rate of malignancy was 11% in surgically resected lesions and less than 1% among patients undergoing surveillance.[58]

Oncologic Outcomes

Prognosis after surgical resection of PCNs depends on whether an invasive component is present, as well as the subtype, grade of dysplasia, margin, and lymph node status at resection.[59,60] Recent estimates of overall survival for invasive IPMN are reported as 50% to 70% at 5 years,[61–64] compared with 10% to 20% for resected PDAC.[62–64] Comparative studies suggest the apparent survival benefit is primarily driven by histopathologic features associated with earlier stage at presentation for IPMNs.[65–67] Even noninvasive IPMNs carry a lifetime risk of recurrence after resection and concomitant PDAC in the remnant gland and therefore require long-term postoperative surveillance.[32,68]

Surgical resection of MCNs without an invasive component is curative.[58,69,70] If an invasive component is present but the tumor is contained within the cyst capsule, 5-year survival is as high as 100% even with larger lesions.[69] For patients with mucinous cystadenocarcinoma, prognosis is poor. According to the NCDB, an estimated 16% have spread to lymph nodes at the time of resection, with a 5-year overall survival of only 35%.[71] Large series of resected mucinous cystadenocarcinoma have reported 3-year overall survival of 59%[70] and median survival of 44 months.[72]

Perioperative Mortality

An analysis of the NCDB reported a 90-day mortality rate for pancreatic resections for MCNs and IPMNs of 2.7% nationwide, ranging from 1.5% at academic/research centers to 5.4% at community cancer programs.[12] This is a dramatic improvement over historic mortality rates and is attributed primarily to improvements in surgical safety in expert hands at high-volume centers.[73–75] A population-based study in California similarly revealed in-hospital mortality of pancreatic resection for premalignant disease was 4-fold higher (2.4 vs 0.6%) at hospitals performing 25 or fewer pancreatectomies per year—yet 65% of resections for premalignant disease were still performed at low-volume centers.[76] For total pancreatectomy, postoperative mortality has been reported as 2.1% at high-volume centers[77]; an international registry-based study between 2014 and 2018 found mortality ranging from 2% in the United States up to nearly 11% in the Netherlands and Germany.[78]

Although efforts to restrict performance of high-risk surgery to high-volume centers have implications for disparities in access to care,[79] the argument for care at high-volume centers is especially compelling for premalignant disease. Because the benefit of surgical resection for cancer prevention is directly linked to the mortality risk of surgery, the mortality cost of intervention may be prohibitively high at low-volume centers, particularly for elderly and higher risk surgical candidates.[80]

Short-Term Complications

Analyses of postoperative outcomes in the National Surgical Quality Improvement Project (NSQIP) database found 25% of patients undergoing pancreatoduodenectomy for benign or premalignant lesions experienced a postoperative complication, with 18% major morbidity. Among elderly patients aged older than 80 years, the rate of major complication was 30%.[81] For patients undergoing distal pancreatectomy, overall morbidity was lower (17%); major morbidity was not reported.[82]

A comparison of outcomes for total pancreatectomy including the NCDB and registries in Germany, the Netherlands and Sweden found 27% of patients experienced major morbidity.[78] This is comparable to series at high-volume centers in which overall morbidity was up to 60% with 23% major morbidity.[77,83]

Postoperative pancreatic fistula

Patients with benign or premalignant pathologic condition are 3 times as likely to develop POPF than those with PDAC.[84] Despite decades of research investigating strategies to reduce POPF, it remains the primary driver of major morbidity and mortality after pancreatic surgery.[85] An estimated 24% of patients undergoing pancreatoduodenectomy and 20% undergoing distal pancreatectomy for premalignant or benign indications will develop a POPF. Of those, 5% experiencing a clinically significant, or International Study Group for Pancreatic Surgery grade B or C fistula, including POPF with persistent drainage for more than 3 weeks, signs of infection, need for additional procedures including percutaneous or endoscopic drainage, angiographic procedure for bleeding, reoperation, organ failure, or death.[81,82,85] By contrast, the frequency of POPF after parenchymal-sparing resection has been reported up to 60% overall with 27% clinically significant POPF.[13,40,44]

Delayed gastric emptying

Delayed gastric emptying (DGE) is one of the most common postoperative complications of pancreatic surgery, affecting approximately 40% of patients.[86,87] DGE is a major contributor to prolonged hospitalization, impacting patients' recovery and quality of life by preventing oral intake, requiring gastric decompression, and in severe cases alternative nonoral or parenteral nutrition for weeks after surgery.[86,88]

Long-Term Complications

Common long-term sequelae of pancreatic resection include endocrine and exocrine pancreatic insufficiency, gastrointestinal dysfunction, diarrhea, weight loss, peptic ulcer disease, malnutrition, recurrent hepatopancreatobiliary disorders (stricture, cholangitis, pancreatitis), and other conditions warranting hospitalization or reoperation.[89,90] In one study of 628 long-term survivors of pancreatoduodenectomy, 32% experienced a postoperative complication in the period between 90 days and median follow-up 5 years after surgery, including biliary stricture or cholangitis (8%), pancreatitis (6%), peptic ulcer disease (3%), incisional hernia (18%), and small bowel obstruction (4%). One in 6 patients required at least 1 reintervention more than 90 days after surgery, which included percutaneous intervention for biliary stricture, endoscopy for biliary complication or peptic ulcer, and reoperation for incisional hernia, SBO, or hepaticojejunostomy revision.[90] Another survey of long-term survivors found similarly high rates of additional hospitalizations (41%) and operative intervention (29%) after full recovery, and found 8% of patients had developed chronic pain requiring long-term use of analgesics, including dependence on narcotics.[89]

Pancreatic exocrine insufficiency

The most common long-term sequela of pancreatic resection is exocrine insufficiency. Loss of pancreatic parenchyma and hormonal function of the duodenum reduces the release of pancreatic fluid and neutralizing bicarbonate, leading to suboptimal pH and inadequate pancreatic enzyme activity for digestion.[91] Malabsorption secondary to exocrine insufficiency leads to steatorrhea, weight loss, and deficiencies of fat-soluble vitamins A, D, E, and K and is associated with nonalcoholic fatty liver disease.[92] In addition to clinical and quality of life implications, pancreatic exocrine insufficiency is costly. A recent analysis of Medicare Part D coverage listed the point-of-sale price for a 1-month supply of pancreatic enzyme replacements up to US$4800, with an initial expected out-of-pocket cost for Medicare beneficiaries of US$1000 per month.[93]

A pooled estimate of prevalence of long-term pancreatic exocrine insufficiency after pancreatoduodenectomy for benign disease was 25%[94]; however, a prospective study found 100% of patients experienced exocrine insufficiency at 6 months after pancreatoduodenectomy, with 30% to 65% persisting long-term.[91] Deficiencies of vitamins D and K were present in up to 80% of patients. The prevalence of exocrine insufficiency depends on the type of segmental resection; 53% of patients undergoing pancreatoduodenectomy are prescribed pancreatic enzyme supplementation within 2 years of surgery compared with 17% after distal pancreatectomy.[95] Surveys of long-term survivors of pancreatoduodenectomy in the United States indicate 50% to 65% of patients require pancreatic enzyme supplementation long-term.[96,97]

Pancreatic endocrine insufficiency

Diabetes after pancreatic surgery is classified by the WHO[98] and American Diabetes Association[99] as pancreatogenic (type 3c) diabetes. Unlike type 1 and 2 diabetes, pancreatogenic diabetes involves the loss of counterregulatory hormones glucagon and pancreatic polypeptide and can be associated with peripheral insulin sensitivity.[34] Consequently, patients are prone to severe fluctuations in glucose levels in response to exogenous insulin, or "brittle" diabetes.[100,101] These can be exacerbated by exocrine insufficiency, in which rapid intestinal transit due to steatorrhea makes carbohydrate absorption and blood glucose response to oral intake less predictable.

Diabetes has been postulated as the most impactful long-term sequelae on quality of life after pancreatectomy, and the negative impact is particularly pronounced among patients who undergo surgery for PCNs rather than cancer.[102] A survey of patients who underwent pancreatic resection and developed new-onset diabetes found those treated for benign pathologic condition consistently reported worse quality of life because of their diabetes than patients treated for cancer. Patients may struggle to accept the unwanted diagnosis and its impact on their social functioning and physical well-being as the cost of cancer prevention, whereas cancer survivors are more accepting of the trade-off. This emphasizes the importance of setting expectations for recovery and long-term health before surgery, and the incorporation of shared decision-making techniques in the surgical management of PCNs to minimize decisional regret.

Systematic reviews have estimated the risk of new-onset diabetes after resection of premalignant lesions as 14% for distal pancreatectomy[103] and 15% for pancreatoduodenectomy, with 45% of those with preexisting diabetes experiencing worsening glycemic control.[94] Maxwell and colleagues prospectively monitored 403 nondiabetic patients' endocrine function after pancreatoduodenectomy and found diabetes developed in 17%.[104] The authors developed the postpancreatectomy diabetes index to categorize patients as low, medium, or high risk of pancreatogenic diabetes based on their preoperative hemoglobin A1c, age, Body Mass Index (BMI), and whether the planned procedure is distal pancreatectomy.[105]

Total pancreatectomy guarantees diabetes and exocrine insufficiency and carries a higher risk of related complications. According to a 2019 systematic review, nearly 1 out of 5 patients is hospitalized for endocrine-related complications after total pancreatectomy with a mortality risk of 2%.[101] A bi-institutional series found 63% of patients experienced hypoglycemic events weekly, with 11% requiring hospital admission.[77] Mortality improved in more recent years, reflecting advances in insulin management and glycemic control.[33,78]

Quality of Life

Many studies have examined the influence of partial pancreatic resection on quality of life.[106] Generally, patients experience a reduction in quality of life immediately after surgery, recovering to approximate baseline 6 to 12 months after surgery.[107–109] A survey of 1102 patients recruited from an online pancreatoduodenectomy survivor support group reported frequent gastrointestinal symptoms, which persisted long-term and were associated with a negative impact on quality of life.[96] Other studies have found quality of life rated similarly to age-matched controls, despite persistent gastrointestinal symptoms.[97,110,111]

Quality of life after total pancreatectomy is rated consistently lower than the general population.[77,101] The impact may be commensurate with patients with diabetes due to other causes,[112,113] in line with the hypothesis that diabetes in particular diminishes quality of life after pancreatic surgery.[102] Gastrointestinal symptoms relating to exocrine insufficiency are common but the reported impact of symptom severity on quality of life is variable. Some studies report diarrhea as a driver of impaired quality of life,[101,113,114] whereas others report no impact despite severe symptoms.[77]

MINIMALLY INVASIVE TECHNIQUES

The main technical innovation in pancreatic surgery is the development and adoption of minimally invasive techniques, including laparoscopic and robotic surgery. Laparoscopic surgery has well-established benefits in general surgery for a variety of operations. By reducing the physiologic impact and immunosuppressive effects of abdominal surgery, using a minimally invasive approach can reduce wound infections and expedite functional recovery.[115–118]

The first attempts at laparoscopic pancreatoduodenectomy and distal pancreatectomy were reported in the 1990s,[119] with the first robotic pancreas operation in 2002.[120] Laparoscopic distal pancreatectomy has since been widely adopted, whereas laparoscopic pancreatoduodenectomy remains limited due to the technical challenges of dissection and enteric reconstruction. Analyses of the NSQIP database revealed as of 2016, 50% of distal pancreatectomies were attempted with minimally invasive techniques, with 22% completed laparoscopically and 8% robotically.[82] By contrast, separate NSQIP studies found only 7% of pancreatoduodenectomy (4% robotic, 3% laparoscopic)[121] and 11% of total pancreatectomy (7% laparoscopic, 4% robotic)[78] were attempted minimally invasively in a similar time period.

Randomized trials have demonstrated faster functional recovery and shorter length of stay for laparoscopic distal pancreatectomy, with similar rates of postoperative complications including POPF compared with open.[122,123] Although 2 small trials suggested laparoscopic pancreatoduodenectomy was safe,[124,125] excess 90-day mortality resulted in the early termination of a phase 2/3 trial.[124–126] Attention has since turned to the robotic platform as a more attractive minimally invasive option for pancreatoduodenectomy, with numerous retrospective series reporting feasibility and safety[127–129] and randomized trials underway.[130,131] A recent analysis of the NCDB found no benefit when measuring time to initiation of adjuvant therapy, and the benefit of the minimally invasive approach in pancreatoduodenectomy remains unproven.[132] The outcomes of minimally invasive central pancreatectomy were investigated in 2 recent systematic reviews, with no significant differences found comparing open versus minimally invasive techniques.[133,134]

In 2020, the International Study Group on Minimally Invasive Pancreas Surgery published evidence-based guidelines addressing laparoscopic and robotic approaches, endorsed by multiple surgical societies.[135] The guidelines recommend consideration of minimally invasive over open distal pancreatectomy, citing evidence of shorter hospital stay, reduced blood loss, and equivalent complication rate. Although minimally invasive pancreatoduodenectomy is considered a valid option, data are insufficient to recommend minimally invasive over open techniques. The Miami guidelines[135] also address parenchymal-sparing resections: minimally invasive enucleation is considered an appropriate alternative to open, whereas current data on the safety of minimally invasive central pancreatectomy are considered inadequate.

SHARED DECISION-MAKING

The stakes in the management of PCNs are high, and patients' preferences must be considered along with clinical features in the surgical management of PCNs. Shared decision-making is a model of engagement between patients and clinicians involving a 2-way exchange of information: the clinician shares options and their pros and cons, and the patients shared their preferences. This exchange leads to the patient's ultimate decision, with the clinician in the role of advisor or educator.[136,137] Higher quality shared decision-making has been linked to lower decisional regret, which is present in up to 20% of patients after pancreas surgery.[138,139]

Limited data regarding patients' preferences and satisfaction with surgical management of PCNs exist. One survey involving patients cared for by 2 surgeons offers a limited window into patients' decision-making and concerns.[140] Patients were strongly motivated to undergo surgery due to fear of cancer and were more concerned about the potential for cancer than the potential for postsurgical lifestyle changes. The vast majority of patients thought they were primarily responsible for making their decision (90%), that they did make the decision (87%), that they had the right amount of involvement in the decision-making process (95%), and 89% were satisfied with their choice, regardless of the final pathologic condition.[140]

Although this cohort demonstrated high satisfaction with the decision-making process and outcome, the use of shared decision-making techniques can be highly variable.[141] There are significant barriers to effective shared decision-making in the management of pancreatic cysts, and a paucity of data to guide its implementation.[138] Risk predictors for postoperative major morbidity[142] and diabetes[105] have recently been developed, both of which could help provide tailored assessment of potential outcomes to individual patients. More tools are needed to facilitate the exchange of information with patients in an individualized and accessible way.

SUMMARY

Since the WHO first established definitions of PCNs in 1996,[18] the operations performed to remove IPMNs and MCNs have remained fundamentally the same. The real evolution—and area in need of continued innovation—has been improvements in preoperative risk assessment that have narrowed the indications for operative intervention. Operating selectively is the best way to maximize the benefit of early intervention while reducing the burden of postoperative morbidity. Because the prevalence of PCNs continues to increase, better diagnostics and methods of surveillance are needed to optimize timely intervention and improve the cost-effectiveness of management strategies on a population level.[143] Unified consensus guidelines are needed to reconcile competing recommendations regarding indications for operative resection. For individual patients, a tailored approach incorporating individualized assessment of risks and benefits into shared decision-making is essential to ensure optimal outcomes while navigating uncertainty.

CLINICS CARE POINTS

- Current guidelines limit surgical intervention to high-risk mucinous PCNs where benefits of operative intervention are estimated to outweigh harms
- Only a minority of patients undergo optimally timed resection of PCNs when high-grade dysplasia is present but invasive carcinoma has not yet developed
- The main operations for PCNs are standard pancreatoduodenectomy and distal pancreatectomy, including local lymph node dissection
- As indications for resection have been limited to lesions with a higher risk of high-grade dysplasia or invasive adenocarcinoma, an oncologic approach is required and the role of parenchymal-sparing resection remains limited
- Total pancreatectomy should only be offered in select cases
- Long-term sequelae after pancreatic surgery include but are not limited to diabetes, exocrine insufficiency, gastrointestinal symptoms, peptic ulcer disease, malnutrition, and need for further interventions
- The severity of life-long sequelae after pancreatic surgery is difficult to predict preoperatively
- Age, overall health, baseline exocrine and endocrine function, health literacy and adherence to treatment should all be considered when determining optimal management
- Shared decision-making is essential to incorporate patient preferences and set expectations for recovery and long-term health after surgery
- All patients should be treated by a multidisciplinary group of specialists at a high-volume pancreatic center

DISCLOSURE

The authors have nothing to disclose.

REFERENCES

1. American Cancer Society. Survival Rates for Pancreatic Cancer. March 2, 2022. Available at: https://www.cancer.org/cancer/pancreatic-cancer/detection-diagnosis-staging/survival-rates.html. Accessed October 31, 2022.
2. Zerboni G, Signoretti M, Crippa S, et al. Systematic review and meta-analysis: Prevalence of incidentally detected pancreatic cystic lesions in asymptomatic individuals. Pancreatology 2019;19(1):2–9.
3. Gardner TB, Glass LM, Smith KD, et al. Pancreatic cyst prevalence and the risk of mucin-producing adenocarcinoma in US adults. Am J Gastroenterol 2013; 108(10):1546–50.
4. Horvath KD, Chabot JA. An aggressive resectional approach to cystic neoplasms of the pancreas. Am J Surg 1999;178(4):269–74.
5. Valsangkar NP, Morales-Oyarvide V, Thayer SP, et al. 851 resected cystic tumors of the pancreas: a 33-year experience at the Massachusetts General Hospital. Surgery 2012;152(3 Suppl 1):S4–12.
6. Tanaka M, Chari S, Adsay V, et al. International consensus guidelines for management of intraductal papillary mucinous neoplasms and mucinous cystic neoplasms of the pancreas. Pancreatology 2006;6(1–2):17–32.

7. Tanaka M, Fernández-Del C, Adsay V, et al. International consensus guidelines 2012 for the management of IPMN and MCN of the pancreas. Pancreatology 2012;12(3):183–97.

8. Tanaka M, Fernández-Del Castillo C, Kamisawa T, et al. Revisions of international consensus Fukuoka guidelines for the management of IPMN of the pancreas. Pancreatology 2017;17(5):738–53.

9. European Study Group on Cystic Tumours of the Pancreas. European evidence-based guidelines on pancreatic cystic neoplasms. Gut 2018;67(5):789–804.

10. Megibow AJ, Baker ME, Morgan DE, et al. Management of incidental pancreatic cysts: A white paper of the ACR incidental findings committee. J Am Coll Radiol 2017;14(7):911–23.

11. Vege SS, Ziring B, Jain R, et al. Clinical Guidelines Committee, American Gastroenterology Association. American gastroenterological association institute guideline on the diagnosis and management of asymptomatic neoplastic pancreatic cysts. Gastroenterology 2015;148(4):819–22, quize12.

12. Ahmad M, Maegawa FB, Ashouri Y, et al. Facility type affects treatment outcomes for patients with mucinous cystic neoplasms and intraductal papillary mucinous neoplasms of the pancreas. Pancreas 2021;50(10):1422–6.

13. Ratnayake CB, Biela C, Windsor JA, et al. Enucleation for branch duct intraductal papillary mucinous neoplasms: a systematic review and meta-analysis. HPB 2019;21(12):1593–602.

14. Scholten L, van Huijgevoort NCM, Bruno MJ, et al. Surgical management of intraductal papillary mucinous neoplasm with main duct involvement: an international expert survey and case-vignette study. Surgery 2018. https://doi.org/10.1016/j.surg.2018.01.025. Published online May 16.

15. Moris M, Bridges MD, Pooley RA, et al. Association Between Advances in High-Resolution Cross-Section Imaging Technologies and Increase in Prevalence of Pancreatic Cysts From 2005 to 2014. Clin Gastroenterol Hepatol 2016;14(4):585–93.e3.

16. Laffan TA, Horton KM, Klein AP, et al. Prevalence of unsuspected pancreatic cysts on MDCT. Am J Roentgenol 2008;191(3):802–7.

17. Kromrey M-L, Bülow R, Hübner J, et al. Prospective study on the incidence, prevalence and 5-year pancreatic-related mortality of pancreatic cysts in a population-based study. Gut 2018;67(1):138–45.

18. Kloppel G, Solcia E, Longnecker DS, et al. Histological typing of tumours of the exocrine pancreas. Berlin: World Health Organization; 1996.

19. Gill AJ, Klimstra DS, Lam AK. Tumors of the Pancreas. In: WHO classification of tumors editorial board. 5th edition. World Health Organization Classification Of Tumors; 2019. p. 296.

20. Scheiman JM, Hwang JH, Moayyedi P. American gastroenterological association technical review on the diagnosis and management of asymptomatic neoplastic pancreatic cysts. Gastroenterology 2015;148(4):824–48,e??

21. Nilsson LN, Keane MG, Shamali A, et al. Nature and management of pancreatic mucinous cystic neoplasm (MCN): A systematic review of the literature. Pancreatology 2016;16(6):1028–36.

22. Malagelada J, Guda N, Goh K-L, et al. Pancreatic cystic lesions. World Gastroenterology Organisation; 2019. Available at: https://www.worldgastroenterology.org/guidelines/pancreatic-cystic-lesions. Accessed November 15, 2022.

23. Roldán J, Harrison JM, Qadan M, et al. Evolving Trends in Pancreatic Cystic Tumors: A 3-Decade Single-Center Experience with 1290 Resections. Ann Surg 2021. https://doi.org/10.1097/SLA.0000000000005142.

24. Aziz H, Acher AW, Krishna SG, et al. Comparison of society guidelines for the management and surveillance of pancreatic cysts: A review. JAMA Surg 2022;157(8):723–30.
25. Elta GH, Enestvedt BK, Sauer BG, et al. ACG clinical guideline: diagnosis and management of pancreatic cysts. Am J Gastroenterol 2018;113(4):464–79.
26. Expert Panel on Gastrointestinal Imaging, Fábrega-Foster K, Kamel IR, et al. ACR appropriateness criteria® pancreatic cyst. J Am Coll Radiol 2020;17(5S): S198–206.
27. Crippa S, Fogliati A, Valente R, et al. A tug-of-war in intraductal papillary mucinous neoplasms management: Comparison between 2017 International and 2018 European guidelines. Dig Liver Dis 2021;53(8):998–1003.
28. Xu M-M, Yin S, Siddiqui AA, et al. Comparison of the diagnostic accuracy of three current guidelines for the evaluation of asymptomatic pancreatic cystic neoplasms. Medicine (Baltim) 2017;96(35):e7900.
29. Allen PJ. Current Controversy of Radiographic Surveillance of Patients With Branch-duct IPMN and Pancreatic Cysts: Commentary on: Ductal Carcinoma Arising in a Largely Unchanged Presumed Branch Duct IPMN After 10 Years of Surveillance. Ann Surg 2017;266(6):e41.
30. Khannoussi W, Vullierme MP, Rebours V, et al. The long term risk of malignancy in patients with branch duct intraductal papillary mucinous neoplasms of the pancreas. Pancreatology 2012;12(3):198–202.
31. Oyama H, Tada M, Takagi K, et al. Long-term Risk of Malignancy in Branch-Duct Intraductal Papillary Mucinous Neoplasms. Gastroenterology 2020;158(1): 226–37.e5.
32. Lawrence SA, Attiyeh MA, Seier K, et al. Should Patients With Cystic Lesions of the Pancreas Undergo Long-term Radiographic Surveillance?: Results of 3024 Patients Evaluated at a Single Institution. Ann Surg 2017;266(3):536–44.
33. Griffin JF, Poruk KE, Wolfgang CL. Is it time to expand the role of total pancreatectomy for IPMN? Dig Surg 2016;33(4):335–42.
34. Andrén-Sandberg Å, Segersvärd R. Risk/benefit of total pancreatectomy for pancreatic cancer: are there indications?. In: Beger HG, Nakao A, Neoptolemos JP, et al, editors. Pancreatic cancer, cystic neoplasms and endocrine tumors: diagnosis and management. John Wiley & Sons, Ltd; 2015. p. 54–8. https://doi.org/10.1002/9781118307816.ch7.
35. Crippa S, Pergolini I, Rubini C, et al. Risk of misdiagnosis and overtreatment in patients with main pancreatic duct dilatation and suspected combined/main-duct intraductal papillary mucinous neoplasms. Surgery 2016;159(4):1041–9.
36. Blair AB, Beckman RM, Habib JR, et al. Should non-invasive diffuse main-duct intraductal papillary mucinous neoplasms be treated with total pancreatectomy? HPB 2022;24(5):645–53.
37. Shi C, Klein AP, Goggins M, et al. Increased prevalence of precursor lesions in familial pancreatic cancer patients. Clin Cancer Res 2009;15(24):7737–43.
38. Nehra D, Oyarvide VM, Mino-Kenudson M, et al. Intraductal papillary mucinous neoplasms: does a family history of pancreatic cancer matter? Pancreatology 2012;12(4):358–63.
39. Fong ZV, Ferrone CR, Lillemoe KD, et al. Intraductal papillary mucinous neoplasm of the pancreas: current state of the art and ongoing controversies. Ann Surg 2016;263(5):908–17.
40. Sauvanet A, Gaujoux S, Blanc B, et al. Parenchyma-sparing pancreatectomy for presumed noninvasive intraductal papillary mucinous neoplasms of the pancreas. Ann Surg 2014;260(2):364–71.

41. Sperti C, Beltrame V, Milanetto AC, et al. Parenchyma-sparing pancreatectomies for benign or border-line tumors of the pancreas. World J Gastrointest Oncol 2010;2(6):272–81.
42. Iacono C, Verlato G, Ruzzenente A, et al. Systematic review of central pancreatectomy and meta-analysis of central versus distal pancreatectomy. Br J Surg 2013;100(7):873–85.
43. Beger HG, Siech M, Poch B, et al. Limited surgery for benign tumours of the pancreas: a systematic review. World J Surg 2015;39(6):1557–66.
44. Xiao W, Zhu J, Peng L, et al. The role of central pancreatectomy in pancreatic surgery: a systematic review and meta-analysis. HPB 2018;20(10):896–904.
45. Zhang R-C, Zhang B, Mou Y-P, et al. Comparison of clinical outcomes and quality of life between laparoscopic and open central pancreatectomy with pancreaticojejunostomy. Surg Endosc 2017;31(11):4756–63.
46. Giuliani T, De Pastena M, Paiella S, et al. Pancreatic Enucleation Patients Share the Same Quality of Life as the General Population at Long-Term Follow-Up: A Propensity-Score Matched Analysis. Ann Surg 2021. https://doi.org/10.1097/SLA.0000000000004911. Published online April 14.
47. Kaiser J, Alhalabi KT, Hinz U, et al. Enucleation for low-grade branch duct intraductal papillary mucinous neoplasms: Long-term follow-up. Surgery 2022;172(3):968–74.
48. Tol JAMG, Gouma DJ, Bassi C, et al. Definition of a standard lymphadenectomy in surgery for pancreatic ductal adenocarcinoma: a consensus statement by the International Study Group on Pancreatic Surgery (ISGPS). Surgery 2014;156(3):591–600.
49. Hirono S, Shimizu Y, Ohtsuka T, et al. Recurrence patterns after surgical resection of intraductal papillary mucinous neoplasm (IPMN) of the pancreas; a multicenter, retrospective study of 1074 IPMN patients by the Japan Pancreas Society. J Gastroenterol 2020;55(1):86–99.
50. Noë M, Niknafs N, Fischer CG, et al. Genomic characterization of malignant progression in neoplastic pancreatic cysts. Nat Commun 2020;11(1):4085.
51. Schweber AB, Agarunov E, Brooks C, et al. Prevalence, Incidence, and Risk of Progression of Asymptomatic Pancreatic Cysts in Large Sample Real-world Data. Pancreas 2021;50(9):1287–92.
52. Del Chiaro M, Segersvärd R, Lohr M, et al. Early detection and prevention of pancreatic cancer: is it really possible today? World J Gastroenterol 2014;20(34):12118–31.
53. Yachida S, Jones S, Bozic I, et al. Distant metastasis occurs late during the genetic evolution of pancreatic cancer. Nature 2010;467(7319):1114–7.
54. Tjaden C, Sandini M, Mihaljevic AL, et al. Risk of the Watch-and-Wait Concept in Surgical Treatment of Intraductal Papillary Mucinous Neoplasm. JAMA Surg 2021;156(9):818–25.
55. Takuma K, Kamisawa T, Anjiki H, et al. Predictors of malignancy and natural history of main-duct intraductal papillary mucinous neoplasms of the pancreas. Pancreas 2011;40(3):371–5.
56. Roch AM, Ceppa EP, Al-Haddad MA, et al. The natural history of main duct-involved, mixed-type intraductal papillary mucinous neoplasm: parameters predictive of progression. Ann Surg 2014;260(4):680–8 ; discussion 688.
57. Daudé M, Muscari F, Buscail C, et al. Outcomes of nonresected main-duct intraductal papillary mucinous neoplasms of the pancreas. World J Gastroenterol 2015;21(9):2658–67.

58. Marchegiani G, Andrianello S, Crippa S, et al. Actual malignancy risk of either operated or non-operated presumed mucinous cystic neoplasms of the pancreas under surveillance. Br J Surg 2021;108(9):1097–104.
59. Kobari M, Egawa S, Shibuya K, et al. Intraductal papillary mucinous tumors of the pancreas comprise 2 clinical subtypes: differences in clinical characteristics and surgical management. Arch Surg 1999;134(10):1131–6.
60. Mino-Kenudson M, Fernández-del Castillo C, Baba Y, et al. Prognosis of invasive intraductal papillary mucinous neoplasm depends on histological and precursor epithelial subtypes. Gut 2011;60(12):1712–20.
61. Marchegiani G, Andrianello S, Dal Borgo C, et al. Adjuvant chemotherapy is associated with improved postoperative survival in specific subtypes of invasive intraductal papillary mucinous neoplasms (IPMN) of the pancreas: it is time for randomized controlled data. HPB 2019;21(5):596–603.
62. Aronsson L, Bengtsson A, Torén W, et al. Intraductal papillary mucinous carcinoma versus pancreatic ductal adenocarcinoma: A systematic review and meta-analysis. Int J Surg 2019;71:91–9.
63. Gavazzi F, Capretti G, Giordano L, et al. Pancreatic ductal adenocarcinoma and invasive intraductal papillary mucinous tumor: Different prognostic factors for different overall survival. Dig Liver Dis 2022;54(6):826–33.
64. Yamada S, Fujii T, Hirakawa A, et al. Comparison of the survival outcomes of pancreatic cancer and intraductal papillary mucinous neoplasms. Pancreas 2018;47(8):974–9.
65. Poultsides GA, Reddy S, Cameron JL, et al. Histopathologic basis for the favorable survival after resection of intraductal papillary mucinous neoplasm-associated invasive adenocarcinoma of the pancreas. Ann Surg 2010;251(3):470–6.
66. Holmberg M, Ghorbani P, Gilg S, et al. Outcome after resection for invasive intraductal papillary mucinous neoplasia is similar to conventional pancreatic ductal adenocarcinoma. Pancreatology 2021;21(7):1371–7.
67. Takeda Y, Imamura H, Yoshimoto J, et al. Survival comparison of invasive intraductal papillary mucinous neoplasm versus pancreatic ductal adenocarcinoma. Surgery 2022;172(1):336–42.
68. Hirono S, Kawai M, Okada K-I, et al. Long-term surveillance is necessary after operative resection for intraductal papillary mucinous neoplasm of the pancreas. Surgery 2016;160(2):306–17.
69. Liang H, Xie W, Lin X, et al. Pathologic T1 and T2 encapsulated invasive carcinomas arising from mucinous cystic neoplasms of the pancreas have favorable prognosis and might be treated conservatively. J Pathol Clin Res 2021;7(5):507–16.
70. Postlewait LM, Ethun CG, McInnis MR, et al. Association of preoperative risk factors with malignancy in pancreatic mucinous cystic neoplasms: A multicenter study. JAMA Surg 2017;152(1):19–25.
71. Ahmad M, Maegawa FB, De La Rosa E, et al. Mucinous cystic neoplasms of the pancreas in the modern era. Experience with 707 patients. Am J Surg 2020;220(6):1433–7.
72. Keane MG, Shamali A, Nilsson LN, et al. Risk of malignancy in resected pancreatic mucinous cystic neoplasms. Br J Surg 2018;105(4):439–46.
73. Cameron JL, Riall TS, Coleman J, et al. One thousand consecutive pancreaticoduodenectomies. Ann Surg 2006;244(1):10–5.

74. Lieberman MD, Kilburn H, Lindsey M, et al. Relation of perioperative deaths to hospital volume among patients undergoing pancreatic resection for malignancy. Ann Surg 1995;222(5):638–45.

75. Brennan MF, Allen PJ, Jarnagin WR. Fifty years of pancreas cancer care. J Surg Oncol 2022;126(5):876–80.

76. Callahan AF, Ituarte PHG, Goldstein L, et al. Prophylactic Pancreatectomies Carry Prohibitive Mortality at Low-Volume Centers: A California Cancer Registry Study. World J Surg 2019;43(9):2290–9.

77. Pulvirenti A, Pea A, Rezaee N, et al. Perioperative outcomes and long-term quality of life after total pancreatectomy. Br J Surg 2019;106(13):1819–28.

78. Latenstein AEJ, Mackay TM, Beane JD, et al. The use and clinical outcome of total pancreatectomy in the United States, Germany, the Netherlands, and Sweden. Surgery 2021;170(2):563–70.

79. Blanco BA, Kothari AN, Blackwell RH, et al. Take the Volume Pledge" may result in disparity in access to care. Surgery 2017;161(3):837–45.

80. Aquina CT, Becerra AZ, Fleming FJ, et al. Variation in outcomes across surgeons meeting the Leapfrog volume standard for complex oncologic surgery. Cancer 2021;127(21):4059–71.

81. Aizpuru M, Starlinger P, Nagorney DM, et al. Contemporary outcomes of pancreaticoduodenectomy for benign and precancerous cystic lesions. HPB 2022;24(9):1416–24.

82. Daniel FE, Tamim HM, Hosni MN, et al. Short-term surgical morbidity and mortality of distal pancreatectomy performed for benign versus malignant diseases: a NSQIP analysis. Surg Endosc 2020;34(9):3927–35.

83. Hartwig W, Gluth A, Hinz U, et al. Total pancreatectomy for primary pancreatic neoplasms: renaissance of an unpopular operation. Ann Surg 2015;261(3):537–46.

84. Callery MP, Pratt WB, Kent TS, et al. A prospectively validated clinical risk score accurately predicts pancreatic fistula after pancreatoduodenectomy. J Am Coll Surg 2013;216(1):1–14.

85. Bassi C, Marchegiani G, Dervenis C, et al. The 2016 update of the International Study Group (ISGPS) definition and grading of postoperative pancreatic fistula: 11 Years After. Surgery 2017;161(3):584–91.

86. Wente MN, Bassi C, Dervenis C, et al. Delayed gastric emptying (DGE) after pancreatic surgery: a suggested definition by the International Study Group of Pancreatic Surgery (ISGPS). Surgery 2007;142(5):761–8.

87. Hanna MM, Gadde R, Allen CJ, et al. Delayed gastric emptying after pancreaticoduodenectomy. J Surg Res 2016;202(2):380–8.

88. Smits FJ, Verweij ME, Daamen LA, et al. Impact of complications after pancreatoduodenectomy on mortality, organ failure, hospital stay, and readmission: analysis of a nationwide audit. Ann Surg 2022;275(1).e222–8.

89. Mayeux SE, Kwon W, Rosario VL, et al. Long-term health after pancreatic surgery: the view from 9.5 years. HPB 2021;23(4):595–600.

90. Brown JA, Zenati MS, Simmons RL, et al. Long-Term Surgical Complications After Pancreatoduodenectomy: Incidence, Outcomes, and Risk Factors. J Gastrointest Surg 2020;24(7):1581–9.

91. Kroon VJ, Daamen LA, Tseng DSJ, et al. Pancreatic exocrine insufficiency following pancreatoduodenectomy: A prospective bi-center study. Pancreatology 2022;22(7):1020–7.

92. Tsunematsu M, Gocho T, Yanagaki M, et al. The impact of postoperative exocrine index on non-alcoholic fatty liver disease following pancreaticoduodenectomy. Ann Gastroenterol Surg 2022;6(5):704–11.
93. Gupta A, Premnath N, Beg MS, et al. Projected 30-day out-of-pocket and total spending on pancreatic enzyme replacement therapy under Medicare Part D. J Clin Orthod 2021;39(3_suppl):401.
94. Beger HG, Poch B, Mayer B, et al. New Onset of Diabetes and Pancreatic Exocrine Insufficiency After Pancreaticoduodenectomy for Benign and Malignant Tumors: A Systematic Review and Meta-analysis of Long-term Results. Ann Surg 2018;267(2):259–70.
95. Thomas AS, Huang Y, Kwon W, et al. Prevalence and risk factors for pancreatic insufficiency after partial pancreatectomy. J Gastrointest Surg 2022;26(7):1425–35.
96. Allen CJ, Yakoub D, Macedo FI, et al. Long-term Quality of Life and Gastrointestinal Functional Outcomes After Pancreaticoduodenectomy. Ann Surg 2018;268(4):657–64.
97. Fong ZV, Alvino DM, Castillo CF-D, et al. Health-related Quality of Life and Functional Outcomes in 5-year Survivors After Pancreaticoduodenectomy. Ann Surg 2017;266(4):685–92.
98. World Health Organization. Definition, Diagnosis and Classification of Diabetes Mellitus and Its Complications : Report of a WHO Consultation. Part 1, diagnosis and classification of diabetes mellitus. World Health Organization; 1999.
99. American Diabetes Association. 2. classification and diagnosis of diabetes. Diabetes Care 2016;39(Suppl 1):S13–22.
100. Tran TCK, van Lanschot JJB, Bruno MJ, et al. Functional changes after pancreatoduodenectomy: diagnosis and treatment. Pancreatology 2009;9(6):729–37.
101. Scholten L, Stoop TF, Del Chiaro M, et al. Systematic review of functional outcome and quality of life after total pancreatectomy. Br J Surg 2019;106(13):1735–46.
102. Shaw K, Thomas AS, Rosario V, et al. Long term quality of life amongst pancreatectomy patients with diabetes mellitus. Pancreatology 2021;21(3):501–8.
103. De Bruijn KMJ, van Eijck CHJ. New-onset diabetes after distal pancreatectomy: a systematic review. Ann Surg 2015;261(5):854–61.
104. Maxwell DW, Jajja MR, Tariq M, et al. Development of Diabetes after Pancreaticoduodenectomy: Results of a 10-Year Series Using Prospective Endocrine Evaluation. J Am Coll Surg 2019;228(4):400–12.e2.
105. Maxwell DW, Jajja MR, Galindo RJ, et al. Post-Pancreatectomy Diabetes Index: A Validated Score Predicting Diabetes Development after Major Pancreatectomy. J Am Coll Surg 2020;230(4):393–402.e3.
106. Toms C, Steffens D, Yeo D, et al. Quality of life instruments and trajectories after pancreatic cancer resection: A systematic review. Pancreas 2021;50(8):1137–53.
107. Heerkens HD, Tseng DSJ, Lips IM, et al. Health-related quality of life after pancreatic resection for malignancy. Br J Surg 2016;103(3):257–66.
108. van Dijk SM, Heerkens HD, Tseng DSJ, et al. Systematic review on the impact of pancreatoduodenectomy on quality of life in patients with pancreatic cancer. HPB 2018;20(3):204–15.
109. Park JW, Jang JY, Kim EJ, et al. Effects of pancreatectomy on nutritional state, pancreatic function and quality of life. Br J Surg 2013;100(8):1064–70.

110. Shaw K, Thomas AS, Rosario VL, et al. Long-term quality of life and global health following pancreatic surgery for benign and malignant pathologies. Surgery 2021;170(3):917–24.
111. van der Gaag NA, Berkhemer OA, Sprangers MA, et al. Quality of life and functional outcome after resection of pancreatic cystic neoplasm. Pancreas 2014; 43(5):755–61.
112. Billings BJ, Christein JD, Harmsen WS, et al. Quality-of-life after total pancreatectomy: is it really that bad on long-term follow-up? J Gastrointest Surg 2005; 9(8):1059–66 ; discussion 1066.
113. Wu W, Dodson R, Makary MA, et al. A Contemporary Evaluation of the Cause of Death and Long-Term Quality of Life After Total Pancreatectomy. World J Surg 2016;40(10):2513–8.
114. Barbier L, Jamal W, Dokmak S, et al. Impact of total pancreatectomy: short- and long-term assessment. HPB 2013;15(11):882–92.
115. Novitsky YW, Litwin DEM, Callery MP. The net immunologic advantage of laparoscopic surgery. Surg Endosc 2004;18(10):1411–9.
116. Jaschinski T, Mosch CG, Eikermann M, et al. Laparoscopic versus open surgery for suspected appendicitis. Cochrane Database Syst Rev 2018;11(11): CD001546.
117. Keus F, de Jong JAF, Gooszen HG, et al. Laparoscopic versus open cholecystectomy for patients with symptomatic cholecystolithiasis. Cochrane Database Syst Rev 2006;4:CD006231.
118. Amodu LI, Howell RS, Daskalaki D, et al. Oncologic benefits of laparoscopic and minimally invasive surgery: a review of the literature. Ann Laparosc Endosc Surg 2022;7:5.
119. Gagner M, Pomp A. Laparoscopic pancreatic resection: Is it worthwhile? J Gastrointest Surg 1997;1(1):20–5 ; discussion 25.
120. Melvin WS, Needleman BJ, Krause KR, et al. Computer-enhanced robotic telesurgery. Initial experience in foregut surgery. Surg Endosc 2002;16(12):1790–2.
121. Vining CC, Kuchta K, Berger Y, et al. Robotic pancreaticoduodenectomy decreases the risk of clinically relevant post-operative pancreatic fistula: a propensity score matched NSQIP analysis. HPB 2021;23(3):367–78.
122. de, Rooij T, van Hilst J, et al. Minimally Invasive Versus Open Distal Pancreatectomy (LEOPARD): A Multicenter Patient-blinded Randomized Controlled Trial. Ann Surg 2019;269(1):2–9.
123. Björnsson B, Larsson AL, Hjalmarsson C, et al. Comparison of the duration of hospital stay after laparoscopic or open distal pancreatectomy: randomized controlled trial. Br J Surg 2020;107(10):1281–8.
124. Palanivelu C, Senthilnathan P, Sabnis SC, et al. Randomized clinical trial of laparoscopic versus open pancreatoduodenectomy for periampullary tumours. Br J Surg 2017;104(11):1443–50.
125. Poves I, Burdío F, Morató O, et al. Comparison of perioperative outcomes between laparoscopic and open approach for pancreatoduodenectomy: the PADULAP randomized controlled trial. Ann Surg 2018;268(5):731–9.
126. van Hilst J, de Rooij T, Bosscha K, et al. Laparoscopic versus open pancreatoduodenectomy for pancreatic or periampullary tumours (LEOPARD-2): a multicentre, patient-blinded, randomised controlled phase 2/3 trial. Lancet Gastroenterol Hepatol 2019;4(3):199–207.
127. Boone BA, Zenati M, Hogg ME, et al. Assessment of quality outcomes for robotic pancreaticoduodenectomy: identification of the learning curve. JAMA Surg 2015;150(5):416–22.

128. Müller PC, Kuemmerli C, Cizmic A, et al. Learning curves in open, laparoscopic, and robotic pancreatic surgery. Annals of Surgery Open 2022;3(1):e111.
129. Shi Y, Wang W, Qiu W, et al. Learning Curve From 450 Cases of Robot-Assisted Pancreaticoduocectomy in a High-Volume Pancreatic Center: Optimization of Operative Procedure and a Retrospective Study. Ann Surg 2021;274(6): e1277–83.
130. Jin J, Shi Y, Chen M, et al. Robotic versus Open Pancreatoduodenectomy for Pancreatic and Periampullary Tumors (PORTAL): a study protocol for a multi-center phase III non-inferiority randomized controlled trial. Trials 2021;22(1):954.
131. Klotz R, Dörr-Harim C, Bruckner T, et al. Evaluation of robotic versus open partial pancreatoduodenectomy-study protocol for a randomised controlled pilot trial (EUROPA, DRKS00020407). Trials 2021;22(1):40.
132. Naffouje SA, Kamarajah SK, Denbo JW, et al. Surgical Approach does not Affect Return to Intended Oncologic Therapy Following Pancreaticoduodenectomy for Pancreatic Adenocarcinoma: A Propensity-Matched Study. Ann Surg Oncol 2022;29(12):7793–803.
133. Farrarons SS, van Bodegraven EA, Sauvanet A, et al. Minimally invasive versus open central pancreatectomy: Systematic review and meta-analysis. Surgery 2022;172(5):1490–501.
134. Rompianesi G, Montalti R, Giglio MC, et al. Robotic central pancreatectomy: a systematic review and meta-analysis. HPB 2022;24(2):143–51.
135. Asbun HJ, Moekotte AL, Vissers FL, et al. The Miami International Evidence-based Guidelines on Minimally Invasive Pancreas Resection. Ann Surg 2020; 271(1):1–14.
136. Stiggelbout AM, Pieterse AH, De Haes JCJM. Shared decision making: Con-cepts, evidence, and practice. Patient Educ Couns 2015;98(10):1172–9.
137. Charles C, Gafni A, Whelan T. Shared decision-making in the medical encounter: what does it mean? (or it takes at least two to tango). Soc Sci Med 1997;44(5):681–92.
138. Trobaugh J, Fuqua W, Folkert K, et al. Shared Decision-Making in Pancreatic Surgery. Annals of Surgery Open 2022;3(3):e196.
139. Wilson A, Winner M, Yahanda A, et al. Factors associated with decisional regret among patients undergoing major thoracic and abdominal operations. Surgery 2017;161(4):1058–66.
140. Puri PM, Watkins AA, Kent TS, et al. Decision-Making for the Management of Cystic Lesions of the Pancreas: How Satisfied Are Patients with Surgery? J Gastrointest Surg 2018;22(1):88–97.
141. Baggett ND, Schulz K, Buffington A, et al. Surgeon Use of Shared Decision-making for Older Adults Considering Major Surgery: A Secondary Analysis of a Randomized Clinical Trial. JAMA Surg 2022;157(5):406–13.
142. Marchegiani G, Crippa S, Perri G, et al. Surgery for Intraductal Papillary Mucinous Neoplasms of the Pancreas: Preoperative Factors Tipping the Scale of Decision-Making. Ann Surg Oncol 2022;29(5):3206–14.
143. Sharib J, Esserman L, Koay EJ, et al. Cost-effectiveness of consensus guideline based management of pancreatic cysts: The sensitivity and specificity required for guidelines to be cost-effective. Surgery 2020;168(4):601–9.